Complications in Cutaneous Surgery

Complications in Cutaneous Surgery

Hugh M. Gloster, Jr., MD

Associate Professor, Director of Dermatologic Surgery, Department of Dermatology, University of Cincinnati, Cincinnati, Ohio, USA

Editor

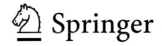 Springer

Hugh M. Gloster, Jr., MD
Associate Professor
Director of Dermatologic Surgery
Department of Dermatology
University of Cincinnati
Cincinnati, OH
USA

Library of Congress Control Number: 2007930545

ISBN: 978-0-387-73151-3   e-ISBN: 978-0-387-73152-0

Printed on acid-free paper.

9 8 7 6 5 4 3 2 1

springer.com

Preface

The demand for outpatient cutaneous surgery procedures has increased at a rapid rate over the last several decades. Cosmetic, excisional, and reconstructive procedures are being performed by primary care physicians and a variety of specialists in different disciplines, such as dermatology, plastic surgery, ophthalmology, and otolaryngology. As the number of cutaneous surgery procedures rises, so will the rate of complications, which are inevitable and occur even with the most skilled, careful, and meticulous surgeons.

In the practice of medicine, we often learn more from complications than triumphs. The authors of the chapters in this book were recruited based on their experience and respective areas of expertise. To my knowledge, no book exists that summarizes the medical literature regarding complications in cutaneous surgery. The goal of this book is to provide a comprehensive text that will enable the practicing physician to formulate a preoperative strategy to prevent complications before they occur and to properly diagnose and manage complications when they arise in order to provide a better service to the patient.

This book is divided into three sections: acute surgical complications, chronic surgical complications, and complications of cosmetic procedures. Each chapter discusses a different complication and outlines proper preventative, diagnostic, and management strategies based on the medical literature and the experience of the author. Acute complications, some of which may be associated with serious morbidity and mortality, are those experienced within the first few weeks of surgery. Chronic complications primarily are the result of suboptimal scarring. Scar revision techniques are reviewed in detail. Psychological complications, which no longer can be overlooked with the growing popularity of cosmetic procedures, are also discussed in this section. Finally, the section on complications of cosmetic procedures covers a wide variety of pertinent topics such as lasers, chemical peels, dermabrasion, liposuction, filler substances, botulinum toxin, and sclerotherapy. This section was included because of the recent increase in cosmetic surgery as physicians look for new ways to expand their practices in the current healthcare market.

All physicians performing cutaneous surgery will experience complications. Each complication should serve as a learning experience that should enable the surgeon to make arrangements to prevent the same complication from occurring again in the future. Hopefully, this book will enhance patient care by allowing the reader to benefit from the collective experience of others instead of learning "the hard way".

Hugh M. Gloster, Jr., MD

Contents

Contributors

Sumaira Z. Aasi, MD
Assistant Professor, Department of Dermatology, Yale University, New Haven, CT, USA

Shawn Allen, MD
Director, Dermatology Specialists of Boulder, Boulder, CO, USA

Tina S. Alster, MD
Director, Washington Institute of Dermatologic Laser Surgery, Clinical Professor of Dermatology, Georgetown University, Washington DC, USA

Steven C. Bernstein, MD, CM, FRCP(C)
Assistant Professor, Department of Medicine, University of Montreal, Montreal, Quebec, Canada

Elizabeth M. Billingsley, MD
Associate Professor, Department of Dermatology, Penn State University College of Medicine, Hershey Medical Center, Hershey, PA, USA

Ross M. Campbell, MD
Total Skin and Beauty Dermatology Center, Birmingham, AL, USA

Betty Davis, MD
Arizona Medical Clinic, Sun City West, AZ, USA

Raymond G. Dufresne, Jr., MD
Professor, Department of Dermatology, Brown Medical School, Rhode Island Hospital, Providence, RI, USA

Darrell J. Fader, MD
Clinical Assistant Professor, Division of Dermatology, Department of Medicine, University of Washington, Seattle, WA, USA

Gregory John Fulchiero, Jr., MD, MS BioEng
Fellow in Dermatologic Surgery, Department of Dermatology, University of Texas, Southwestern, Dallas, TX, USA

Hayes B. Gladstone, MD
Director, Division of Dermatologic Surgery, Department of Dermatology and Otolaryngology, Stanford University, Stanford, CA, USA

Dee Anna Glaser, MD
Associate Professor, Department of Dermatology, St. Louis University, St. Louis, MO, USA

Hugh M. Gloster, Jr., MD
Associate Professor, Director of Dermatologic Surgery, Department of Dermatology, University of Cincinnati, Cincinnati, OH, USA

C. William Hanke, MD, MPH, FACP
Visiting Professor, Department of Dermatology, Carver College of Medicine, University of Iowa Hospitals and Clinics, Iowa City, IA, USA

Christopher B. Harmon, MD
Clinical Instructor, Department of Dermatology, University of Alabama at Birmingham, Birmingham, AL, USA

Nathaniel J. Jellinek, MD
Assistant Professor, Brown Medical School, Providence, RI, USA

Evan C. Jones, MD, MPH
Clinical Instructor, Department of Dermatology, St. Louis University, St. Louis, MO, USA

A. Paul Kelly, MD
Professor and Chief, Division of Dermatology, Charles R. Drew University of Medicine and Science, Department of Internal Medicine, King/Drew Medical Center, Los Angeles, CA, USA

David Leffell, MD
Professor and Surgery Chief, Department of Dermatology, Section of Dermatologic Surgery and Cutaneous Oncology Director, Yale School of Medicine, New Haven, CT, USA

Mary E. Maloney, MD
Professor, Department of Dermatology, Chief, Division of Dermatology, University of Massachusetts Medical School, Worcester, MA, USA

Greg S. Morganroth, MD
Assistant Clinical Professor, Department of Dermatology, University of California, San Francisco, San Francisco, CA, Adjunct Clinical Assistant Professor, Department of Otolaryngology, Head and Neck Surgery, Stanford University, Stanford, CA, USA

Girish S. Munavalli, MD, MHS
Clinical Instructor, Department of Dermatology, Johns Hopkins University School of Medicine, Charlotte, NC, USA

Marcy Neuburg, MD
Associate Professor, Department of Dermatology, Medical College of Wisconsin, Milwaukee, WI, USA

Isaac M. Neuhaus, MD
Assistant Professor, Department of Clinical Dermatology, University of California, San Francisco, San Francisco, CA, USA

Tri H. Nguyen, MD
Associate Professor, Department of Dermatology and Otorhinolaryngology, M. D. Anderson Cancer Center, University of Texas, Houston, TX, USA

Michelle Pipitone, MD
Department of Dermatology, University of Cincinnati, Cincinnati, OH, USA

Deborshi Roy, MD
772 Parks Avenue, New York, NY, USA

Neil Scott Sadick, MD
Clinical Professor, Department of Dermatology, Weill Medical College of Cornell University, New York, NY, USA

Roberta Sengelmann, MD
Assistant Professor, Department of Dermatology and Otolaryngology, Department of Internal Medicine and Dermatology, Washington University School of Medicine, St. Louis, MO, USA

J. Barton Sterling, MD
Cosmetic and Procedural Dermatology Cernter, Spring Lake, NJ, USA

Elizabeth L. Tanzi, MD
Co-Director, Wahington Institute of Dermatologic Laser Surgery, Clinical Instructor of Dermatology, Johns Hopkins Medical Center, Washington DC, USA

Robert A. Weiss, MD
Associate Professor, Department of Dermatology, Johns Hopkins University School of Medicine, Director, Maryland Laser, Skin, and Vein Institute, Hunt Valley, MD, USA

Section I
Acute Surgical Complications

1
Preoperative Evaluation

Marcy Neuburg

Any comprehensive text of complications in cutaneous surgery should begin with a review of the preoperative evaluation. Complications in surgery are generally defined as unanticipated morbid events or occurrences leading to suboptimal outcomes. Consequently, if physicians could accurately anticipate such untoward events, they might be effectively minimized or even prevented. A comprehensive preoperative evaluation will often allow the surgeon to accurately identify patients at risk for intraoperative and postoperative problems. The physician may thus have an opportunity prevent surgical complications and optimize surgical outcomes. This chapter discusses the essential elements of the psychological, physical, and medical profiles, which together comprise the preoperative evaluation.

Psychological Profile

Cutaneous surgery covers a broad spectrum of conditions ranging from surgical enhancement of normal structures to treatment of life-threatening malignancies. The psychological issues experienced by our patients are similarly broad and varied. The vast majority of cutaneous surgical procedures do not require a formal psychological evaluation prior to surgery. However, surgeons whose practice is concentrated on cosmetic procedures may occasionally find it necessary to refer patients for such evaluations preoperatively. Indeed, some larger cosmetic practices actually employ or affiliate with a psychologist for this purpose.

A preoperative, face-to-face consultation is particularly important for patients undergoing cosmetic procedures or cancer surgery. These patients typically have a number of concerns that are best discussed prior to surgery. Addressing these issues early in the physician–patient relationship will put the patient at ease and establish a pattern of open communication. An informal psychological profile can easily be constructed during this meeting.

The main elements of the psychological profile, which are outlined in detail by Goin and Goin,[1] include appearance, affect, mood, orientation, thought processing, judgment, and insight. Patients whose behaviors fall outside the norms of these elements are in most cases easily identified by simple observation and conversation.

Appearance

The patient's clothing and manner of dress should be appropriate to the occasion. Odors suggestive of poor hygiene or problems with self-care should be noted. These individuals may be prone to postoperative infections and/ or require extra assistance if postoperative care of a surgical site is anticipated. An extremely neat or disheveled appearance may be suggestive of underlying psychological issues. Nonverbal cues observed during the patient interview, such as excessive sweating, tremulousness, tearfulness, or poor eye contact, might indicate increased anxiety in a patient with an otherwise calm demeanor.

Affect/Mood

Like appearance, a patient's mood and affect should be appropriate to the setting and the conversation. The clinician should be aware of signs of depression or other mood disorders that may interfere with the patient's ability to actively participate in their care. The overly anxious patient may talk excessively and/or exhibit nonverbal cues such as sweating, hand wringing, or tremulousness. Similarly, poor eye contact or monosyllabic responses to open-ended questions may signal the presence of an underlying mood or affect pathology.

Orientation

Orientation to person, place, and time are usually apparent from normal conversation. Lack of appropriate orientation is relatively rare and occurs most often in the elderly or brain-injured individuals. Use of open-ended questions during the interview process may allow the physician to recognize underlying problems of orientation. Establishment of normal orientation is important because it is required for informed consent. Patients who are not oriented may not legally give consent for surgical procedures. In these situations, the surgeon must identify the individual who holds the legal power of attorney for medical issues in order to obtain legal consent prior to planned surgical intervention.

Thought Processing

Disordered thought processing is usually manifest during the patient interview, but the signs may be subtle. The most commonly encountered disorders are associated with early dementia and include confabulation and loss of short-term memory. Indeed, high-functioning patients with early Alzheimer's disease may confabulate in an attempt to mask short-term memory loss. Such patients will often be noted to ask the same questions repeatedly. These problems will only become manifest during a more extended interaction. Flight of ideas, paranoia, or tangential thinking in a person suffering from schizophrenia may not be readily apparent during a brief encounter with the physician or office staff.

Judgment and Insight

Patients exhibiting faulty judgment or lack of insight into their disease process or its proposed treatment may not be able to give informed consent. Preoperative identification of these individuals may aide in postoperative care planning.

The importance of the various elements of the psychological profile is not the same for all cutaneous surgical procedures. Widespread psychological pathology is not necessarily a contraindication for cancer surgery as long as there is informed consent or a medical power of attorney that is positioned to make medical decisions on behalf of the patient. On the other hand, surgical procedures that are purely cosmetic in nature are, in most cases, not appropriate in individuals exhibiting pathological behaviors in any one or more of the above categories. Accordingly, the face-to-face preoperative interview is of premier importance for individuals considering cosmetic surgery. Simply reviewing a form that arrives in the mail will not allow the physician to preoperatively identify the young woman with the clinical eating disorder seeking liposuction or the young man seeking scar revision for self-inflicted wounds. In the case of cosmetic surgery, it is critical that the patient and the physician have shared expectations concerning the outcome of the planned procedure both in terms of what it will look like and how the patient's specific needs will be met.

Medical and Surgical History

The concept that "history repeats itself" is uniquely appropriate to surgery. Patients who are most likely to have problems are those who have had problems. An accurate and thorough medical and surgical history will allow the physician to correctly identify patients who are most likely to experience intraoperative and/or postoperative complications.

Gathering of the medical and surgical history can be accomplished using a variety of formats. A form filled out by the patient is commonly used for this purpose. Alternatively, the physician or allied health personnel can gather this information during the initial interview (Fig. 1-1). The purpose of the medical and surgical history is to allow the preoperative identification of high-risk patients, thus allowing the surgeon to appropriately alter the surgical plan in order to minimize risk and potential complications.

Patient Demographics

The initial documentation of the patient visit should include complete patient demographics, including name, age, address, phone contact, referring physician, and primary care physician. The names and phone numbers of specialists who might need to be contacted regarding the plan of care should also be listed. For example, if the patient is being treated for a platelet disorder, the hematologist may need to be consulted regarding the patient's suitability for surgery. It is also helpful to identify special issues like medical power of attorney (name and contact information) or family members who will be involved in the patient's care.

Allergies

An accurate history of allergies to medications is essential. Many of the antibiotics used in cutaneous surgery are common sources of medical allergies. To this end, patients should be specifically queried regarding a history of reactions to penicillin and its derivatives as well as other antibiotics. Local anesthetics are probably the most common medications used in cutaneous surgery. True allergies to local anesthetics are extremely rare. However, patients will commonly report allergies to these preparations. Careful questioning often suggests that the reaction was likely mediated by a vagal rather than allergic phenomenon. These patients often have experienced palpitations or lightheadedness and attribute this to an "allergic" reaction. It is may be advisable to obtain testing by an allergist prior to surgery, which allows the safe use of local anesthetics and dispels the notion of allergy held by the patient. The subject of local anesthetic reactions and toxicities is covered in detail in the following chapter.

MOHS SURGERY PRE-OPERATIVE CONSULTATION

Lesion # _____

Name _____ DOB _____ Hosp. # _____

Address _____ Phone # _____

Referring MD _____ Med. MD _____

History of Present Illness:

Location   _____

Size   _____

Diagnosis   _____

Previous rx   _____

Duration   _____ Radiation_____

Family History   _____

Medications   _____

                              _____

         ASA   ☐ No ☐ Yes   D/C 2 wks pre-op   ☐ Yes ☐ No

Allergies   _____

Supplements   _____

Tobacco _____ Ethanol _____

Review of Systems/Diseases

Hepatic	☐ No ☐ Yes_____		Glaucoma	☐ No ☐ Yes_____
Cardiac	☐ No ☐ Yes_____		Bleeding	☐ No ☐ Yes_____
Hypertension	☐ No ☐ Yes_____		Healing	☐ No ☐ Yes_____
Renal	☐ No ☐ Yes_____		Scarring	☐ No ☐ Yes_____
Respiratory	☐ No ☐ Yes_____		Prosthesis	☐ No ☐ Yes_____
CNS	☐ No ☐ Yes_____		HSV	☐ No ☐ Yes_____
Diabetes	☐ No ☐ Yes_____		Prophylaxis	☐ No ☐ Yes_____
			Rx	_____

Previous surgeries _____

General health and nutrition _____   Consult appointment   ☐ No ☐ Yes_____

Other _____   Medical Clearance   ☐ No ☐ Yes_____

                                                  ☐ Pre-op photo taken

                                                  ☐ Pre-op instructions given

DOS: _____

             _____

Above findings reviewed and confirmed by:

MD _____ Date _____

FIGURE 1-1. A preoperative questionnaire is often a useful way to obtain information about the patient's medical and surgical history.

Medications and Supplements

The medication list is probably the single most useful element of the patient's medical history. The astute clinician can discern much of the pertinent medical history from this list. A complete listing of medications should include prescribed as well as over-the-counter preparations. The latter should be inclusive of various dietary supplements (vitamins, herbal remedies, etc.), many of which have been reported to interfere with normal blood clotting. Details of dosage and frequency should be included. Special attention must be directed to medications that have the potential to contribute to intraoperative or postoperative bleeding, including aspirin or aspirin-containing products, nonsteroidal anti-inflammatory agents, warfarin, certain antibiotics (beta lactam group), and many dietary supplements (garlic, feverfew, ginko).[2,3]

Systemic steroids in therapeutic doses (nonmaintenance) may predispose patients to postoperative infections and/or interfere with wound healing. Similarly, problems with wound healing have been described in patients taking systemic retinoids or newer antirejection medications taken by organ transplant recipients. Patients who take medications that interfere with planned conscious sedation agents or anxiolytics should be identified and instructed when and if their prescribed medications should be taken on the day of surgery. For example, a patient taking a cold remedy containing a sedative antihistamine might require a reduced dose of diazepam for intraoperative anxiolysis or sedation.

Tobacco and Alcohol

Both smoking and alcohol consumption have the potential to adversely affect surgical outcomes. Thus, patients should be carefully questioned as to their smoking and drinking habits. Smoking causes relative tissue hypoxia, which may contribute to a number of complications including delayed wound healing, wound infections, compromise of flap or graft viability, and overall reduction of long-term cosmetic outcomes. Closure of wounds under excessive tension in smokers is more likely to result in healing complicated by necrosis and dehiscence. The acute and chronic affects of alcohol consumption on hemostasis are well recognized. Excessive intraoperative bleeding can be an acute effect of alcohol (as a direct effect on platelets) or a chronic effect caused by hepatic insufficiency and its associated clotting dysfunction. In addition, heavy drinkers may require larger doses of sedatives in order to achieve conscious sedation. The decision to discontinue use of tobacco products for a period prior to surgery is largely individual. In patients who are undergoing surgery that is purely cosmetic, cessation of smoking should be considered, as failure to do so may adversely affect cosmetic results. Consumption of alcohol just prior to surgery should be discouraged.

Social/Family History

Knowledge of a patient's social and family history is often critical to surgical planning. Patients with certain familial syndromes may require multiple surgical procedures throughout their lifetime, thus influencing reconstructive options chosen by the surgeon. A patient who has a lip cancer and plays the trombone for a living will need to know how long to be off work after the surgery. A professional fashion model seeking cosmetic enhancement will likely have different expectations in terms of surgical outcomes than an individual whose livelihood is not closely linked to their physical appearance. A good understanding of the patient's normal level of activity (especially exercise habits) will help prevent postoperative

complications in that postoperative wound care instructions and activity restrictions can be appropriately tailored to the individual patient.

Medical History/Review of Systems

The level of detail that is required in the patient's medical history and review of systems is directly proportional to the complexity of both the planned procedure and the proposed type of anesthesia. For simple excisions under local anesthesia, a comprehensive review would be unnecessary and excessive. For larger, more prolonged procedures or those involving conscious sedation or general anesthesia, such a complete review would be entirely appropriate. As a general rule, the complexity of the planned procedure, the possible complications, and their implications should be reflected in the extent of the medical history the physician chooses to elicit from the patient.

The organization of the medical history and review of systems is best approached by organ systems. This can be done during a patient interview or using a checklist filled out by the patients. It is best to query patients regarding their history of specific conditions rather than general disease states. For example, rather than asking, "How is your heart?" more useful information will be gleaned from, "Have you ever been told that you had a heart attack? Heart murmur? Heart failure? Have you ever been told that you should take antibiotics before going to the dentist because of your heart?"

Central Nervous System

Previous thromboembolic or hemorrhagic disease of the central nervous system (CNS) places patients at increased risk for future CNS events. Preoperative identification of patients with a history of stroke or transient ischemic event is important, particularly when it comes to perioperative management of antiplatelet regimens. If the patient has had a recent stroke, elective surgery should be delayed until appropriate medical clearance is obtained from the patient's treating physician. A history of vertebrobasilar insufficiency, more common in the elderly, usually requires alterations in patient positioning in order to avoid diminished flow associated with this condition.

In patients with a history of seizures, it is helpful to know the frequency and quality of the seizures including when the patient last had a seizure. Preoperative confirmation that blood levels of antiepileptics are in the therapeutic range should be considered for more complex surgical procedures.

Cardiovascular

In general, patients with a history of cardiac disease are at higher risk for perioperative cardiac complications.

The risk of cardiac complications associated with surgical procedures is stratified according to the complexity and invasiveness of the procedure. Cutaneous surgery falls within the lowest risk group.[4,5]

Patients should be specifically queried (in layman's terms) regarding a previous history of heart attack, heart murmur, irregular heartbeat, heart failure, mitral valve prolapse, chest pain, or shortness of breath. Patients with chest pain of cardiac origin should be further questioned as to the frequency of their symptoms, whether it occurs at rest and whether it responds to nitrates. All elective surgery should be delayed in patients with recent myocardial infarction or signs and symptoms suggestive of unstable angina. Similarly, patients who have recently had a coronary stent placed should have elective surgery delayed 4 weeks. At this time interval, antiplatelet agents typically used following stent placement can be safely stopped with little risk of thrombosis. Re-stenosis following coronary angioplasty (with or without stenting) usually occurs, if at all, within 8 to 12 months of the procedure. Noncardiac elective surgery in patients who have been symptom-free with normal exercise tolerance after this period pose no increased risk of cardiac complications related to the previous percutaneous procedure.

Implanted pacemakers and implantable cardiac defibrillators (ICDs) are common in patients being considered for cutaneous surgery. The American College of Cardiology has not developed formal guidelines addressing the potential interactions of these devices with electrical/magnetic activity commonly found in the surgical suite. However, bipolar electrocautery is generally recommended wherever possible. If monopolar electrocautery is used, the dispersive unit should be placed away from the implanted device in a position where the path of electricity does not intersect the leads of the implanted device. Turning off the ICD is also an option; however caution should be exercised if this is done in a setting where cardiac monitoring is not available. A complete and updated discussion of this subject can be accessed online at the website of the American College of Cardiology (http://www.acc.org).

Patients with valvular heart disease may be at increased risk for perioperative complications, including thromboembolic disease or endocarditis. These conditions and their management are covered in subsequent chapters.

A diagnosis of claudication or Raynaud's disease may complicate healing of surgical wounds in affected areas. Acral sites are most at-risk and epinephrine should be used judiciously, if at all.

Uncontrolled hypertension is associated with a risk of several surgical complications including bleeding/hemorrhage, cardiac events, and stroke. While it is not the purview of the dermatologic surgeon to treat hypertension, it is reasonable to perform preoperative measurement of blood pressure to rule out this potentially hazardous entity. Care should be exercised in treatment of the elderly individual with systolic hypertension. Acute reduction of systolic pressure may cause hypoperfusion.

Pulmonary

The primary concern in patients with pulmonary disease is whether or not they will tolerate the planned surgery. Pulmonary disease is generally grouped into acute and chronic conditions. Surgery in patients with acute upper or lower airway disease, including acute asthmatics and patients with upper respiratory infections, should be delayed until their disease is abated. Performing an elective surgical procedure on the nose of a patient with sinusitis, bronchitis, or other upper respiratory infection should similarly be delayed. In an elderly patient with poorly compensated chronic lung disease requiring supplemental oxygen, a nonsurgical treatment should be considered. Patients who cannot lie flat may require altered surgical planning to accommodate their disability. A patient who gives no history of pulmonary disease but appears clinically short of breath during the interview should probably be referred for medical evaluation.

Hepatic

Patients should be specifically asked if they have ever had jaundice or hepatitis. A history of liver disease may predispose the affected patient to bleeding complications. Additionally, patients with known hepatic dysfunction may require dose adjustment of anesthetic agents.[6] Easy bruising, bleeding gums, or unexplained bruising may indicate a clinically significant bleeding diathesis. Hepatic dysfunction may interfere with the normal metabolism of lidocaine, the most commonly used local anesthetic. Procedures involving potentially larger amounts of lidocaine, such as tumescent liposuction, should be approached with extreme caution in these patients.

Renal

Intact renal function is not a prerequisite for safely undergoing cutaneous surgery.[7] However, uremia interrupts the normal hemostatic pathways so extra bleeding precautions may be necessary in such patients. When possible, patients on hemodialysis should be scheduled for surgery immediately after rather than just before their regular dialysis session. Transplant recipients with a functioning graft are not normally at increased risk of perioperative bleeding. The primary issue in these patients is the increased risk of infection related to chronic immunosuppression. The use of antibiotics in this patient population is discussed in a later chapter.

Endocrine

The most common endocrine issues encountered by the dermatologic surgeon are diabetes and thyroid disease.[8] Diabetic patients are more likely to have small vessel disease that may impair wound healing. Additionally, diabetic patients are predisposed to wound infection. Epinephrine should be used judiciously in these patients and administration of perioperative antibiotics should be considered. Hard candy or sweetened juices should be readily available for patients experiencing episodes of hypoglycemia. Thyroid disease is common, particularly in patients who were treated with ionizing radiation for skin conditions (e.g., acne) as teens or young adults. Medically managed thyroid disease is not a problem for minor surgical procedures.

Skin

While often taken for granted, the cutaneous history is very important. A previous history of skin cancers should be documented, as well as a history of previous radiation, especially to the area of planned surgery. Previous surgical scars should be examined for evidence of abnormal wound healing. Scars that are spread, hypertrophic, or keloidal should be noted. It is very important to always directly visualize patients' mature scars. Frequently, patients will mistake visible scars for abnormal scarring when in fact the scar is normal for the age, location, and clinical setting.

Surgical History

The best indicator of surgical complications is a history of previous surgical complications. The surgical history should include a complete list of previous surgical procedures along with indications and dates. Patients should be carefully questioned regarding problems with anesthesia, infections, bleeding, or wound healing related to these surgeries. Tooth extractions, which may be the only surgery to have been performed on healthy individuals, should also be included. A complete surgical history will also reveal the presence of prosthetic devices. The use of perioperative antibiotics in patients with implanted prostheses is covered in a later chapter.

Physical Exam

The physical exam required prior to cutaneous surgical procedures is for the most part dictated by the planned surgery. If the patient is undergoing preoperative evaluation for a skin cancer on the temple, the surgeon will want to perform an exam that will address the surgical issues unique to that location. If the cancer under consideration is large and fixed to underlying structures, preoperative imaging might be in order. A tumor of the eyelid might require the participation of an occuloplastic surgery colleague for optimal care. A thorough physical exam specifically tailored to the patient's indication for surgery will greatly enhance appropriate surgical planning and the overall quality of surgical outcomes. This is even more critical for cosmetic procedures. The preoperative evaluation must assure that the patient is not only psychologically and medically well suited for the procedure, but that the cosmetic correction or enhancement is both indicated and possible and that the expectations are realistic.

Patient Education

A last element of the preoperative evaluation is patient education, which is an opportunity for the surgeon to confirm that the patient's expectations can be met by the planned procedure. Well-educated patients who know precisely what to expect before, during, and after their surgery tend to be less apprehensive and better able to participate in their care. They are also fully prepared to provide informed consent, a requisite of any surgical intervention. The physician, ancillary personnel, or a well-constructed handout can provide patient education. The advantage of a face-to-face encounter is that the patient will have an opportunity to ask questions and have their concerns addressed in a straightforward manner. Appropriate documentation is also an important component of patient education.

References

1. Goin JM, Goin MK. Changing the body: psychological effects of plastic surgery. Baltimore: Williams & Wilkins; 1981.
2. Burroughs SF, Johnson GJ. Beta-lactam antibiotic-induced platelet dysfunction: evidence for irreversible inhibition of platelet activation in vitro and in vivo after prolonged exposure to penicillin. Blood 1990;75:1473–1480.
3. Pribitkin ED, Boger G. Herbal therapy: what every facial plastic surgeon must know. Arch Facial Plast Surg 2001;3:127–132.
4. Eagle KA, Berger PB, Calkins H, et al. ACC/AHA guideline update for perioperative cardiovascular evaluation for noncardiac surgery–executive summary: a report of the American College of Cardiology/American Heart Association Task Force on Practice Guidelines (Committee to Update the 1996 Guidelines on Perioperative Cardiovascular Evaluation for Noncardiac Surgery). J Am Coll Cardiol 2002;39(3):542–553.
5. Mukherjee D, Eagle KA. Cardiac risk in noncardiac surgery. Minerva Cardioangiol 2002;50:607–619.
6. Conn M. Preoperative evaluation of the patient with liver disease. Mt Sinai J Med 1991;58:75–80.
7. Gilbert PL, Stein R. Preoperative evaluation of the patient with chronic renal disease. Mt Sinai J Med 1991;58:69–74.
8. Gilbert PL. Preoperative evaluation of the patient with endocrine disease. Mt Sinai J Med 1991;58:58–68.

2
Acute Emergencies in the Dermatology Office

Darrell Fader

The dermatologic office emergency is often dismissed as medical oxymoron. The medications administered or procedures performed rarely precipitate a crisis. Nevertheless, certain medical questions and emergencies are relevant to the dermatologic physician, regardless of their low frequency. Based upon the limited literature available and clinical experience, this chapter is designed to offer a practical approach to selected emergency issues that are potentially encountered in the practice of medical and surgical dermatology.

The Emergency Plan

Emergency Medical Services

Ischemic heart disease and sudden cardiac death remain the leading cause of death in the United States and most developed nations.[1] Approximately two thirds of those deaths (about 1000 cases a day) occur outside the hospital setting.[2] Most of these deaths are reversible if acted upon promptly and systematically, according to the American Heart Association's Cardiac Care Committee. The American Red Cross's health and safety committee further avers that roughly one third to one half of sudden cardiac arrests are preventable if an organized chain of survival resuscitation plan and defibrillation were initiated within the first 5 minutes of arrest.[3–6] While the vast majority of cardiac arrests occur at home, outdoors, or in cars, some inevitably occur in a physician's office.

While ventricular fibrillation is no longer thought to be the most common presenting rhythm in patients who suffered sudden cardiac death, it is the most common initial rhythm in survivors of cardiac arrest.[7] Terminating ventricular fibrillation can be achieved by electrical defibrillation, and the time from arrest to defibrillation is the most important factor predicting survival. Defibrillation delivered within 1 minute of arrest is associated with a >70% survival rate, dropping by 10% for each minute defibrillation is delayed.[7–9]

Emergency medical services (EMS) have emerged over the past few decades to increase the chances of survival for victims of cardiac arrest outside the hospital setting. The American Heart Association's four-step chain of survival system includes (1) early access to an emergency medical system; (2) early initiation of cardiopulmonary resuscitation (CPR); (3) early defibrillation; and (4) an early advanced life support system.[10] The highest hospital discharge rate for cardiac arrest has occurred in victims treated with basic life support (BLS) within 4 minutes of arrest and advanced cardiac life support (ACLS), including defibrillation, within 8 minutes.[11]

Level of Training

For the dermatologist formulating an emergency plan, the primary considerations are: What kind of EMS system exists in the area? How fast can it be mobilized? These questions directly relate to the level of emergency training and equipment necessary for the office. A dermatology unit located within an academic medical center may lie yards away from a level one trauma emergency room. Similarly, a hospital code team may be available by page within minutes. Alternatively, an office may be situated in a city such as Seattle, Washington, with a well-established and pioneering EMS system with an average response time of 4 minutes.[3,12] In such settings, extensive emergency equipment and ACLS training may be redundant. More practical approaches would then include making sure the patient is placed on the surgical table in the Trendelenberg position. Alternatively, the patient could be placed supine on the floor with arms alongside the body. Loosening or removing clothing and providing materials for obtaining intravenous access facilitate the efforts of the EMS team. If necessary, CPR should be initiated early and continue until the code team is ready to take over. A dermatologist located in a more rural setting, where an EMS system is not able to respond within minutes of an arrest, should have a more self-sufficient emergency plan. In this scenario, ACLS certification and more emergency equipment would be appropriate (see below).

Anesthesia Considerations

Class I facilities are those in which cutaneous surgical procedures are performed under topical, local, or regional anesthesia (nerve blocks). Anesthesia may be supplemented with oral or intramuscular analgesics (e.g., meperidine) or sedatives (e.g., benzodiazepines). Class II facilities offer the intravenous administration of sedatives or analgesics in addition to Class I anesthesia. Class III facilities offer general anesthesia with the external support of vital body functions.[13] BLS certification is recommended for class I facilities, whereas at least one staff member in a class II or III facility should be ACLS trained.[14] General dermatology and most surgical dermatology suites fall under the class I designation. Therefore, ACLS training is not routinely indicated for these facilities. It is possible, however, that some hospitals or health care centers may require ACLS certification regardless of office category to confer privileges.

Should more than 8 minutes transpire from the time EMS is called until they can provide defibrillation, if necessary, then the office should be prepared to initiate ACLS. If EMS can be mobilized more quickly, then the facility classification should determine ACLS certification needs. Nevertheless, contacting your local EMS for training and equipment and training recommendations appears prudent.

Against the background of these guidelines, it is useful to review several surveys regarding the preparedness and certification of family practitioners and pediatricians. In a survey of several dozen Michigan physicians, half of whom were family practitioners, Kobernick found that over 70% of the respondents had seen at least one case of chest pain, dyspnea, and seizures in their office.[15] Over half had witnessed anaphylaxis and syncope. However, only 11% of the group had adequate equipment to manage all of these emergencies. Of all practitioners surveyed, approximately 70% were BLS certified and 35% were ACLS certified.

Fuchs and colleagues studied 280 pediatricians and family practitioners in the Chicago area.[16] Certification in BLS was achieved by 88% and in ACLS by 16%. Fewer than one third of the offices in which physicians reported seeing a child each week with asthma, anaphylaxis, sickle-cell crisis, status epilepticus, and sepsis were fully equipped to treat these emergencies. Finally, Altieri and colleagues analyzed responses from 175 pediatricians in the Washington, DC, metropolitan area. A total of 77% of office practices included a member with BLS training, 25% included a member with ACLS. Less than half of the

offices felt adequately equipped for life-threatening emergencies.[17] These surveys were in predominantly urban settings where the EMS system was readily accessible. The initial task of improving such statistics would seem to belong to the primary care providers whose medical purview includes these emergencies on a more regular basis. Dermatologists should at least concentrate on increasing BLS certification and developing an emergency plan.

The Office Team

Each staff member should have a prearranged clearly defined role for an effective office emergency plan. The ultimate goal is to stabilize the patient until the EMS support arrives. The patient is assessed by the physician and nurse. CPR is initiated if indicated, while an assigned staff member activates the EMS system. Another staff member can serve as the designated recorder of event times, serial vital sign measurements, and administered medications. Further roles can include obtaining intravenous access, greeting and escorting the arriving EMS team to the patient, and communicating with family. The crash cart inventory should be periodically reviewed and renewed as necessary. Mock codes can be helpful to further refine the office team emergency plan. Such a plan should be documented and distributed to the staff. Figure 2-1 outlines a sample office plan during such a code. For a more detailed review of BLS and ACLS implementation, the reader is advised to consult other sources, including American Heart Association texts, for appropriate guidelines.[18-20]

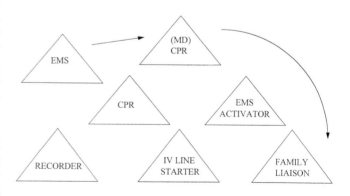

EMS-Emergency Medical Services
CPR-Cardiopulmonary Resuscitation

FIGURE 2-1. By clearing defining each staff member's role during a medical emergency, the physician can stabilize a patient until emergency medical services (EMS) support arrives. Various roles are illustrated above, with the physician as the main coordinator. When EMS arrives, the physician can assume the role of communicating with the patient's family.

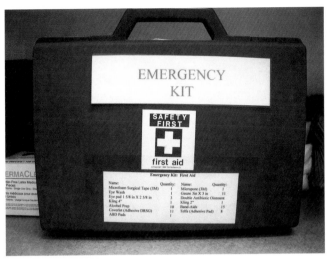 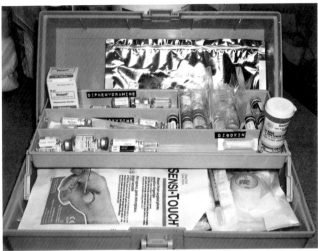

FIGURE 2-2. An office crash cart should be readily accessible, with clearly labeled and updated contents.

Equipment

The telephone remains the most important piece of emergency equipment in the dermatologist's office, as it provides the first link in the chain of initiating the EMS process. The use of 911 systems has simplified the process, although it is not universally available in the United States. Enhanced 911 systems provide dispatchers with the address and phone number of the caller automatically.[20,21] An office crash cart should be readily available. Sometimes pictures of each drawer or compartment in a crash cart can be displayed across the top of the cart to minimize last-minute frenetic searching for supplies. Equipment and medications are described elsewhere.[22,23] Reasonable basic equipment would include a portable oxygen tank with mask or nasal cannula, oral or nasopharyngeal airway, intravenous catheters, tubing, fluids, and suction. Medications include epinephrine 1 : 1000, lorazepam (Ativan), diazepam (Valium), diphenylhydramine (Benadryl), dextrose 50%, nitroglycerin tablets, and baby aspirin (Fig. 2-2).

Automatic External Defibrillators

To enhance the survival rate of sudden cardiac arrest in the community, the American Heart Association began a more concerted effort in the past decade to promote the use of the automated external defibrillator (AED).[24–26] The goal is to provide critically important prompt defibrillation from first responders with minimal training (police officers, firefighters, security guards, flight attendants, some laypeople) until further help arrives. While such devices were first introduced for clinical use in the late 1970s, technological advances in the past two decades have greatly increased the safety and efficacy of AEDs by nonmedical personnel.[27,28,33–36]

Automatic external defibrillatoris are computerized devices consisting of adhesive electrodes which recognize cardiac rhythms and deliver an electrical shock across the chest wall to terminate ventricular fibrillation. If ventricular fibrillation or rapid, pulseless ventricular tachycardia is detected by the electrode/defibrillator pads placed over the cardiac apex and upper right chest, then the operator is advised by audible and/or visual prompts to deliver a shock by pressing a button. The operator does not need to know how many joules to use because it is preprogrammed. Because an operator is required to activate the shock switch, these devices are considered "automated" rather than "automatic."[27,33–36]

Following shock delivery, the AED will reanalyze the rhythm and advise additional shocks if fibrillation persists. Following three unsuccessful shocks, the AED will recommend resuming CPR. The AED will cease shocks if it detects that ventricular fibrillation has terminated. Trained first responders can often deliver the first defibrillation shock within 30 seconds of turning on the device. Current AED models are portable, lightweight (under 10 lbs.), and cost approximately $2500 to $3000 (Fig. 2-3). A variety of studies show that the ability of AEDs to detect ventricular fibrillation approaches 100% sensitivity and specificity.[27–36]

It should be stated that AEDs are only one part of an effective EMS system. Concomitant bystander CPR and the rapid mobilization of an advanced cardiac life support team are also important factors in patient survival. Given the emerging presence of AEDs in non–hospital settings, it seems reasonable for dermatologists practicing in more remote communities with limited or no EMS service to consider including an AED among their emergency equipment.

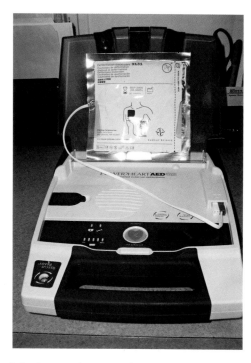

FIGURE 2-3. Automatic external defibrillators have been made increasingly more portable and user friendly. Adhesive electrodes are placed over the patient's cardiac apex and upper right chest to detect the cardiac rhythm. With audible and visual prompting, the device advises the operator to deliver a defibrillating shock by pressing a button.

Anaphylaxis

Anaphylaxis is a generalized multiorgan allergic reaction characterized by rapid evolution. Reactions may begin with a prodrome of cutaneous features that include diffuse erythema, pruritus, or urticaria, followed by inspiratory stridor, laryngoedema, bronchospasm, hypotension, cardiac arrhythmias, or hyperperistalsis. Systemic reactions can be mild, moderate, or severe because any combination of the above signs and symptoms can occur.[37,38] Anaphylaxis is a potentially life-threatening event, accounting for approximately 1500 deaths annually in the United States.[39]

In classic anaphylaxis, the offending antigen binds to immunoglobin E (IgE) on mast cells and basophils, initiating the release of preformed mediators such as histamine and newly formed mediators such as prostaglandins and leukotrienes. Vascular permeability is increased and vascular smooth muscle is relaxed, leading to hypotension. Pulmonary smooth muscle constriction results in the characteristic bronchospasm.[40,41] Onset of symptoms is usually immediate, occurring within seconds to minutes of exposure to the offending antigen. Peak severity then progresses over the next 5 to 30 minutes. Some reactions,

however, may present up to 4 hours after antigen ingestion (e.g., medication or food).[39,41]

Etiologies include a variety of microorganisms, medications, foods, physical factors, and exercise. For many, no cause can be identified.[42] Implicated foods in adults include peanuts, shellfish, tree nuts (e.g., almonds, hazelnets, walnuts, pecans), and other fish.[41–44] In children, eggs, peanuts, milk, soy, tree nuts, shellfish, and wheat are most commonly responsible.[41,44] The most common antibiotics causing anaphylaxis are penicillins, cephalosporins, sulfonamides, and vancomycin.[44–46] Penicillin in particular accounts for 75% of anaphylactic mortalities in the United States, with fatalities occurring in 1 in 50,000 to 1 in 100,000.[39,46] Insect stings, particularly from the fire ant or Hymenoptera (bee, wasp, hornet, yellow jacket, sawfly), result in approximately 40 to 100 anaphylactic deaths per year in the United States.[39,43,47] A subset of anaphylactic reactions are exercise induced. These reactions can occur after ingestion of a specific food (exercising within 4–6 hours after eating a particular food) or several hours following ingestion of any food. Alternatively, reaction to exercise alone without any temporal relationship to meals can occur.[41]

Anaphylactoid reactions are clinically similar, but are not IgE mediated. Therefore, they are not allergic reactions. They occur by directly stimulating mast cells and basophils, provoking the release of the same histamines, leukotrienes, and prostaglandins implicated in the clinical presentation of anaphylaxis. Anaphylaxis and anaphylactoid reactions are often referred to collectively as *anaphylaxis*. An important distinction is that the latter can often be prevented by pretreatment with steroids and antihistamines. Anaphylactoid reactions are most commonly caused by radiocontrast media, aspirin, nonsteroidal anti-inflammatory agents, opioids, and muscle relaxants.[39,41,43]

The incidence of anaphylactic reactions in the dermatology office is likely very low because the most common etiologies are not often directly relevant to the typical office encounter. Nevertheless, etiologies could include preoperative antibiotic prophylaxis with a penicillin or cephalosporin, local anesthesia infiltration with an ester anesthetic or lidocaine with methylparaben (see Lidocaine "Allergy" below), an insect sting, or an ill-fated sampling of displayed waiting room food. Bacitracin, neomycin, and topical nitrogen mustard–induced anaphylaxis have been reported.[48–54] Many of these cases exhibited concomitant stasis dermatitis and/or ulceration, presumably providing more rapid systemic absorption of the offending agent. Similarly, the medical disinfectant chlorhexidine has been shown to rarely cause anaphylactic symptoms during or shortly following surgical procedures, with specific IgE and positive skin test reactions demonstrated.[45,55–57] Avoiding mucous membrane application and using lower concentrations of chlorhexidine (0.05%) may minimize these reactions.

Similarly, while natural rubber latex allergies are becoming increasingly more recognized, a small percentage of patients can manifest anaphylactic reactions. Such patients usually have undergone multiple surgeries, require long-term bladder care, or are health workers more habitually exposed to such materials than the average patient. Alternatively, atopic individuals have an enhanced risk of anaphylaxis to natural rubber latex.[45] In the acutely bronchospastic, hypotensive patient, the dermatologist should therefore consider latex or topical medication–induced anaphylaxis.

Prompt recognition is the key to anaphylaxis management. While the history and clinical presentation are often diagnostic, sometimes laboratory evaluation can be helpful, consisting of elevated plasma or urinary histamine levels or plasma tryptase levels drawn after the onset of symptoms.[39,41,57] The patient should be placed supine on the examining table, preferably in the Trendelenberg position, and tight clothing should be loosened. Vital signs can be assessed while low-flow oxygen (1–2 L/min) by face mask is initiated. Efforts to eliminate or minimize antigen exposure include wiping off the antigen (e.g., bacitracin) or applying a tourniquet proximal to the injection site (e.g., anesthetic or insect sting), which is loosened every 5 minutes for at least 3 minutes.[57] The designated staff member can then activate the EMS system according to office protocol. Intravenous access may be needed for fluid resuscitation in cases of persistent hypotension.

The essential medication for the initial treatment of anaphylaxis is epinephrine. Its α1-agonist properties increase peripheral vascular resistence and decrease urticaria, its β1-agonist activities increase cardiac rate and contractility, and the β2-agonist component relaxes bronchial smooth muscles. As soon as anaphylaxis is suspected, 0.3 to 0.5 mL of epinephrine 1:1000 is administered subcutaneously or intramuscularly, usually into the upper arm. Gentle massage of the injection site facilitates absorption. A patient taking a β-blocker should be started on a lower dose (0.2 mL). The pediatric dose is 0.01 mL/kg, up to a maximum of 0.3 to 0.5 mL.[37,39–41,58] Rapid inactivation of epinephrine may require repeat dosing two or three times at 5 to 10 minute intervals. Severe hypotension may require intravenous epinephrine (1:10,000 at 1 mcg/min, increased to 10 mcg/min as needed).[39] This would be best managed by the summoned EMS team because more thorough cardiac monitoring is required.

Nebulized β-adrenergic agents such as albuterol with or without intravenous aminophylline may be considered in patients with severe bronchoconstriction. Simultaneous H1 and H2 blockade may be used early on (within the first 20 minutes) to prevent reactions (e.g., a maximum of Benadryl 50 mg IM and ranitidine 1 mg/kg IV), while steroids may prevent a delayed reaction that could occur 3 to 6 hours later.[39–41,58]

While waiting for epinephrine to take effect, the physician should ensure that an open airway is maintained by appropriate head tilt or jaw thrust maneuvers. The office team should be prepared to initiate BLS if respiratory failure and shock develop.[58] The summoned EMS team can then arrive prepared for possible ACLS initiation prior to transport to a hospital. All patients with anaphylaxis should be monitored for up to 8 to 24 hours following the initial attack, depending on episode severity, due to the possibility of recurrent symptoms after initial resolution.[37,39–41] Ultimately, a referral to an allergist–immunologist for further evaluation and management appears prudent.

Vasovagal Syncope

Vasovagal syncope is the most common cause of acute brief unconsciousness. It is far more prevalent than anaphylaxis. There are often no associated cardiac or neurological abnormalities. Emotional stress, acute pain, or fear are precipitating factors, although frequently no cause is identified.[59]

The characteristic prodrome of a vasovagal reaction includes anxiety, diaphoresis, nausea, tachypnea, tachycardia, and/or confusion. The skin becomes pale and cool. Vagal-induced bradycardia in the setting of decreased systemic vascular resistance can initiate collapse. Pseudo-seizure activity can occur, characterized by brief clonic activity. Blood pressure may initially decrease but is restored with recumbency. Conversely, anaphylaxis features warm, erythematous, dry, pruritic skin with tachycardia and recumbent hypertension.[37,58]

Vasovagal events can be minimized by performing procedures such as injections and biopsies with the patient placed in a supine position. Occasionally, the simple act of a prior explanation of the procedure may allay anxiety. For patients with a known history of vasovagal syncope, it may be wise to place a towel over their eyes to avoid sights of blood, surgical trays, and biopsy specimens. A distracting conversation ("talkesthesia") can be similarly beneficial. Following the procedure, the patient should slowly sit up and be watched for several minutes while postoperative instructions are discussed. Should a vasovagal reaction develop, the patient is promptly restored to recumbency, preferably in the Trendelenberg position. A cool water wash cloth placed on the forehead with a low power fan directed toward the face is often helpful. Patients should be educated as to the difference between this benign condition and true allergy. In summary, early recognition, restoration of recumbency, and reassurance constitute the management approach to vasovagal events.[58,59]

Lidocaine "Allergy"

Lidocaine is extensively used in the dermatology office. Occasionally, a patient will claim an allergy to local anesthetics, including lidocaine. The first report of allergy to a local anesthetic was published in the early 20th century, involving a case of a contact dermatitis on the provider's (dentist) hand.[60] Subsequent similar reports all concerned reactions to the ester types of anesthetics. This group of agents, which include procaine, tetracaine, and benzocaine, are derivatives of para-aminobenzoic acid (PABA), an established allergen.[61] Occasionally, more serious clinical presentations, including the urticaria and dyspnea seen in anaphylaxis, may be elicited when obtaining a patient's medical history. Evaluating this history and managing such patients can be a very frustrating and cumbersome endeavor for the clinician and patient because alternatives, such as general anesthesia in an operating room, are disproportionately expensive and morbid for simple office procedures.

Toxic reactions to lidocaine resulting from overdosage (central nervous system or myocardial depression or excitation, perioral numbness, nausea, seizures, or coma) or vasovagal reactions should be distinguished to avoid confusion with allergy. True allergic reactions to pure lidocaine are extremely rare, although there is a case report literature that supports this phenomenon.[62–64] Lidocaine belongs to the amide class of anesthetics, which do not cross-react with ester anesthetics. It is estimated that less than 1% of reported "allergic" reactions to local anesthetics are immune mediated, and that amide anesthetics comprise of very small percentage of those reactions.[62,65,66] A growing case report literature of type IV (delayed type) sensitivity to lidocaine, in which a pruritic erythematous eruption develops 2 days following exposure, has emerged, indicating that such reactions may occur more frequently than previously thought.[61,67–72]

Methyl- and propylparaben are preservatives added to a variety of lotions, cosmetics, foodstuffs, and lidocaine bottles to extend their shelf life. There is some cross-reactivity with PABA. Similarly, sulphite preservatives added to lidocaine and ester anesthetics are structural analogs of PABA. Sulpha-allergic patients should therefore avoid use of anesthetics containing methylparaben and sulfite preservatives.[62,73]

Anxiety regarding the use of needles, and/or the effects of the frequently added epinephrine in lidocaine vials, can lead to palpitations, "panic attacks," and vasovagal events that the patient may long remember as an allergic reaction.

Finally, there are a couple of other issues that should be considered in the differential diagnosis of a lidocaine allergy. Concurrent drug exposures, such as nonsteroidal anti-inflammatory drugs and antibiotics, may be the real culprits. Latex allergies should also be included as a possibility.[45]

Skin prick and intradermal tests with various concentrations of lidocaine with methylparaben and appropriate controls have been advocated in the workup of a lidocaine allergy. Patch testing and intradermal challenge assist in the evaluation of type IV sensitivity.[66,74,75] Such investigations are best performed by allergists. Negative results with the above screening tests may lead to a challenge with subcutaneous injections of lidocaine. Skin testing results are often equivocal, however. In vitro testing is recommended for those patients with a history of anaphylaxis.[62,74,75]

If the surgical procedure is minor, one can consider intralesional antihistamines (diphenylhydramine or chlorpheniramine) with the appropriate postoperative sedation precautions. Temporary anesthesia may also be achieved by the intradermal injection of normal saline or a topical cold spray (Frigiderm). Even nondrug approaches such as acupuncture or hypnosis have been offered.[76] Ultimately, patients may require referral to a surgeon for general operating room excision and closure or other analgesics/sedatives, such as nitrous oxide, meperidine, or ketamine.[76]

It should be recalled that the intravenous administration of lidocaine for ventricular arrhythmias or the induction of anesthesia for surgery (with propofol) is routinely and countlessly performed. Allergic reactions to lidocaine in those settings is extremely rare.[73] Consequently, a patient claim of lidocaine allergy should be met with a thorough history evaluation and possible allergy consultation to more fully establish its validity. Adverse drug reactions to local anesthetics, lidocaine in particular, have an established differential diagnosis with "allergy" appearing low on the list.

Acute Stroke

Stroke is the third leading cause of death in the United States (after coronary heart disease and cancer), and the leading cause of adult brain injury. Each year approximately 500,000 Americans suffer a stroke, nearly 25% of which are fatal.[77] A stroke occurs when the blood supply to a portion of the brain is disrupted, resulting in a sudden neurologic deficit from inadequate oxygen delivery. Roughly 85% of strokes are ischemic, in which a blood clot arising within a cerebral vessel or traveling from elsewhere (an embolism) completely occludes a cerebral artery. The remainder are hemorrhagic strokes, where a cerebral artery ruptures, causing bleeding into the surface of the brain (e.g., from an aneurysm) or within the brain substance (e.g., from hypertension).[77–80]

While historically little treatment was available to alter the course of the stroke, the potential role of early surgery for hemorrhagic strokes and the established role of fibrinolytic therapy for ischemic strokes has now justified the rapid evaluation and management of the acute stroke victim.[81–85]

The American Heart Association and American Stroke Association have established stroke management guidelines for physicians, EMS personnel, and the general public. A seven D's mnemonic had been offered: detection, dispatch, delivery, door, data, decision, and drug.[86] The first three D's are the purview of the BLS providers in the community, including the dermatology office and EMS responders. **Detection** occurs when the signs and symptoms of a stroke are recognized and the EMS system is activated. The EMS team is **dispatched** and the victim is **delivered** to a hospital appropriate for acute stroke care. Once at the hospital, the patient is quickly evaluated and triaged at the **door** (emergency department), where **data** (a head computerized tomography scan) is obtained and the decision to proceed with fibrinolysis (**drug**) is made.

The dermatologist's role chiefly concerns the detection phase of a sudden neurologic deficit. This may include an alteration in consciousness (confusion, coma, seizures), aphasia, dysarthria, facial weakness or asymmetry, extremity weakness, paralysis, sensory loss, ataxia, visual loss (particularly in one eye), or vertigo. A severe headache, nausea, or vomiting generally suggests hemorrhage rather than ischemia. Signs and symptoms can develop in clusters or in isolation and may wax and wane or advance rapidly.[87,88]

A quick and practical exam tool to evaluate a stroke is the Cincinatti Prehospital Stroke Scale. It focuses on three major physical findings: facial droop, arm drift, and abnormal speech. The patient is asked to show teeth or smile. Asymmetry may be abnormal. The patient is asked to close eyes and extend both arms straight out front for 10 seconds. If one arm does not move at all or one arms drifts down, this is considered abnormal. The patient is then asked to repeat a phrase. Slurred words, using wrong words, or the failure to speak are abnormal results. An abnormality in any one of these exercises is strongly suggestive of a stroke.[89]

The primary function of the dermatologist who suspects a patient is having a stroke is to immediately activate the EMS system. In most cases, definitive hospital-based intervention (i.e., fibrinolysis) must occur within 3 hours of the onset of stroke symptoms to be beneficial.[84] The time-critical nature of stroke management means that the patient should be transported rapidly. In the interim, the medical office should attend to the ABCs (airway, breathing, circulation) of basic life support as needed until the EMS responders arrive.

Status Epilepticus

Dermatologists encounter patients whose cutaneous disease has potential epileptic manifestations, most notably those with tuberous sclerosis, neurofibromatosis, Sturge–Weber syndrome, and lupus erythematosis. The theoretical risk of office seizures, therefore, merits brief mention of a responsible approach.

Of the million Americans who suffer from recurrent seizures, approximately 3% to 8% of them will manifest at least one episode of status epilepticus, characterized by general tonic-clonic seizures lasting longer than 20 minutes, or a series of recurrent seizures lasting more than 30 minutes with a loss of consciousness. There may be no previous history of seizures. Status epilepticus is associated with a 6% to 18% mortality and higher morbidity.[90]

The dermatologist's first priority is the maintenance of a patent airway while the EMS is notified. An oral or nasopharyngeal airway may be useful. If available, oxygen can be delivered by face mask. Vital signs should be monitored. The ideal area to place the patient is a soft, flat surface away from sharp objects.[90,91] Objects and fingers should not be placed in the victim's mouth. If seizure activity has abated and the patient is breathing and has a pulse, placing him/her in a recovery position (a modified lateral position) will allow the clearance of any pooled airway secretions.[20,92,93] In all likelihood, EMS personnel should have arrived by this point to continue management.

If EMS has not arrived within 5 minutes, a peripheral intravenous line should be placed and blood sampled for serum glucose, calcium, electrolytes, and relevant anticonvulsant levels. Subsequently, a bolus of 50 cc 50% glucose is injected prior to a maintenance infusion of normal saline if available.[91] If EMS is still absent at 10 minutes, then seizure control is necessary. The benzodiazepine lorazepam (Ativan) administered at a dose of 1 to 2 mg intravenously will stop seizures within minutes in the vast majority of patients.[90] Lorazepam has emerged as the seizure drug of choice with a longer action time, 10- to 12-hour half-life, and lower risk of respiratory depression and hypotension than 5 to 10 mg of diazepam (Valium).[90,94] Regardless of whether or not seizure activity has ceased, patients should be evaluated in an emergency room for seizure etiology and management options.

Electrosurgery and Pacemakers/Defibrillators

The increasing prevalence of implantable pacemakers and defibrillators has raised questions regarding the safety during electrosurgical procedures. Standard dermatologic electrosurgery consists of a high-frequency, high-voltage, low-amperage alternating current that generates an intense heat at the electrode, dehydrating and coagulating tissue.[95] Electrodesiccation (direct tissue contact) and electrofulguration (1–2 mm separation of tip from tissue) are monoterminal techniques for which a dispersive plate is not required. The patient's body acts as its own relative ground. In electrocoagulation, the amperage is greater and voltage lower with a biterminal arrangement. A dispersive plate can enhance its effect. Electrocutting is another high-frequency modality with an undamped sine wave, as opposed to the damped waves of the techniques just described. The net effect is a higher energy current that separates tissue ("cuts"). Electrodesiccation, fulguration, coagulation, and cutting current have been thought to involve a potentially significant transfer of electrical activity to patients with pacemakers.[96]

Fixed-rate pacemakers have no theoretical basis for harmful interaction because they lack a sensing device with which bursts of electrosurgery could interfere. They fire continuously at a programmed rate. A patient's intrinsic heart rate may compete with this arrangement and initiate ventricular tachycardia or fibrillation.[97,98] Subsequently, more patient-concordant pacemakers were developed.

Demand pacemakers have both a sensing and pacing function. Ventricular-inhibited pacemakers fire when the patient's intrinsic heart rate is slower than the programmed heart rate. A ventricular-triggered type fires at a preset rate when no spontaneous heartbeats are detected. It fires with each spontaneous beat as well, yet has no effect then because cardiac muscle has already been depolarized by the patient's own heartbeat. Many pacemakers have a safety system in which the pacemaker functions in fixed-rate mode in the event of sensory failure. In addition, a switch can be activated via an externally applied magnet to switch from demand to fixed-rate function.[95,98]

Concerns regarding pacemaker/electrosurgery interactions have evolved from two theoretical scenarios. If a ventricular-inhibited pacemaker misinterprets electrical interference as a spontaneous beat, bradycardia or asystole may ensue if the patient's spontaneous rate is slow or nonexistent. Alternatively, a ventricular-triggererd pacer may sense such interference as instrinsic beats and fire inappropriately, provoking tachyarrhythmias.[95]

The practice of electrosurgical restraint with pacemakers originated in the urologic literature of the 1970s, in which very high-energy electrocutting was used during transurethral prostatic surgery. Reports of pacemaker battery depletion featured one device that failed several weeks after electrocutting and another that malfunctioned after 45 minutes of electosurgery.[99,100] Others described bradycardia from electrosurgical interference in patients with demand pacemakers.[101,102] Pacemaker inhibition with electrocutting but not electrocoagulation has been noted.[99,103] O'Donoghue reported asystole from 5-second bursts of electrocutting. The pacemaker was converted to fixed-rate mode by applying an external magnet, and the patient fully recovered.[104] By 1975, Krull and colleagues offered dermatologists a set of recommendations based on these experiences. Electrosurgery should be avoided in pacemaker patients if an alternative, equally effective modality existed. Prior consultation with a cardiologist, emergency backup, short bursts of electosurgery (under 5 seconds), and good grounding away from the heart were all recommended.[98] Finally, considerations should be given to magnetically converting the pacemaker to fixed-rate mode for the procedure. Several subsequent reports questioned the practice of magnetic conversion, citing cases where electrosurgery caused a program change in certain specific pacemaker models while the magnet was on.[105,106]

Improvements in pacemaker shielding and filtering systems were reflected in Schultz's series of 33 patients who endured transurethral electrosurgery without incident.[107] Yet despite technological advances in cardiac pacer protective circuitry and reprogrammability, electrosurgery remains cited as a common external cause of transient pacemaker malfunction, even in the 1990s.[108,109] Levine and colleagues described a pacemaker patient who developed two episodes of electrosurgically induced ventricular fibrillation during a coronary revascularization. During chest closure following the procedure, electrosurgery was used for hemostasis without incident.[108] Kellow recalled a patient in whom a transurethral resection of the prostate was performed. His pacemaker failed to capture due to an altered threshold after at least 5 to 10 minutes of electrocutting.[110] Goodman urged fellow anesthesiologists to transcend anectodal discussions and identify the overall incidence of pacemaker failure during electrosurgery.[111]

Implantable cardioverter-defibrillators (ICDs) are implantable electronic devices that sense cardiac electrical activity and terminate ventricular fibrillation and ventricular tachyarrhythmias. Electromagnetic interference could potentially damage/deactivate the ICD device or trigger the device to deliver a defibrillatory discharge. There are some reports of interference with ICDs, but not in a dermatologic surgical context.[112–115]

It is therefore important to realize that guidelines for the dermatology patient with a pacemaker or ICD have evolved from a case report literature largely irrelevant in surgical procedure, pacemaker era, electrosurgical modality, procedure duration, and/or energy level. Even more recent reviews in the dermatologic literature persist in referencing nondermatologic literature to justify very cautious management guidelines, including detailed preoperative cardiac clearance, programmer availability for deactivation of the ICD or conversion of pacemaker to fixed-rate mode, continuous cardiac monitoring with electrocardiogram (ECG) and/or pulse oximetry, ACLS equipment availability including resuscitative drugs if necessary, cardiology/hospital access, and a postprocedure plan to coordinate the reactivation or functional assessment of the device by the patient's cardiologist.[116]

The most recent survey of dermatologic surgeons corroborates a previous survey regarding the heterogeneity in approach to the electrosurgical precautions taken with cardiac devices.[117,118] While most surgeons responding indicated that they use short bursts of electrocautery (71%), use minimal power (61%), and avoid use directly around the pacemaker/ICD (57%), the use of heat cautery (34%) or bipolar forceps (19%) to avoid any electrical current passing to the patient is less commonly employed. Finally, obtaining cardiology consultation (11%), deactivating the ICD (15%), or changing the pacemaker to fixed-rate mode (1%), and postoperative evaluation of the device by a cardiologist (2%) are very infrequently utilized.[118]

Of the 166 Mohs surgeons who responded to the survey, there were six reported incidences of pacemaker reprogramming and four incidences of ICD firing during the surgical procedures. There were 18 patients with "adverse effects," including syncope, altered mental status, palpitations, and one case of hemodynamic instability (no further information known). There were no acute resuscitative efforts needed nor long-term morbidities or mortalities related to the use of electrosurgery in the survey. The overall complication rate thought to result from electrosurgery was calculated to be 0.8 patients/100 years of surgical practice, or roughly one case per three surgical careers of at least 30 years each.

It should be noted that surveys are recall based, and a definitive cause-and-effect relationship between electrosurgery and these events is not certain.

Ultimately, definitive recommendations regarding the use of electrosurgery in patients with pacemakers or ICDs awaits studies that prospectively measure adverse events and compare this to the rate of pacemaker and ICD malfunction in those not undergoing the use of electrosurgery. Each dermatologist needs to pursue a strategy that he/she is comfortable with. It appears prudent at this point to recommend some basic guidelines until more enlightening studies emerge[116–120]:

1. Consider electrocautery or bipolar instruments that minimize or eliminate the theoretical risk of interference.
2. Carefully place the dispersive electrode ("ground plate") so that the pacemaker or ICD is not in the path of current flow between the electrosurgical instrument and the ground plate.
3. Ensure that electrical equipment is functioning properly with adequate grounding.
4. Maintain current flow to 3- to 5-second bursts, with pauses between bursts to minimize any prolonged potential interference.
5. Use the lowest electrosurgical current necessary for hemostasis.
6. Have an emergency plan, including defibrillation equipment, if necessary.
7. Consider consulting with the patient's cardiologist prior to surgery for perioperative and postoperative management suggestions.

References

1. Guidelines for cardiopulmonary resuscitation and emergency cardiac care. Emergency Cardiac Care Committee and Subcommittees, American Heart Association. Part I Introduction. JAMA 1992;268:2171–2183.
2. Heart and stroke facts: 2000 statistical update. American Heart Association; 1999.
3. Weaver WD, Hill D, Fahrenbruch CE, et al. Use of automated external defibrillator in the management of out-of-hospital cardiac arrest. N Engl J Med 1988;319:661–666.
4. Bayes de Luna A, Coumel P, Leclercq JF. Ambulatory sudden cardiac death; mechanisms of production of fatal arrhythmia on the basis of data from 157 cases. Am Heart J 1989;117:151–159.
5. White RD, Hankins DG, Bugliosi TF. Seven years' experience with early defibrillation by police and paramedics in an emergency medical services system. Resuscitation 1998;39:145–151.
6. Kellermann AL, Hackman BB, Somes G, Kreth TK, Nail L, Dobyns P. Impact of first-responder defibrillation in an urban emergency medical services system. JAMA 1993;270:1708–1713.
7. Varon J, Marik P. Treatment of cardiac arrest with automatic external defibrillators: impact on outcome. Am J Cardiovasc Drugs 2003;3:265–270.
8. Holmberg M, Holmberg S, Herlitz J. The problem of out-of-hospital cardiac arrest prevalence of sudden death in Europe today. Am J Cardiol 1999;83:88D–90D.
9. Auble TE, Menegazzi JJ, Paris PM. Effect of out-of-hospital cardiac defibrillation by basic life support providers on cardiac arrest mortality; a metaanalysis. Ann Emerg Med 1995;25:642–648.
10. Cummins RO, Ornato JP, Thies WH, Pepe PE. Improving survival from sudden cardiac arrest: the "chain of survival" concept. A statement for health professionals from the Advanced Cardiac Life Support Subcommittee and the Emergency Cardiac Care Committee, American Heart Association. Circulation 1991;83:1832–1847.
11. Eisenberg MS, Bergner L, Hallstrom A. Cardiac resuscitation in the community: importance of rapid provision and implications for program planning. JAMA 1979;241:1905–1907.
12. Weaver WD, Copass MK, Hill D, Fahrenbruch C, Hallstrom AP, Cobb L. Cardiac arrest treated with a new automatic external defibrillator by out-of-hospital first responders. Am J Cardiol 1986;57:1017–1021.

13. Guidelines of care for office surgical facilities: part I. J Am Acad Dermatol 1992;26:763–765.

14. Guidelines of care for office surgical facilities: part II. J Am Acad Dermatol 1995;33:265–270.

15. Kobernick MS. Management of emergencies in the medical office. J Emerg Med 1986;4:71–74.

16. Fuchs S, Jaffe DM, Christoffel KK. Pediatric emergencies in office practices: prevalence and office preparedness. Pediatrics 1989;83:931–939.

17. Altieri M, Bellet J, Scott H. Preparedness for pediatric emergencies encountered in the practitioner's office. Pediatrics 1990;85:710–714.

18. Emergency Cardiac Care Committee and subcommittees, American Heart Association. Guidelines for cardiopulmonary resuscitation and emergency cardiac care, II: adult basic life support. JAMA 1992;268:2184–2198.

19. Emergency Cardiac Care Committee and subcommittees, American Heart Association. Guidelines for cardiopulmonary resuscitation and emergency cardiac care, III: adult advanced cardiac life support. JAMA 1992;268:2199–2241.

20. BLS for healthcare providers. American Heart Association; 2001.

21. Emergency Cardiac Care Committee and subcommittees, American Heart Association. Guidelines for cardiopulmonary resuscitation and emergency cardiac care, IX; ensuring effectiveness of communitywide emergency cardiac care. JAMA 1992;268:2289–2295.

22. Thomas RM, Amonette RA. Emergencies in skin surgery. In: Roenigk RK, Roenigk HH, eds. Dermatologic surgery, principles and practice. 2nd ed. New York: Marcel Dekker; 1996:77–89.

23. Nagi C, Thomas RM. Recognition and management of office medical and surgical emergencies. In: Wheeland RG, ed. Cutaneous surgery. Philadelphia: Saunders; 1994:150–158.

24. Cummins RO. From concept to standard-of-care? Review of the clinical experience with automated external defibrillators. Ann Emerg Med 1989;18:1269–1275.

25. Cummins RO, Thies W. Encouraging early defibrillation: the American Heart Association and automated external defibrillators. Ann Emerg Med 1990;19:1245–1248.

26. Weisfeldt ML, Kerber RE, McGoldrick RP, et al., for the American Heart Association Task Force on automatic external defibrillation. Public access to defibrillation. Circulation 1995;92:2763.

27. Marenco JP, Wang PJ, Link MS, et al. Improving survival from sudden cardiac arrest: the role of the automated external defibrillator. JAMA 2001;285:1193–1200.

28. Cummins RO, Eisenberg M, Bergner L, Murray JA. Sensitivity, accuracy, and safety of an automatic external defibrillator. Lancet 1984;2:318–320.

29. Liner BE, Jorgenson DB, Poole JE, et al., for the LIFE Investigators. Treatment of out-of-hospital cardiac arrest with low-energy impedance-compensating biphasic waveform automatic external defibrillators. Biomed Instrum Technol 1998;32:631–644.

30. Stults KR, Brown DD, Cooley F, et al. Self-adhesive monitor/defibrillator pads improve pre-hospital defibrillation success. Ann Emerg Med 1987;16:872–877.

31. Carlson MD, Freeman CS, Garan H, Ruskin JN. Sensitivity of an automatic external defibrillator for ventricular tachyarrhythmias in patients undergoing electrophysiologic studies. Am J Cardiol 1988;61:787–790.

32. Poole JE, White RD, Kanz KG, et al. Low-energy impedance-compensating biphasic waveforms terminate ventricular fibrillation at high rates in victims of out-of-hospital cardiac arrest. J Cardiovasc Electrophysiol 1997;8:1373–1385.

33. Ramaswamy K, Page RL. The automated external defibrillator: critical link in the chain of survival. Ann Rev Med 2003;54:235–243.

34. Varon J, Marik PE. Treatment of cardiac arrest with automatic external defibrillators: impact on outcome. Am J Cardiovasc Drugs 2003;3:265–270.

35. Das MK, Zipes DP. Sudden cardiac arrest and automated external defibrillators. Circ J 2003;67:975–982.

36. Liddle R, Davies CS, Colquhoun M, Handley AJ. ABC of resuscitation: the automated external defibrillator. BMJ 2003;327:1216–1218.

37. Soto-Aguilar MC, deShazo RD, Waring NP. Anaphylaxis: why it happens and what to do about it. Postgrad Med 1987;82:154–170.

38. McLean-Tooke APC, Bethune CA, Fay AC, Spickett GP. Adrenaline in the treatment of anaphylaxis: what is the evidence? BMJ 2003;327:1332–1334.

39. Tang AW. A practical guide to anaphylaxis. Am Fam Physician 2003;68:1325–1332.

40. Bochner BS, Lichtenstein LM. Anaphylaxis. N Engl J Med 1991;324:1785–1790.

41. Malde B, Ditto AM. Anaphylaxis. Allergy Asthma Proc 2004;25:S52–S53.

42. Kemp SF, Lockey RF, Wolf BL, et al. Anaphylaxis — a review of 266 cases. Arch Intern Med 1995;155:1749–1754.

43. Lieberman P. Anaphylaxis and anaphylactoid reactions. In: Middleton E, ed. Allergy: principles and practice. 5th ed. St. Louis: Mosby; 1998:1079–1089.

44. Ditto AM, Grammer LG. Food allergy. In: Grammer LG, Greenberger PA, eds. Patterson's allergic diseases. 6th ed. Philadelphia: Lippincott Williams & Wilkins; 2002:260.

45. Thong BY, Chan Y. Anaphylaxis during surgical and interventional procedures. Ann Allergy Asthma Immunol 2004;92:619–628.

46. Joint Task Force on Practice Parameters. The diagnosis and management of anaphylaxis. J Allergy Clin Immunol 1998;101:S465–S528.

47. Neugut A, Ghatak, AT, Miller RL. Anaphylaxis in the United States: an investigation into its epidemiology. Arch Intern Med 2001;161:15–21.

48. Pippen R. Anaphylactoid reaction after Chymacort ointment. BMJ 1966;1:1168–1172.

49. Comaish JS, Cunliffe WJ. Absorption of drugs from various ulcers: a cause of anaphylaxis. Br J Clin Pract 1967;21:97.

50. Roupe G, Strennegard O. Anaphylactic shock elicited by topical administration of bacitracin. Arch Dermatol 1969;100:450–452.

51. Daughters D, Zackheim H, Maibach H. Urticaria and anphylactoid reactions after topical application of mechlorethamine. Arch Dermatol 1973;107:429–430.

52. Vale MA, Connolly A, Epstein AM, et al. Bacitracin-induced anaphylaxis. Arch Dermatol 1978;114:800.

53. Schechter JF, Wilkison RD, Carpio JD. Anaphylaxis following the use of bacitracin ointment. Arch Dermatol 1984;120:909–911.

54. Phillips TJ, Rogers GS, Kanj LF. Bacitracin anaphylaxis. J Geriatr Dermatol 1995;3:83–85.

55. Okano M, Nomura M, Hata S, et al. Anaphylactic symptoms due to chlorhexidine gluconate. Arch Dermatol 1989;125:50–52.

56. Pharm NH, Weiner JM, Reisner GS, Baldo BA. Anaphylaxis to chlorhexidine: case report: implication of immunoglobulin E antibodies and identification of an allergenic determinant. Clin Exp Allergy 2000;30:1001–1007.

57. Garvey LH, Roed-Petersen J, Husum B. Anaphylaxis I anesthetized patients: four cases of chlorhexidine allergy. Acta Anaesthesiol Scand 2001;45:1290–1294.

58. Gordon BR. Prevention and management of office allergy emergencies. Otolaryngol Clin North Am 1992;25:119–134.

59. Martin JB, Ruskin J. Faintness, syncope, and seizures. In: Wilson JD, et al., eds. Harrison's principles of internal medicine. 12th ed. New York: McGraw-Hill; 1991:134–140.

60. Mook WH. Skin reactions to apothesin and quinine in susceptible persons. Arch Dermatol 1920;1:651–655.

61. Mackley CL, Marks JG. Lidocaine hydrochloride. Am J Contact Dermat 2003;14:221–223.

62. Chiu C, Lin T, Hsia S, et al. Systemic anaphylaxis following local lidocaine administration during a dental procedure. Ped Emerg Care 2004;20:178–180.

63. Giovannitt J, Bennett CR. Assessment of allergy to local anesthetics. J Am Dent Assoc 1979;98:701–706.

64. Chin TM, Fellner MJ. Allergic hypersensitivity to lidocaine hydrochloride. Int J Dermatol 1980;19:147–148.

65. Verrill PJ. Adverse reactions to local anesthetics and vasoconstrictor drugs. Practitioner 1975;214:380–387.

66. Amsler E, Flahault A, Mathelier-Fusade P, Aractingi S. Evaluation of re-challenge in patients with suspected lidocaine allergy. Dermatology 2004;208:109–111.

67. Curley RK, Macfarlane AW, King CM. Contact sensitivity to the amide anesthetics lidocaine, prilocaine, and mepivacaine: case report and review of the literature. Arch Dermatol 1986;122:924–926.

68. Bircher AJ, Messmer SL, Surber C, Rufli T. Delayed-type hypersensitivity to subcutaneous lidocaine with tolerance to articaine: confirmation by in vivo and in vitro tests. Contact Dermatitis 1996;24:387–389.

69. Whalen JD. Delayed-type hypersensitivity after subcutaneous administration of amide anesthetic. Arch Dermatol 1996;132:1256–1257.

70. Briet S, Rueff F, Przybilla B. "Deep impact" contact allergy after subcutaneous injection of local anesthetics. Contact Dermatitis 2001;45:296–297.

71. Downs AM, Lear JT, Wallington TB, Sansom JE. Contact sensitivity and systemic reaction to pseudoephedrine and lignocaine. Contact Dermatitis 1998;39:33.

72. Kaufman JM, Hale EK, Ahinoff RA, Cohen DE. Cutaneous lidocaine allergy confirmed by patch testing. J Drugs Dermatol 2002;2:192–194.

73. Finucane BT. Allergies to local anesthetics — the real truth. Can J Anesth 2003;50:869–874.

74. Macy E. Local anesthetic adverse reaction evaluations: the role of the allergist. Ann Allergy Asthma Immunol 2003; 91:319–320.

75. Chandler MJ, Grammer LC. Provocative challenge with local anesthetics in patients with a prior history of reaction. J Allergy Clin Immunol 1987;79:883–886.

76. Lu D. Managing patients with local anesthetic complications using alternative methods. Penn Dent J 2002;69(3): 22–29.

77. Bronner LL, Kanter DS, Manson JE. Primary prevention of stroke. N Engl J Med 1995;333:1392–1400.

78. Pepe PE. The chain of recovery from brain attack: access, pre-hospital care, and treatment. In: Proceedings of the National Symposium on Rapid Identification and Treatment of Acute Stroke. Bethesda, MD: The National Institute of Neurological Disorders and Stroke; 1996:20–42.

79. Broderick JP, Brott T, Tomsick T, et al. The risk of subarachnoid and intracerebral hemorrhages in blacks as compared with whites. N Engl J Med 1992;326:733–736.

80. Brott T, Thalinger K, Hertzberg V. Hypertension as a risk factor for spontaneous intracerebral hemorrhage. Stroke 1986;17:1078–1083.

81. Broderick JP, Brott TG, Tomsick T, et al. Ultra-early evaluation of intracerebral hemorrhage. J Neurosurg 1990;72: 195–199.

82. The NINDS rt-PA Stroke Study Group. Tissue plasminogen activator for acute ischemic stroke. N Engl J Med 1995;333:1581–1587.

83. Hacke W, Kaste M, Fieschi C, et al. Intravenous thrombolysis with recombinant tissue plasminogen activator for acute hemispheric stroke: the European Cooperative Acute Stroke Study (ECASS). JAMA 1995;274:1017–1025.

84. Kwiatkowski TG, Libman RB, Frankel M, et al. Effects of tissue plasminogen activator for acute ischemic stroke at one year. N Engl J Med 1999;340:1781–1787.

85. Albers GW, Bates VE, Clark WM, et al. Intravenous tissue-type plasminogen activator for treatment of acute stroke: the Standard Treatment with Alteplase to Reverse Stroke (STARS) Study. JAMA 2000;283:1145–1150.

86. Hazinki MF. Demystifying recognition and management of stroke. Curr Emerg Cardiac Care 1996;7:8.

87. Barsan WG, Brott TG, Broderick JP, et al. Time of hospital presentation in patents with acute stroke. Arch Intern Med 1993;153:2558–2561.

88. Feldmann E, Gordon N, Brooks JM, et al. Factors associated with early presentation of acute stroke. Stroke 1993;24:1805–1810.

89. Kothari R, Pancioli A, Liu T, et al. Cincinnati Prehospital Stroke Scale: reproducibility and validity. Ann Emerg Med 1999;33:373–378.

90. Selbst SM. Office management of status epilepticus. Pediatr Emerg Care 1991;7:106–109.

91. Delgado-Escueta AV, Wasterlain C, Treiman DM, et al. Management of status epilepticus. N Engl J Med 1982;306: 1337–1340.

92. Handley AJ, Becker LB, Allen M, et al. Single-rescuer adult basic life support: an advisory statement from the Basic Life Support Working Group of the International Liaison Committee on Resuscitation. Resuscitation 1997; 34:101–108.

93. Turner S, Turner I, Chapman D, et al. A comparative study of the 1992 and 1997 recovery positions for use in the UK. Resuscitation 1998;39:153–160.

94. Emergency Cardiac Care Committee and subcommittees, American Heart Association. Guidelines for cardiopulmonary resuscitation and emergency cardiac care, IV: special resuscitation situations. JAMA 1992;268:2242–2250.

95. Sebben JE. Electrosurgery and cardiac pacemakers. J Am Acad Dermatol 1983;9:457–463.

96. Popkin GL. Electrosurgery. In: Epstein E, ed. Skin surgery. Springfield, IL: Thomas; 1982:385–404.

97. Escher DJW. Types of pacemakers and their complications. Circulation 1973;47:1119–1129.

98. Krull EA, Pickard SD, Hall JC. Effects of electrosurgery on cardiac pacemakers. J Derm Surg 1975;1:43–45.

99. Wajszezak WJ, Mowry RM, Dugan WL. Deactivation of a demand pacemaker by transurethral electrocautery. N Engl J Med 1969;280:34–35.

100. Schwingshackl H, Maurer R, Amor H. Interfering influence of low frequency alternating currents on asynchronous and controlled pacemaker systems during the use of electrosurgical devices. Schweiz Med Wochenschr 1971; 101:46–52.

101. Green LF, Merideth J. Transurethral operations employing high frequency electrical currents in patients with demand cardiac pacemakers. J Urol 1972;108:446–448.

102. Smith BR, Wise WS. Pacemaker malfunction from urethral electrocautery. JAMA 1971;218:256.

103. Batra YK, Bali IM. Effect of coagulation and cutting current on a demand pacemaker during transurethral resection of the prostate. A case report. Can Anaesth Soc J 1978;25:65.

104. O'Donoghue JK. Inhibition of a demand pacemaker by electrocautery. Chest 1973;64:664–666.

105. Parsonnet V, Furman S, Smyth NPD, et al. Optimal resources for implantable cardiac pacemakers. Intersociety commission for heart disease resources. Circulation 1980;68:226A.

106. Domino KB, Smith TC. Electrocautery-induced reprogramming of a pacemaker using a precordial magnet. Anesth Analg 1983;62:609–612.

107. Schultz W. Transurethral electro-resection in patients with cardiac pacemakers. Urologe 1979;18:247–249.

108. Levine PA, Balady GJ, Lazar HL, et al. Electrocautery and pacemakers: management of the paced patient subject to electrocautery. Ann Thorac Surg 1986;41: 313–317.

109. Hayes DL, Vlietstra RE. Pacemaker malfunction. Ann Intern Med 1993;119:828–835.

110. Kellow NH. Pacemaker failure during transurethral resection of the prostate. Anaesthesia 1993;48:136–138.

111. Goodman NW. Diathermy and failure of cardiac pacemakers. Anaesthesia 1993;48:824.

112. Furman S. Electrosurgical device interference with implanted pacemakers. JAMA 1978;239:1910.

113. Pinski SL. Emergencies related to implantable cardioverter-defibrillators. Crit Care Med 2000;28(Suppl):N174–N180.

114. Niehaus M, Tebbenjohanns J. Electromagnetic interference in patients with implanted pacemakers or cardioverter-defibrillators. Heart 2001;86:246–248.

115. Madigan JD, Choudhri AF, Chen J, et al. Surgical management of the patient with an implanted cardiac device: implications of electromagnetic interference. Ann Surg 1999;230:639–647.

116. LeVasseur JG, Kennard CD, Finly EM, Muse RK. Dermatologic electrosurgery in patients with implantable cardioverter-defibrillators and pacemakers. Dermatol Surg 1998;24:233–240.

117. Sebben JE. The status of electrosurgery in dermatologic practice. J Am Acad Dermatol 1988;19:542–549.

118. El-Gamal HM, Dufresne RG, Saddler K. Electrosurgery, pacemakers and ICDs: a survey of precautions and complications experienced by cutaneous surgeons. Dermatol Surg 2001;27:385–390.

119. Riordan AT, Gamache C, Fosko SW. Electrosurgery and cardiac devices. J Am Acad Dermatol 1997;37:250–255.

120. Martinelli PT, Schultze KE, Nelson BR. Mohs micrographic surgery in a patient with a deep brain stimulator: a review of the literature on implantable electrical devices. Dermatol Surg 2004;30:1021–1030.

3
Nerve Injury

Shawn Allen and Roberta Sengelmann

A detailed knowledge of neuroanatomy is essential to performing safe and effective head and neck cutaneous surgery. Damage to underlying nerves may result in functional and cosmetic compromise. Both sensory and motor nerves are vulnerable to injury during the course of surgery, and consequences of nerve injury in the head and neck region can range from minor and temporary to debilitating and permanent. A comprehensive understanding of seven neurological anatomic danger zones of the head and neck helps to avoid unwelcome nerve injury, as well as ensure a thorough preoperative informed consent. This chapter discusses the different types of nerve injury, the location of important anatomic danger zones, injury prevention strategies, the consequences of nerve injury, and the approach to management of nerve injuries.

Different Types of Nerve Injury and Their Consequences

Motor nerves terminate in motor endplates at their target muscles, while sensory nerves end in free nerve endings in the skin, mucosa, or other target organs. Motor nerve injuries may result in paralysis (complete loss of movement) or paresis (partial loss of movement). Sensory nerve injury may result in anesthesia (absence of sensation), paresthesia (abnormal sensation), and or dysesthesia (painful sensation). Consequences of nerve injuries will vary based largely on the following three factors: the type or extent of the injury, which nerve is injured, and the location of the injury along the nerve.

First, the type of nerve injury can be classified into three categories: neuropraxia, axonotmesis, and neurotmesis. *Neuropraxia* is a temporary localized block in nerve conduction without structural injury to the nerve cell body. Generally, this is seen after a nerve compression injury such as a "Saturday night palsy." Ischemia

from inadvertent intraforamenal regional nerve blocks or blunt trauma from tumescent liposuction can also produce similar temporary consequences. *Axonotmesis* is defined as damage to the axon and myelin sheath with preservation of the endoneurium, perineurium, and epineurium. This often occurs with partial surgical transection of the nerve. In either of the above two types of injuries, spontaneous recovery most often follows. By contrast, *neurotmesis*, the most severe type of injury, occurs when the nerve has been completely transected. This type of injury has a poor prognosis for spontaneous recovery and reinnervation may require surgical intervention.

Second, the specific nerve injured and its function (motor or sensory) will determine the general clinical outcome. Motor nerve injuries may result in muscular dysfunction and cosmetic asymmetry, while sensory nerve injury may result in altered sensation in the affected area. Both of these clinical outcomes can be concerning to both the patient and the surgeon.

Finally, injuries occurring more distally along the nerve will result in more limited impairment and are also more likely to spontaneously resolve. In distal nerve injuries, the proximity of the injury to the nerve target allows for more rapid and more precise reinnervation. Conversely, proximal injuries will likely result in more widespread and more permanent impairment and carry a greater risk for partial or inadequate spontaneous reinnervation.

Avoiding Nerve Injury: "An Ounce of Prevention Is Worth a Pound of Cure"

Superficial Musculoaponeurotic System

The best way to manage nerve injury is to avoid it in the first place. Operating in the appropriate surgical plane is crucial when performing cutaneous surgery. Facial motor nerve branches course above the deep fascia but below the fibromuscular sheath, known as the superficial musculoaponeurotic system (SMAS). The contiguity of this fibrous sheath helps to organize and coordinate movement of the muscles of facial expression. In the pretragal area, the SMAS is connected to the parietal fascia via dense connective tissue and attaches to the temporalis muscle superiorly, the orbicularis oculi anteriorly, and the platysma inferiorly. In areas where facial musculature is absent, such as the scalp and temple, the SMAS provides a thick inelastic sheath identifiable as the galea aponeurotica and temporoparietal fascia, respectively. Because facial motor nerves travel below the SMAS, blunt dissection in a plane superficial to the SMAS will help prevent inadvertent facial motor nerve damage.

While motor nerves course deep to the SMAS, sensory nerves are often found in neurovascular bundles, which penetrate the SMAS as they rise superficially toward the dermis. They course more randomly and superficially in the skin as they travel in a plane between the SMAS and the subcutaneous fat to terminate in dermal or mucosal free nerve endings. Some degree of damage to smaller branches of sensory nerves is inevitable in nearly all incisional surgery, but symptoms usually spontaneously resolve. Damage to the larger proximal sensory nerve trunks should be carefully avoided as spontaneous reinnervation is more unlikely and the area of diminished or absent sensation may be significant and permanent.

Recognizing the location of the anatomic danger zones for the facial motor and sensory nerve trunks will help to avoid nerve injury. In all cutaneous surgical procedures, the risks of motor and sensory nerve injury should be included as part of a comprehensive preoperative consent.

Knowledge of the Seven Anatomic Danger Zones

In addition to observing a supra-SMAS surgical plane, there are seven neurological head and neck anatomic danger zones where either the motor and or sensory nerves course more superficially or large sensory nerve trunks originate from the skull. The risks and consequences of nerve injury during cutaneous surgery are greatest in these locations.

In these danger zones, branches of three cranial nerves and a branch of the upper cervical plexus are of primary concern and include: the facial nerve (seventh cranial nerve), the trigeminal nerve (fifth cranial nerve), the spinal accessory nerve (eleventh cranial nerve), and the great auricular nerve (upper cervical plexus). Although the facial and trigeminal nerves carry both motor and sensory fibers, the facial nerve primarily controls facial motor movements, while the trigeminal nerve primarily provides sensory innervation to the face. The spinal accessory nerve provides motor function to muscles in the neck and shoulder, while the great auricular nerve provides sensory innervation to the neck and periauricular area.

Overview of Facial and Cervical Motor Nerves: The Facial Nerve and Spinal Accessory Nerve

The Facial Motor Nerve (Cranial Nerve 7)

The facial nerve is derived from the second embryonic arch and its five major facial branches carry motor fibers to control the muscles of facial expression. In addition to its motor function, the facial nerve also carries visceral motor fibers providing secretomotor stimulation of the submandibular, sublingual, intralingual, and lacrimal glands, and provides taste to the lateral anterior two thirds of the tongue and palate via the nervus intermedius.

The facial nerve emerges from the skull via the stylomastoid foramen. In the infant and preadolescent children, the mastoid process is not fully developed and the main facial nerve trunk is exposed and susceptible to injury deep in this area. After exiting the foramen and giving off the posterior auricular nerve (which innervates the posterior auricular, intrinsic auricular, and occipitalis muscles and provides sensation to the external auditory canal and skin of the concha) as well as a branch to the digastric muscles, it travels upwards into and through the parotid gland. Once invested in the parotid gland, it partitions into the temporofacial and cervicofacial divisions followed by further separation into the five facial motor nerve branches: the temporal, zygomatic, buccal, marginal mandibular, and cervical nerves. These branches exit the parotid gland superiorly, anteriorly, and inferiorly to innervate their target muscles from an inferolateral direction (the exception to this is the buccal branch of the facial nerve which innervates the buccinator muscle from a superficial aspect). Surgical danger zones exist for four of these five major facial branches (the temporal, zygomatic, buccal, and marginal mandibular nerves).

The Spinal Accessory Nerve (Cranial Nerve 11)

In the cervical region, the spinal accessory nerve provides motor innervation to the sternocleidomastoid and trapezius muscles. It facilitates shoulder, head, and neck movements. The nerve travels in the posterior triangle of the neck, from the posterior border of the sternocleidomastoid muscle inferolaterally toward the trapezius muscle in the shoulder. The corresponding danger zone exists for this nerve and is described in a later section on danger zone 7.

Danger Zone 1: Temporal Branch of the Facial Nerve

Course of Temporal Nerve and Location of the Anatomic Danger Zone

The most cephalad of the facial nerve motor branches, the temporal (frontal) branch, courses from a point located 0.5 cm inferior to the tragus to a point 2.0 cm superior and lateral to the tail of the eyebrow before it dives beneath the frontalis muscle. The temporal branch innervates the frontalis, corrugator supercilii, orbicularis oculi, and the anterior and superior auricular muscles. This first danger zone is identified as a triangle outlined by drawing a line from 0.5 cm inferior to the tragus to 2.0 cm above the lateral brow (this overlaps with the path of the main branch of the nerve) then down through the lateral brow to the lateral orbital rim. The triangle is completed by a horizontal line drawn from the point at the orbital rim, along the zygoma, to the intersection of the first line. It should be noted that the nerve is most susceptible to injury over the zygomatic arch, where it travels most superficially (Fig. 3-1).

Avoidance of Temporal Nerve Injury

In order to avoid damage during surgery in this area, the surgeon should bluntly dissect in a plane above the SMAS. Importantly, when approaching the zygoma and temporal

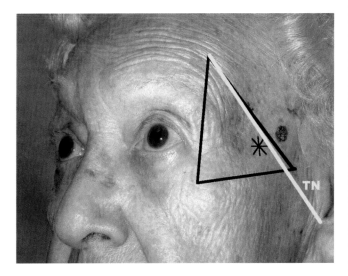

FIGURE 3-1. Danger zone 1 outlined. The course of the temporal nerve (TN in yellow) is shown. The asterisk indicates the location along the zygoma where the temporal nerve courses most superficially and is at greatest risk to injury.

region there is loss of the subcutaneous layer and the SMAS is found closer to the skin surface. Careful dissection is mandatory in this area. Additionally, when performing a facelift procedure, the surgeon may also choose a much deeper plane of dissection to avoid temporal nerve injury. This deep plane is created by dissecting below the deep temporal fascia, from the temporal scalp downward toward the supraorbital rim and zygomatic arch. Marino has described this "mesotemporalis" flap, which is then completed by dissecting a supra-SMAS layer in the deep subcutaneous plane from the ramus of the mandible to the zygoma.[1] Where these two planes meet at the zygomatic arch defines the SMAS and the nerve can be identified within it.

Consequences of Temporal Nerve Injury

Consequences of nerve injury to the temporal branch of the facial nerve may include paresis or paralysis of the frontalis, corrugator supercilii, orbicularis oculi, and anterior and superior auricularis muscles. At rest, brow ptosis and forehead asymmetry, as well as diminished forehead rhytides and a weakened frown, may result. Impaired and asymmetrical facial expression may result from the inability to elevate the ipsilateral brow, and significant lateral brow hooding may cause a visual field impairment (Fig. 3-2). Rarely, an inability to tightly close the eye can result, but this is uncommon due to redundant innervation of the orbicularis oculi via the zygomatic branches of the facial nerve.

Management of Temporal Nerve Injury

Management of temporal branch injury may require suspensory surgical intervention (i.e., brow lift) to elevate the ipsilateral forehead and or brow in an effort to reverse brow ptosis. Botulinum toxin injections to the unaffected forehead can also improve symmetry both at rest and with animation. However, the potential for bilateral brow ptosis and a "frozen forehead" appearance from contralateral botulinum injections must be considered.

If the patient has lost the ability to fully close the eye, they may be at risk for a secondary keratopathy and corneal irritation. Lubricating eye drops and punctual plugs may help alleviate dryness symptoms during a period of observation. If necessary, surgical management of an unresolved paralytic lagophthalmos may include tarsorrhaphy and or the implantation of palpebral springs, magnets, or gold weights in order to facilitate closure of the eye.[2] In our experience, spontaneous regeneration and partial to total functional recovery is the rule when temporal nerve injury occurs distally (Fig. 3-2C). In these cases, we recommend symptomatic treatment accompanied by an observation period of approximately 6 to 12 months before further surgical intervention is attempted.

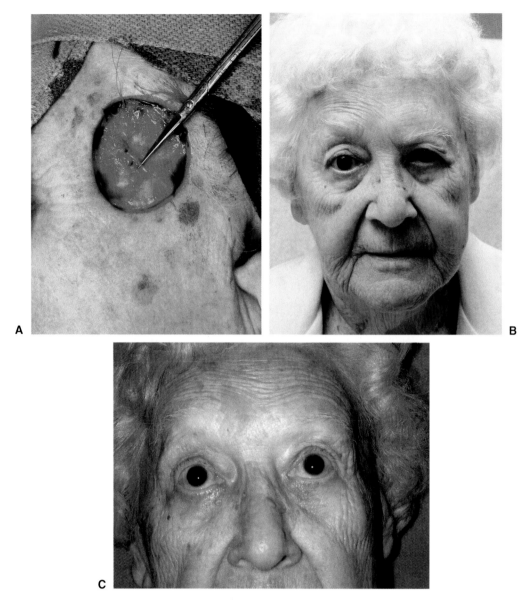

FIGURE 3-2. (A) An intraoperative picture of the left temporal nerve (surgical scissors elevating nerve) during Mohs surgery for a neurotropic moderately differentiated squamous cell carcinoma. (B) This patient temporarily lost function to the ipsi- lateral frontalis muscle (notice left brow droop and absent left forehead rhytides). (C) Near complete spontaneous recovery was seen 8 months postoperatively.

Danger Zone 2: Zygomatic and Buccal Branches of the Facial Nerve

Course of the Zygomatic and Buccal Nerves and Location of the Anatomic Danger Zone

The second danger zone contains both the zygomatic and buccal branches of the facial nerve. Proximally, after exist- ing the parotid parenchyme, these branches course deep in the mid-cheek just over the masseter muscle, then dis- tally branch and rise more superficially sending rami both above and below the zygomaticus muscles and lip leva- tors. The parotid duct also can be found in this danger zone, traveling parallel to the major buccal nerve branch.

The zygomatic branch exits the superomedial aspect of the parotid gland and courses in the direction of the lateral canthus. As it journeys along its course, it sends branches to innervate the numerous upper facial muscles including the lower orbicularis oculi, procerus, zygomati- cus major and minor, levator labii superioris alaeque nasi, and part of the buccinator muscle.

The buccal branch emerges caudad to the zygomatic branch and travels in an inferomedial path from the parotid gland, along the surface of the masseter muscle

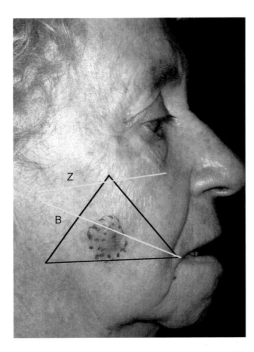

FIGURE 3-3. Danger zone 2 outlined. The course of the zygomatic nerve (Z) and buccal nerve (B) are shown.

and below the lip levators, in the direction of the oral commissure. Its main branch courses parallel to the parotid duct (Stensen's duct) in an imaginary line drawn from the tragus to the oral commissure. Both the buccal branch of the facial nerve and the parotid duct are at risk of injury before they pierce the buccinator muscle. The buccal branch innervates the buccinator muscle from this superficial position before it penetrates the muscle. It also inferolaterally innervates the orbicularis oris, zygomaticus muscles, levator labii superioris, levator anguli oris, levator labii superioris alaeque nasi, nasalis, and the depressor septi muscles and does so inferolaterally.

This second danger zone is defined by the zygomaticus major anteriorly, the parotid gland posteriorly, and the mandibular body inferiorly. A line from the angle of the mandible to the mid-zygoma down to the oral commissure and back to the angle of the mandible forms the triangular danger zone (Fig. 3-3). Included in this area are the zygomatic and buccal nerves as well as the parotid duct and part of the facial artery and vein.

Avoidance of Zygomatic and Buccal Nerve Injuries

When operating in this area, undermining in the subcutaneous layer above the SMAS will ensure avoidance of damage to both the zygomatic and buccal branches, as well as the parotid duct. By contrast, operating in a plane that is deep to the platysmal SMAS and parotid fascia, as might occur during deep facelifts or with resection of deeply invasive cutaneous malignancies, places the patient at increased risk for nerve and duct injury (Fig. 3-4A). In addition, small rami of the zygomatic branch innervating the orbicularis oculi, at the superomedial aspect of the danger zone, course superficially above the zygomaticus major and minor muscles and may be at increased risk of injury in this area.

Consequences of Zygomatic and Buccal Nerve Injuries

Depending on how proximally the nerve injury occurs, damage to the zygomatic branch of the facial nerve can result in denervation of some or all of the muscles it innervates. Weakness or paralysis of the lower orbicularis oculi, procerus, zygomaticus major and minor, levator labii superioris alaeque nasi, as well as part of the buccinator muscle may occur. Clinical manifestations may include an inability to fully close the lower eye, decreased ability to scowl, and difficulty elevating the corner of the mouth and flaring the nose. At rest, a droop of the ipsilateral lower eyelid, oral commissure, and upper lip may be evident (see Fig. 3-4B).

Damage to the buccal branch may also result in pronounced perioral weakness or paralysis but with a more pronounced effect, as well as a decreased ability to flare the ipsilateral nose. For example, pronounced dysfunction of the buccinator muscle may result in an oral droop, a flaccid cheek, and difficulty eating, accompanied by frequent biting of the buccal mucosa (Fig. 3-4B).

Cosmetically, the resulting asymmetry from damage to either of these facial nerve branches can be concerning and becomes exaggerated when the patient attempts to smile. When smiling, the asymmetry resulting from a buccal nerve injury becomes apparent as the contralateral unaffected lip angle elevates while the affected side remains static (see Fig. 3-4C). In addition, a flattening of the nasolabial furrow is often seen with buccal nerve injuries.

Management of Zygomatic and Buccal Nerve Injuries

Spontaneous resolution of functional impairment is rare when the proximal large motor nerve branches have been completely transected. The distal terminal branches of the zygomatic and buccal nerves are often very small and they may go unnoticed during surgery. Many times injury to these branches is only appreciated postoperatively and may often have minimal consequences and resolve spontaneously. In addition, because individual patients will vary in the extent of innervation and cross-innervation occurring between the zygomatic and buccal branches, nerve injuries in this danger zone may present with various clinical outcomes. This built-in neurological redundancy allows for preservation of some of the functions of the mid-face when an injury occurs to either of

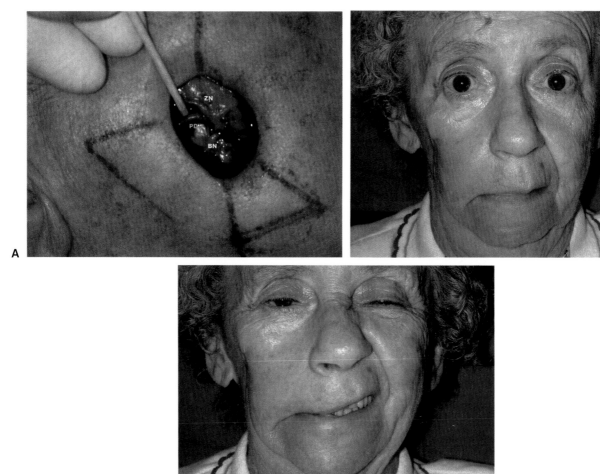

FIGURE 3-4. (A) The anastomoses of the buccal nerve (BN, yellow) and zygomatic nerve (ZN, yellow) seen anterior to applicator stick and the parotid duct (PD, green) inferior to applicator stick were exposed during Mohs surgery. (B) Damage resulted in ipsilateral lip droop, difficulty eating, and (C) an asymmetrical smile.

these facial nerve branches. Fortunately, due to their deeper anatomic location damage to one or both of these nerves is rare.

In clinical practice, it is often unclear whether injury in this area will be temporary and minor or become permanent and significant. As such, particularly with central to medial face injuries, it is recommended that the patient be followed for at least 6 months to determine the degree to which the nerve will regenerate and maintain or regain function without surgical intervention. If progress is seen, it may be advisable to wait at least one full year before proceeding with reinnervation procedures that carry their own inherent additional risks.

When appropriate, nerve anastomosis for the zygomatic or buccal branch can be performed, but it is often a difficult procedure with varying success rates. If significant and permanent zygomatic or buccal nerve injury occurs, nerve repair or grafting or a free muscle flap may

be necessary to restore a more normal appearing smile and restore animation and function to the mid-face. Suspensory surgery may also help restore cosmetic symmetry at rest, but alone will not correct the loss of function or the asymmetry that occurs with animation.

Danger Zone 3: Marginal Mandibular Branch of the Facial Nerve

Course of the Marginal Mandibular Nerve and Location of the Anatomic Danger Zone

The third danger zone parallels the course of the marginal mandibular nerve as it crosses over the body of the mandible, just anterior to the masseter muscle. Proximally, the nerve is somewhat protected by jowl fat and

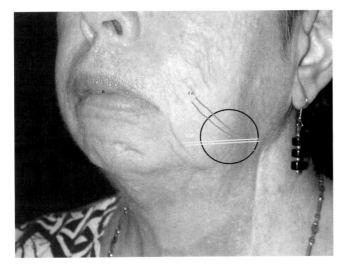

FIGURE 3-5. Danger zone 3 is outlined. The marginal mandibular nerve (MM) runs laterally along the mandible from the masseter muscle toward the chin area. The facial artery (FA) can be palpated at the lateral edge of the danger zone, just anterior to the masseter muscle.

runs perpendicular to the palpable facial artery. It travels laterally along the body of the mandible to innervate the depressors of the mouth: the orbicularis oris, depressor anguli oris, depressor labii inferioris, and mentalis muscles. It also innervates the risorius and upper portion of the platysmal muscles.

This danger zone is defined by a 2-cm-diameter circle centered at the mid-mandible, approximately 2 cm lateral to and 2 cm inferior to the oral commissure. In this location, the protective layer of SMAS thins and the nerve is vulnerable to damage. The facial artery and vein should also be avoided at the lateral edge of this danger zone (Fig. 3-5).

Avoidance of Marginal Mandibular Nerve Injury

Avoidance of nerve injury in this area is assisted by clear visualization of the plane of dissection. It should be noted that the overlying SMAS from the platysmal muscle thins as the muscle nears the depressor anguli oris and penetration of the thinned SMAS occurs easily. Palpating the facial artery, running deep and perpendicular to the nerve in the mid-mandible (at the medial border of a clinched masseter muscle), will help to identify the location of the proximal nerve branch. From this point, the marginal mandibular nerve travels along the body of the mandible toward the mentolabial crease. Importantly, thermal energy from electrodessication of the facial artery or vein in this area may be conducted to and injure the nerve; therefore, careful electrosurgery in this location is advised.

Consequences of Marginal Mandibular Nerve Injury

Damage to the marginal mandibular nerve can result in disfiguring changes. Elevation of the upper lip on the affected side and an asymmetrical smile results due to unopposed action of the ipsilateral zygomaticus muscles and other lip levators. Loss of chin wrinkling will also occur with paralysis of the mentalis muscle. Additionally, protrusion of the ipsilateral lower lip at rest as well as an inability to depress the ipsilateral mouth occurs as a result of an absent sphincter action of the lower orbicularis oris muscle and inactivation of the lip depressors, respectively (Fig. 3-6). Speech impairment may also result as the sphincter action of the orbicularis oris is vital to sounding out certain letters such as *g*, *p*, and *q*.

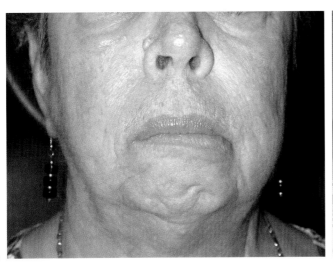
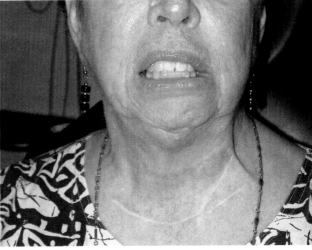

FIGURE 3-6. Surgical injury of the left marginal mandibular nerve resulted in asymmetrical ipsilateral lip elevation and protrusion of the ipsilateral lower lip at rest (A) and the inability to fully show the ipsilateral lower teeth (B).

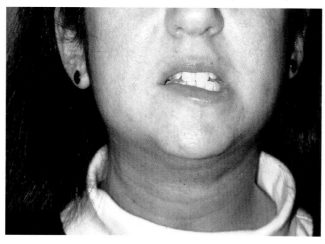 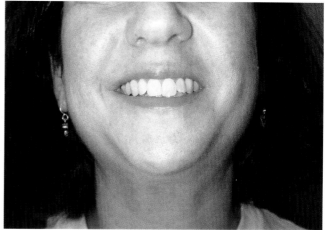

A   B

FIGURE 3-7. (A) Patient revealing injury to the right marginal mandibular nerve 2 months following neck and jowl liposculpturing. (B) Patient with spontaneous resolution 8 months following surgery.

Management of Marginal Mandibular Nerve Injury

Repair of a transected marginal mandibular nerve may require nerve repair or graft with or without a free muscle flap. Again, a waiting period of 6 to 12 months may be advisable to allow for spontaneous recovery of function. The authors have seen a temporary paresis of the marginal mandibular nerve following neck and jowl liposculpturing, which resolved to baseline over the course of 6 months. This injury was due to blunt trauma, and the resulting neuropraxia eventually resolved (Fig. 3-7).

Overview of Facial and Cervical Sensory Nerves: The Trigeminal Nerve and Great Auricular Nerve

The Trigeminal Nerve (Cranial Nerve 5)

The trigeminal nerve, the largest of the cranial nerves, is derived from the first branchial embryonic arch and supplies cutaneous sensation to the facial skin and mucosa as well as motor innervation to the muscles of mastication. This nerve is divided into three major divisions (*trigeminal*, Latin meaning *three twins*): the ophthalmic division (V1), the maxillary division (V2), and the mandibular division (V3). These divisions course superficially toward the skin surface, branching readily and widely. Three major branches of these divisions emerge from the cranium through discrete foramina: from the supraorbital foramen exits the supraorbital nerve (V1), from the infraorbital foramen exits the infraorbital nerve (V2), and from the mental foramen exits the mental nerve (V3). Each foramen and nerve trunk is located on the face, in

the mid-pupillary line, and each identifies the origin of a unique facial danger zone.

The Great Auricular Nerve

The great auricular nerve is a division of the upper cervical nerves (C2, C3) and travels superomedially along the lateral neck toward the auricle. It divides into an anterior and posterior branch to supply cutaneous sensation to the lateral neck, the lateral, pretragal, and mandibular cheek; the external ear and postauricular area; as well as the posterior scalp. It is a pure sensory nerve and travels above the SMAS to terminate in dermal free nerve endings.

These sensory nerves are often found in neurovascular bundles and, as mentioned, they course in a plane between the SMAS and the subcutaneous fat to terminate in free nerve endings in the dermis and mucosa. Knowledge of the locations of the nerves and origination points from the skull assists the surgeon in both avoiding trauma to the large neural trunks as well as establishing effective regional nerve blocks.

Danger Zone 4: Opthalmic Division — Supraorbital Nerve and Supratrochlear Nerve

Course of the Supraorbital and Supratrochlear Nerves and Location of the Anatomic Danger Zone

The ophthalmic division (V1) of the trigeminal nerve subdivides into the frontal, lacrimal, nasociliary, and meningeal branches. The supratrochlear and supraorbital nerves are derived from the frontal branch and are the

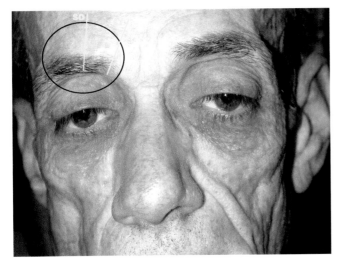

FIGURE 3-8. Danger zone 4 is outlined. The supraorbital nerve (SO) and supratrochlear nerve (ST) are at risk of injury in this location.

branches at greatest risk of injury during cutaneous surgery above the orbit.

The supraorbital nerve emerges from the supraorbital foramen in the mid-pupillary line and courses deep to the corrugator muscle to penetrate the frontalis muscle and SMAS. The supraorbital nerve provides sensation to the central upper eyelid, ipsilateral forehead, and scalp. Damage to the nerve in this area will result in diminished or absent sensation in the corresponding location.

The supratrochlear nerve emerges 1 cm lateral to midline, approximately 1.5 cm medial to and slightly inferior to the supraorbital nerve and foramen. It immediately penetrates the corrugator muscle to provide sensation to the medial upper eyelid, medial forehead, and medial scalp. Transection of the corrugator muscle, such as in a browlift procedure, may result in damage to the supratrochlear nerve accompanied by a corresponding regional anesthesia. In this scenario, however, some degree of eyelid, forehead, and scalp sensation may be preserved because of the overlapping supraorbital nerve branches that may be spared as they course deep to (not through) the corrugator muscle. Detailed knowledge of these locations will avoid injury as well as ensure effective regional nerve blocks of the upper eyelid and forehead.

This fourth danger zone, which includes the supraorbital and supratrochlear nerves, can be found in the eyebrow region by first identifying the supraorbital foramen. Both the supraorbital and supratrochlear nerve can be found in this danger zone. The foramenal notch can be palpated at the underside of the orbital rim in the mid-pupillary line, approximately 2.5 cm lateral to midline. From this point, an imaginary circle with a 3-cm diameter helps to establish the area where trauma to either the supraorbital or supratrochlear nerve is most likely (Fig. 3-8). Nerve damage occurring deep in this area will result in more significant and widespread consequences.

Avoidance of Supraorbital and Supratrochlear Nerve Injuries

When operating in the supraorbital area, avoiding transection of the nerve trunks is facilitated by visualization of the undermining plane at the level of the periosteum. It is important to dissect bluntly in this area in order to avoid nerve transection and loss of sensation to a significant area of the upper face. For example, during endoscopic browlifts, blunt dissection just above the periosteum with clear visualization of the nerves originating from the skull will help to avoid unwanted injury.

Consequences of Supraorbital and Supratrochlear Nerve Injuries

Nerve injury to either of these branches will result in paresthesia, dysesthesia, and or anesthesia to the affected area. The supraorbital nerve is distributed more centrally and laterally, and it supplies sensation to the upper eyelid, mid-forehead and mid-scalp. The supratrochlear nerve projects more medially along the forehead and scalp, supplying sensation to the medial upper eyelid, medial forehead, and medial frontal scalp. Due to some overlap in the sensory distribution between these two nerves, preservation of some degree of sensation may occur with transection of only one of these nerve trunks.

Management of Supraorbital and Supratrochlear Nerve Injuries

Management of sensory nerve injuries may be limited to observation. Spontaneous recovery occurs frequently and full recovery is more likely following a distal nerve injury, while more proximal injuries to larger nerve trunks may result in more permanent and widespread loss of sensation. As the nerve regenerates, the patient may experience a tingling or pins-and-needles sensation in the affected area. The risks of sensory nerve injury, including the symptoms that may occur as the nerve spontaneously regenerates, should be discussed preoperatively with the patient during the process of informed consent.

Although it is true that many trigeminal nerve injuries will spontaneously resolve, as clinicians have become more experienced with trigeminal nerve repair, some have become more aggressive in their recommendations regarding surgical repair and the timing of the repair. For large central trunk injuries, some experienced surgeons now recommend reexploring nerve injuries with no evidence of healing by 12 to 16 weeks.[3] With sensory nerve injuries, however, no studies have been performed to establish whether surgical intervention is more effective than observation alone. It is our practice to observe the patient for at least 6 to 12 months prior to considering surgical intervention.

Danger Zone 5: Maxillary Division — The Infraorbital Nerve

Course of the Infraorbital Nerve and Location of the Anatomic Danger Zone

The maxillary division (V2) of the trigeminal nerve includes the zygomatic, infraorbital, pterygopalatine, and meningeal branches. Although the zygomatic branch does provide important sensory innervation to the lateral face (via the zygomaticofacial and zygomaticotemporal nerves), the infraorbital branch supplies the largest area of clinical importance. The infraorbital nerve emerges from the infraorbital foramen located approximately 1 cm below the infraorbital rim in the mid-pupillary line. It provides sensation to the ipsilateral nasal sidewall, lower eyelid, central cheek, and upper lip.

This fifth danger zone can be demarcated by identifying the infraorbital foramen 1 cm below the infraorbital rim in the mid-pupillary line and above the mandibular second premolar tooth. The foramenal notch can be palpated on the downsloping surface of the maxillary bone. From this point, a 3-cm-diameter circle will outline the danger zone (Fig. 3-9). It should also be noted that the zygomatic branches of the facial nerve, which innervate the nasalis and levator labii superioris muscles, are also found deep in this area.

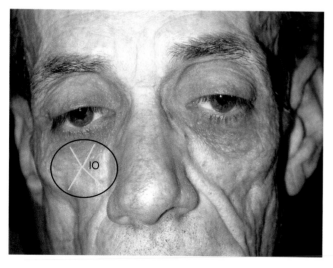

FIGURE 3-9. Danger zone 5 is outlined. The infraorbital nerve (IO) branches widely and is at risk of injury in this location.

Avoidance of Infraorbital Nerve Injury

Avoidance of injury in this area is crucial when performing subperiosteal facelifts or surgery on invasive carcinomas, and when establishing regional nerve blocks. Knowledge of the origination of the nerve trunks will help in visualizing the nerve in this area. In addition, insertion of the needle into the foramen and subsequent injection of anesthesia during a nerve block can result in nerve compression and a neuropraxia. Slight withdrawal of the needle following contact with the maxilla will help to prevent ischemic injury to the nerve. Fortunately, the neuropraxia and alteration in sensation usually resolve spontaneously.

Consequences of Infraorbital Nerve Injury

Either injury or an effective infraorbital nerve block will result in a loss of sensation to the ipsilateral lower eyelid, lateral nasal sidewall and ala, as well as the central cheek and upper cutaneous and mucosal lip. Nerve injury and loss of sensation to the upper lip may result in hot or cold burns or self-inflicted bites to the area while eating. Counseling the patient regarding these risks is important both with invasive surgery and when performing regional nerve blocks in this area.

Management of Infraorbital Nerve Injury

Following nerve damage, spontaneous reinnervation is more likely to occur if the injury occurs more distally along the nerve fibers. Fortunately, many of the injuries encountered in cutaneous surgery occur distally. Recovery may take months to years to reestablish but observation is encouraged. With sensory nerve injuries, no studies have been performed to establish whether surgical intervention is more effective than observation alone.

Danger Zone 6: Mandibular Division — Mental Nerve

Course of the Mental Nerve and Location of the Anatomic Danger Zone

The mandibular division (V3) of trigeminal nerve includes the buccal, auriculotemporal, lingual, inferior alveolar, pterygoid, and meningeal branches. The mental nerve, a ramus of the inferior alveolar branch, exits the body of the mandible in the mid-pupillary line through the mental foramen, approximately 1.5 cm lateral and 1.5 cm inferior to the oral commissure. It supplies sensation to the ipsilateral chin and lower cutaneous and mucosal lip.

This sixth danger zone is recognized by identifying the mental foramen approximately 1.5 cm lateral and 1.5 cm

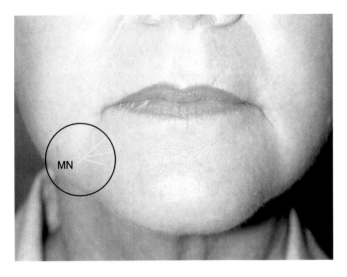

FIGURE 3-10. Danger zone 6 is outlined. The mental nerve (MN) is at risk of injury in this location.

inferior to the oral commissure. It is located along the border of the mandible, in the mid-pupillary line, and creating a 3-cm-diameter circle from this point will define this anatomic danger zone (Fig. 3-10). Additionally, the second mandibular premolar tooth may be used as a landmark to identify the approximate lateral location of the bony exit of the mental nerve. This dental landmark also can be helpful when performing intraoral mental nerve blocks.

Avoidance of Mental Nerve Injury

Locating this danger zone will assist in avoidance of nerve injury, as well as allow for successful regional nerve blocks to the lower chin and lip. Intraforamenal infiltration of anesthesia and an ensuing neuropraxia can be avoided by withdrawing the needle several millimeters after making contact with the mandible prior to injecting anesthesia. If the needle is inserted into the foramen during infiltration, the patient will likely experience a significant amount of discomfort during the injection and immediate withdrawal and redirection of the needle should follow.

Consequences of Mental Nerve Injury

Damage to the mental nerve or an effective nerve block will lead to sensory loss to the inferior cutaneous and mucosal lip as well as the ipsilateral chin area. This may result in difficulty sensing food products inside the mouth vestibule as well as an inability to appreciate drooling in the area. In addition, inadvertent lip biting may occur. Due to lack of sensation, an impaired ability to play certain wind instruments also may result and musicians should be specifically counseled regarding this potential risk.

Management of Mental Nerve Injury

Spontaneous recovery is more likely if the damage occurs distally along the nerve fibers, and this may take months to years to reestablish. No evidence currently exists to support surgical intervention with sensory nerve injuries. An observation period of 6 to 12 months may be acceptable.

Danger Zone 7: Cervical Nerves — The Spinal Accessory Nerve and Great Auricular Nerve

Erb's Point

When operating in the lateral neck region, one must avoid damage to both the spinal accessory nerve and the great auricular nerve (a branch of the upper cervical branches C2 and C3). The spinal accessory nerve supplies motor innervation to the neck and shoulder muscles, while the great auricular nerve supplies sensory innervation to the neck and periauricular area. Both of these nerves are encountered in danger zone 7, near an area known as Erb's point.

With the patient's head turned in the opposite direction, Erb's point can be located along the posterior border of the sternocleidomastoid muscle approximately 6.5 cm directly below the external auditory canal. A 3-cm-diameter circle, centered at Erb's point, establishes danger zone 7 (Fig. 3-11). From this point, the spinal accessory nerve travels inferolaterally toward the shoulder, while the great auricular nerve travels superomedially toward the angle of the mandible.

Course of the Spinal Accessory Nerve

From Erb's point, the spinal accessory nerve runs inferolaterally through the posterior triangle to reach the trapezius muscle. It travels just below the superficial cervical fascia and supplies motor innervation to both the sternocleidomastoid and the trapezius muscles. Rotational movement of the head is largely dependent upon innervation of the sternocleidomastoid muscle via the spinal accessory nerve. In addition, the ability to shrug and abduct the shoulder depends on the innervation of the trapezius muscle via this nerve as well.

Avoidance of Spinal Accessory Nerve Injury

Avoidance of injury requires proper identification of Erb's point and blunt dissection in a supra-SMAS plane. Although the spinal accessory nerve travels deeply into the neck toward the trapezius muscle, this danger zone

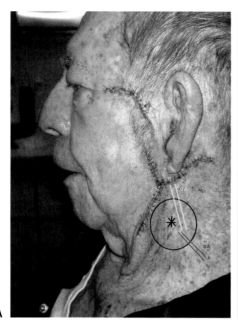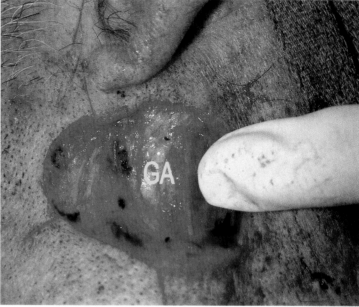

A   B

FIGURE 3-11. (A) Danger zone 7 is outlined. The asterisk indi- located. (B) The ascending trunk of the posterior branch of the
cates Erb's point, where both the spinal accessory nerve (SA, great auricular nerve (GA, in yellow) can be seen anterior to
in blue) and the great auricular nerve (GA, in yellow) are the surgeon's gloved finger.

identifies where it is most superficial in its course. Because good outcome and reinnervation of the muscles after
of the thin cervical fascia in this area, damage to the nerve accessory nerve repair, graft, or transfer.[4,5] A common
may occur during procedures ranging from simple extir- approach is to attempt end-to-end reanastomosis of the
pation of cysts to maneuvering of large cervicofacial flaps injured nerve within the first few days following the
to lower facelifting/necklifting procedures. injury. Early surgical intervention may avoid significant
muscle atrophy and fibrosis.

Consequences of Spinal Accessory Nerve Injury

Damage to the spinal accessory nerve will result in weakness when turning the head in the opposite direction
(sternocleidomastoid muscle), an impaired ability to
shrug the ipsilateral shoulder, as well as a shoulder
droop at rest (trapezius muscle). The ensuing downward
lateral rotation of the scapula is known as the "winged
scapula." Due to the lack of any redundant motor nerve
supply to the sternocleidomastoid and trapezius muscles,
spontaneous recovery of function following spinal accessory nerve injury is unlikely without subsequent nerve
grafting. Therefore, early surgical intervention may be
warranted.

Management of Spinal Accessory Nerve Injury

Management of spinal accessory nerve injury may require
surgical intervention for functional recovery of the trapezius and sternocleidomastoid muscles. Studies have shown

Course of the Great Auricular Nerve

The great auricular nerve provides cutaneous sensation
to the angle of the mandible, lateral neck, and periauricular skin. It courses superiorly and anteriorly from
the posterior edge of the sternocleidomastoid muscle, at
Erb's point, toward the posterior ear (Fig. 3-11). As it
rises superiorly, it divides into an anterior and posterior
branch. The anterior branch largely supplies sensation to
the pretragal and mandibular cheek, while the posterior
branch supplies sensation to the postauricular, external
ear, and occipital scalp areas.

Avoidance of Great Auricular Nerve Injury

When operating around Erb's point as well as in the
infra-auricular area, blunt dissection accompanied by
good visualization will assist in avoiding injury to the
small superficial great auricular branches. Like all sensory
nerves, the great auricular nerve and its branches course
through and above SMAS and are susceptible to injury
just below the dermis if they go unnoticed.

Consequences of Great Auricular Nerve Injury

Patients should be warned of the risk of nerve injury and the potential for paresthesia, dysesthesia, or anesthesia in the periauricular region. Lack of sensation in the periauricular area may be of limited significance but associated dysesthesias can be troublesome. In addition, the anterior branch of the great auricular nerve supplies part of the lateral cheek and paresthesia, dysesthesia, or anesthesia in this area often can be of significant concern to the patient.

Management of Great Auricular Nerve Injury

Although spontaneous resolution following injury often occurs, patients should be warned that temporary paresthesias in the form of a tingling sensation may persist for several months as the nerve regenerates. Surgical intervention often is not recommended due to the limited significance of the areas affected.

Management of Nerve Injuries

The Process of Spontaneous Nerve Recovery

The management of nerve injuries largely depends on the likelihood of spontaneous recovery. Intraoperative damage to peripheral nerves that occurs along the axon may allow for spontaneous regeneration of new distal axonal segments, particularly if the damage is only partial thickness or occurs near the target organ. In more severe types of nerve injury (neurotmesis), a process known as Wallerian degeneration may occur as the distal aspect of the injured axon dies. In this process, Schwann cells and macrophages phagocytose the degenerating axon and an empty endoneural tube remains. Within 24 hours after injury, axonal buds begin to develop from the distal tip of the proximal nerve ending. Although functional, the newly regenerated nerve may contain fewer axons than the original preinjured nerve. Therefore, with certain nerve injuries, spontaneous or near complete muscular and sensory function may return.

Spontaneous regeneration and reinnervation of the nerve may occur as early as several months or as late as several years postinjury. Trauma or ischemia to the facial nerve may result in paralysis despite an intact nerve (a neuropraxia or axonotmesis). In these cases, it is customary to wait an adequate period of time to allow for reinnervation before considering surgical intervention. The spontaneous return of some degree of function may support a continued conservative approach. Electromyography can assist in the evaluation of cases failing to show clinical improvement after a given period of observation. In certain cases, an observation period of 18 to 24

months may be considered appropriate. However, after 1 to 2 years, the possibility of reinnervating the existing facial musculature becomes more difficult due to the atrophy and motor endplate fibrosis that occurs.[6]

Surgical Intervention

Although most sensory nerve injuries are allowed to resolve spontaneously, as clinicians have become more experienced with trigeminal nerve repair, some have begun to perform early surgical repair of sensory nerve injury. For example, with larger nerve trunk injuries showing no spontaneous recovery some experienced surgeons recommend reexploring sensory nerve injuries within 3 to 4 months of the injury.[3] However, because most sensory nerve injuries are generally treated by observation, this discussion will focus on surgical approaches to facial motor nerve injury management.

If facial motor nerve paralysis does occur, the goals of a surgical intervention should include restoration of function, a normal resting appearance, and symmetry with facial animation. To this end, primary nerve repair, nerve grafting, free muscle flaps, and/or suspension surgeries will often be necessary to achieve some or all of these goals.

Early surgical intervention should be attempted within the first 72 hours following facial nerve injury. This early window will allow for the use of a nerve stimulator to identify the proximal and distal limbs of the nerve. After this 72-hour period the neurotransmitter stores necessary to depolarize the nerve trunks are depleted and the usefulness of electrostimulation is diminished.[7] Some experts have reported that with certain motor nerve injuries it may also be advisable to allow a longer waiting period to observe for spontaneous recovery of facial mimetic function.[7] This is particularly true when the nerve injury involves the zygomatic and buccal branches and occurs more distally along the nerve trunk. However, if the repair of a facial nerve injury is delayed greater than 18 to 24 months, fibrosis and atrophy of the muscle may progress to the point of irreversible motor end dysfunction despite eventual nerve repair.[8] When this occurs, muscle transfers, such as a partial temporalis transfer, or free tissue transfers may be the only solution to restore facial reanimation. In addition, suspension surgery may help to restore facial symmetry, but does nothing to reanimate the face.

Different Locations Require Different Approaches

Examining a patient with a unilateral facial nerve palsy helps to appreciate the different presentations associated with injury to the various branches of the facial nerve (Fig. 3-12). For example, the brow droop of the temporal

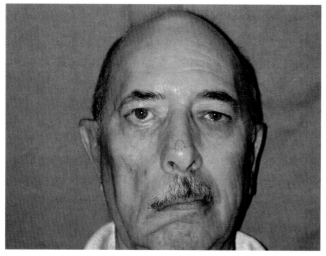

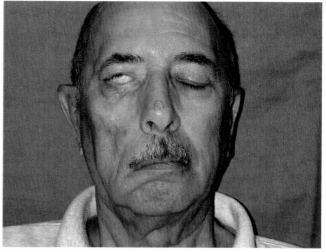

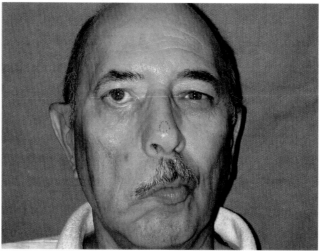

FIGURE 3-12. (A) This patient presented with an iatrogenic, complete, right-sided facial nerve palsy from a childhood surgery. Notice the absent forehead rhytides (temporal nerve), lower eyelid ectropion (zygomatic nerve), and facial droop (zygomatic, buccal, and marginal mandibular nerves) at rest. (B). The patient could not close his right eye (temporal and zygomatic nerves) and (C) shows an asymmetrical pucker (buccal and marginal mandibular nerves).

branch injury, the ectropion and inability to fully close the eye from zygomatic nerve injury, the drooping of the angle of the mouth due to buccal nerve injury, and the asymmetric smile due the marginal mandibular nerve injury all result in different functional and cosmetic compromise and require different surgical approaches for repair (Fig. 3-12). In an attempt to counteract gravity, surgical slings and suspension sutures may be necessary, while restoration of animation will require nerve repair or grafting or the transposition of muscles into the affected areas.

Moreover, when planning a facial nerve injury repair, different areas of the face lend themselves to different approaches. For example, in the periorbital region static suspensory surgery, as opposed to nerve repair, is the most common approach. Here the goal is often to return a normal cosmetic appearance, as significant functional

impairment may be limited. Accordingly, botulinum injections to the uninvolved forehead may restore a more normal resting appearance, but lack of animation with facial expressions will be pronounced.

In the mid-face, masseter muscle transfer may be an effective approach to reanimating and returning function to the oral commissure and smile complex following buccal or zygomatic branch injury of the facial nerve. In addition, free muscle grafts in this area have been performed utilizing the gracilis, serratus, pectoralis minor, latissimus dorsi, extensor hallucis brevis, and extensor carpi radialis brevis muscles.[8–12] Grafted muscles can be surgically positioned, revascularized, and reinnervated using local neurovascular structures to achieve an acceptable functional result. As mentioned above, some experts commonly observe injuries of the buccal and zygomatic nerves, particularly when they occur in the central face

between lines bounded laterally by the lateral canthus and medially by the lateral lip.[7]

With surgical interventions, it may be possible to return to a more normal function and appearance, but success of these techniques depends largely on the skill and experience of the reconstructive surgeon. In addition, it should be noted that obtaining insurance coverage for such procedures may be difficult due to the rare performance of these challenging procedures. Although a consensus is lacking, for most sensory nerve injuries and for certain motor nerve injuries a waiting period may be advisable to allow for spontaneous recovery of function. In the absence of a spontaneous resolution, a surgical approach may be warranted.

Conclusion

An important part of successful cutaneous surgery must include not only a profound knowledge of anatomy but also a thorough preoperative informed consent process. This includes reviewing the risks of motor and sensory nerve injury, especially when operating in the head and neck region. Some degree of sensory nerve injury is inevitable in skin surgery. However, serious motor nerve injuries are rare because cutaneous surgeons are most often operating in a subcutaneous plane above the SMAS. When motor injury does occur, it may often be due to blunt trauma or thermal damage from electrodessication and should spontaneously revert over time. However, for deep tumors, large flaps, rhytidectomy procedures, and novice surgeons, the risks of nerve injury are very real and can have serious consequences for the patient.

A detailed knowledge of the facial and cervical neuroanatomy, accompanied by proper surgical technique with particular attention in the previously described seven anatomic danger zones, will help prevent unwanted nerve injury. Should motor or sensory nerve injury occur, a waiting period is generally advised to ascertain the extent and consequences of the injury. When it is apparent that a motor nerve injury is unlikely to resolve spontaneously intervention with techniques such as suspension procedures, botulinum toxin injections, nerve repair, nerve grafting, or neuromusculocutaneous flaps may be indicated. It is also important to remember that the best management of nerve injuries is prevention. There is no substitute for a strong knowledge base, extensive training with skilled surgeons, and a wealth of surgical experience.

References

1. Marino H. The forehead lift: some hints to secure better results. Aesthetic Plast Surg 1977;1:251.
2. Thomas DA, Khalifa YM. Temporalis fascia in the management of gold eyelid weight extrusion. Ophthalmal Plast Reconstr Surg 2005;21:153–155.
3. Lam NP, Donoff B, et al. Patient satisfaction after trigeminal nerve repair. Oral Surg Oral Med Oral Pathol Oral Radiol Endod 2003;95:538–543.
4. Novak CB, Mackinnon SE. Patient outcome after surgical management of an accessory nerve injury. Otolaryngol Head Neck Surg 2002;127:221–224.
5. Chandawarkar RY, Cervino AL, Pennington GA. Management of iatrogenic injury to the spinal accessory nerve. Plast Reconstr Surg 2003;111:611–617.
6. Byrne PJ. Importance of facial expression in facial nerve rehabilitation. Curr Opin Otolaryngol Head Neck Surg 2004;12:332–335.
7. Myckatyn TM, Mackinnon SE. The surgical management of facial nerve injury. Clin Plast Surg 2003;30:307–318.
8. Crumley RL. Muscle evaluation of facial reanimation surgery. In: Portmann M, ed. Facial nerve. New York: Masson; 1985.
9. Hata Y, Yano K, Matsuba K, et al. Treatment of chronic facial palsy by transplantation of the neurovascularized free rectus abdominus muscle. Plast Reconstr Surg 1990;86:1178–1187.
10. Mackinnon SE, Dellon L. Technical considerations of the latissimus dorsi flap: a segmentally innervated muscle for facial reanimation. Microsurgery 1988;9:36–45.
11. Mayou BJ, Watson JS, Harrison DH, et al. Free microvascular and microneural transfer of the extensor digitorum brevis muscle for the treatment of unilateral facial palsy. Br J Plast Surg 1983;71:510–518.
12. Terzis JK. Pectoralis minor: a unique muscle for correction of facial nerve palsy. Plast Reconstr Surg 1989;83:767–776.

Suggested Further Readings

Achauer B, Eriksson E, Vander Kolk C. Plastic surgery: indications, operations, and outcomes. St. Louis: Mosby; 2000.
Bolognia J, Jorizzo J, Rapini R, et al. Dermatology. St Louis: Mosby; 2003.
Robinson J, Hanke CW, Sengelmann R, et al. Surgery of the skin: procedural dermatology. St. Louis: Mosby; 2005.
Seckel, B. Facial danger zones: avoiding nerve injury in facial plastic surgery. St. Louis: Quality Medical Publishing; 1994.
Wilson-Pauwels L, Akesson EJ, Stewart PA. Cranial nerves: anatomy and clinical comments. Philadelphia: Decker BC; 1998.

4

Hemorrhagic Complications in Cutaneous Surgery

Hugh M. Gloster, Jr.

It is logical to assume that anyone who performs cutaneous surgery has had or will have some sort of hemorrhagic complication, an inevitable event even in the hands of the most careful and skilled surgeon. Therefore, it is important for cutaneous surgeons to not only take precautions to prevent bleeding complications before they occur, but also to be capable of diagnosing and managing these unfortunate events as they arise to provide a better service for patients. This article will focus on the prevention, diagnosis, and management of hemorrhagic complications in cutaneous surgery.

Causes of Persistent Bleeding and Hematoma

The major hemorrhagic complications confronting the cutaneous surgeon are persistent intraoperative and postoperative bleeding, and the development of a hematoma within the first few postoperative days. These complications cause anxiety and discomfort for the patient, result in extra time expenditure for the physician, and greatly increase the risk of infection, dehiscence, and necrosis. The most common causes of persistent bleeding and hematoma are drug-induced coagulopathy and inadequate intraoperative hemostasis.[1,2] Less common factors and conditions that may be associated with an increased risk of perioperative bleeding include hypertension, some herbal supplements, vitamin E, ephedra, certain genodermatoses, bleeding disorders, fibrinolytic disorders, increasing age, atrophy, and chronic steroid use.

A good preoperative patient history and physical exam should identify these potential sources of excessive bleeding. Patients should be asked about all prescription and nonprescription medications (including vitamins and dietary supplements) and whether there is a personal or family history of excessive or prolonged bleeding. Petechiae or eccymoses on physical exam may indicate a bleeding problem. Screening laboratory tests should be performed if a hereditary or acquired coagulopathy is suspected. These tests should include a complete blood count, a platelet count, a prothrombin time, and a partial thromboplastin time.[1] The patient should be referred to their primary care physician or a hematologist for further evaluation if abnormalities are detected.

Drug-Induced Coagulopathy

Anticoagulants and platelet inhibitors each interfere with specific reactions in the coagulation cascade. Anticoagulants inhibit thrombin generation and fibrin formation. Antiplatelet agents block platelet activation and aggregation. The indications for administering anticoagulation therapy are prevention of venous thromboembolism, treatment of deep vein thrombosis, and primary prevention of myocardial ischemia, acute myocardial ischemia, atrial fibrillation, and valvular heart disease. Antithrombotic agents approved for use in the United States are summarized in Table 4-1.[3] Aspirin, nonsteroidal anti-inflammatory drugs (NSAIDS), ticlopidine, clopidogrel, and warfarin are the most likely medications to be encountered by the dermatologist. Platelet glycoprotein inhibitors, unfractionated heparin, direct thrombin inhibitors, low-molecular-weight heparins, and plasminogen activators are less likely to be administered in an outpatient setting. Nevertheless, physicians are currently prescribing an increasing number of sophisticated antithrombotic agents and the interactions between these medications, their tissue effects, and the extent to which they increase hemorrhagic complications after surgical procedures has yet to be determined.

Aspirin may reduce the risk of serious vascular events by one quarter in high-risk patients (e.g., patients with acute myocardial infarction, ischemic stroke, coronary artery disease, peripheral arterial disease, and atrial fibrillation).[4] Aspirin, which is thought to be a major source of intraoperative bleeding problems, irreversibly inhibits the enzyme cyclooxygenase (COX), thereby blocking the

TABLE 4-1. Antithrombotic agents approved for use in the United States.

Class	Subclass	Chemical (brand) name
Antiplatelet agents	Aspirin, NSAIDS	—
	Inhibitors of adenosine diphosphate (ADP)–induced platelet activation	Ticlopidine hydrochloride (Ticlid)
		Clopidogrel (Plavix)
	Platelet glycoprotein IIb/IIIa inhibitors	Abciximab (ReoPro)
		Eptifibatide (Integrilin)
		Tirofiban hydrochloride (Aggrastat)
Antithrombin anticoagulants	Unfractionated heparin	—
	Direct thrombin inhibitors	Hirudin (Refludan)
		Bivalirudin (Hirulog)
		Argatroban (Novastan)
	Low-molecular-weight heparins	Enoxaparin sodium (Lovenox)
		Dalteparin sodium (Fragmin)
		Ardeparin (Centaxarin/Normiflo)
		Danaparoid (Orgaran)
		Tinzaparin (Innohep)
	Coumarins	Warfarin (Coumadin)
Thrombolytic (fibrinolytic) therapy	Plasminogen activators	Streptokinase (Streptase)
		Alteplase (tPA/Activase)
		Reteplase (r-PA/Retavase)
		Tenecteplase (TNL-tPA/TNKase)

Source: Adopted from Alam and Goldberg.[3]

conversion of arachidonic acid to prostanoids like thromboxane A2, leading to impaired platelet aggregation and the formation of platelet plugs.[5] Platelet plugs are responsible for small vessel (e.g., capillaries, arterioles, venules) hemostasis and the prevention of immediate intraoperative bleeding. Aspirin usually does not cause delayed bleeding hours to days after surgery because of its antiplatelet effects. Platelets are inhibited for their entire lifespan of 7 to 10 days. Thus, aspirin must be discontinued 7 to 10 days preoperatively to allow platelet function to return to normal. Aspirin may be resumed 1 day after surgery.

Nonsteroidal anti-inflammatory drugs reversibly inhibit COX and thus have less of a clinical effect than aspirin. Antiplatelet effects last only while the drug is in the circulation, which depends on the half-life of the medication, which is typically less than 3 to 4 days.[6] Thus, NSAIDS should be withheld 1 to 3 days preoperatively (depending on the half-life of the drug) and resumed 1 day postoperatively.

The numerous over-the-counter and prescription medications that contain aspirin and NSAIDS are listed in Table 4-2.[7] Consequently, it is important that physicians obtain a thorough preoperative history of all medications the patient uses prior to surgery in order to decrease the risk of perioperative bleeding.

Certain NSAIDS, such as celecoxib, specifically inhibit COX-2 and may be useful to the dermatologic surgeon by providing an anti-inflammatory and analgesic medication with minimal adverse effects on platelets.[8] Cyclooxygenase exists as two isoenzymes, COX-1 and COX-2.

Cyclooxygenase 1 produces prostaglandins involved in maintaining normal gastric mucosa, regulating renal blood flow, and aiding in clotting through effects on platelet aggregation. Cyclooxygenase 2 produces prostaglandins that mediate pain and inflammation. Traditional NSAIDS inhibit COX-1 and COX-2, thus producing adverse effects on platelets, renal blood flow, and gastric mucosa. Celecoxib selectively inhibit COX-2, thereby maintaining anti-inflammatory and analgesic effects with less risk of bleeding problems or gastritis. Therefore, COX-2 inhibitors may be useful alternative preoperative medications for patients requiring NSAIDS for pain relief of chronic conditions (e.g., arthritis) because it would not be necessary to discontinue these drugs preoperatively to avoid potential hemorrhagic complications. Cyclooxygenase-2 inhibitors may also be a useful postoperative analgesic alternative to narcotics and traditional NSAIDS, particularly after surgery on the ear, an anatomic site that is prone to chondritis and postoperative bleeding problems.[8]

Clopidogrel and ticlopidine, which decrease the risk of morbid events in patients with atherosclerotic cardiovascular disease, irreversibly inhibit adenosine diphosphate (ADP)–induced platelet activation and lead to irreversible inhibition of platelet aggregation for the entire lifespan of the platelet.[9–11] Dipyridamole impairs platelet granule release of ADP and inhibits platelet adhesion.[12] Simultaneous administration of aspirin and either ticlopidine, clopidogrel, or dipyridamole produces additive risk reduction superior to aspirin alone because these medications block complementary pathways in the platelet

Table 4-2. Over-the-counter and prescription products containing aspirin and nonsteriodal anti-inflammatory drugs.

Medication type	Aspirin-containing products	NSAIDs	
Over-the-counter	Alka-Seltzer	Advil	
	Aspirin	Aleve	
	Aspirin Regimen Bayer	Motrin	
	BC Powders	Nuprin	
	Ecotrin	Orudis KT	
	Excedrin Extra Strength		
	Goody's Body Pain Formula Powder		
	Goody's Extra Strength Pain Relief		
	Momentum Backache Relief		
	Vanquish Analgesic Caplets		
Prescription	Easprin	Anaprox	Nalfon
	Excedrin	Arthrotec	Naproxyn
	Disalcid	Cataflam	Oruvail
	Salflex	Clinoril	Ponstel Kapseals
	Trilisate	Daypro	Relafen
		Disalcid	Salflex
		Dolobid	Tolectin
		EC-Naproxyn	Toradol
		Feldene	Trilisate
		Indocin	Voltaren
		Lodine	

Source: Adopted from Chang and Whitaker.[7]
Abbreviation: NSAIDs, nonsteriodal anti-inflammatory drugs.

aggregation cascade.[13] These medications theoretically may also increase the risk of perioperative bleeding, particularly in combination with aspirin, due to synergistic effects. As of yet, however, there have been no reported cases of hemorrhagic complications in cutaneous surgery with these medications. Similarly, pentoxifylline appears unassociated with surgical bleeding complications.[14]

Alcohol, which is a potent vasodilator that also impairs platelet function, may cause perioperative bleeding problems.[1] Patients should be cautioned to avoid alcohol in the immediate perioperative period.

Many patients require chronic anticoagulation with warfarin. Published studies describe the risk of major bleeding or thromboembolic events due to warfarin therapy as between 2% and 12% per year.[15,16] Warfarin, a coumarin derivative, is a structural analog and antagonist of vitamin K that interferes with the cyclic interconversion of vitamin K and its 2,3 epoxide, thereby inhibiting the synthesis of vitamin K–dependent coagulation factors II, VII, IX, and X, as well as the naturally occurring endogenous anticoagulant proteins C and S.[17,18] Antagonism of vitamin K reduces the rate at which these factors and proteins are produced, thus creating a state of anticoagulation. As a result, fibrin formation is impaired. Fibrin is responsible for large vessel hemostasis and the prevention of delayed bleeding hours to days after surgery. Warfarin does not affect platelets, so intraoperative or immediate postoperative bleeding is usually insignificant. Instead, warfarin interferes with the formation of the fibrin plug, which interrupts later steps in the clot-

ting cascade. Warfarin, which impairs hemostasis 72 to 96 hours, should be discontinued 3 to 5 days preoperatively and may be resumed 1 to 3 days after surgery.

If it is not feasible to discontinue warfarin preoperatively, the surgeon may attempt to limit the extent of surgery, obtain meticulous hemostasis, and apply a firm pressure dressing. If the contemplated surgery is extensive, radiation therapy should be considered. Alternatively, the patient may be hospitalized and switched to low-dose heparin 1 week preoperatively. Possible antidotes for the management of copious or persistent warfarin-induced bleeding include oral or parenteral vitamin K, whole blood, or fresh frozen plasma.[19]

Recently, particularly in the dermatology literature, several authors have questioned the benefit of discontinuing anticoagulants (ACA) and platelet inhibitors (PLTI) before cutaneous surgery procedures.[20–28] When contemplating the discontinuation of ACA and PLTI, the crucial factors to consider are the benefits of these drugs to the patient and the risks of briefly withholding medication preoperatively. The benefits of ACA and PLTI are the prevention of myocardial infarction (MI), cerebrovascular accidents (CVA), and deep vein thromboses (DVT). These drugs are also lifesaving for patients with prosthetic valves or hypercoagulable states and provide pain relief of chronic conditions such as arthritis. The main risks of discontinuing ACA and PLTI are major thrombotic complications such as MI, CVA, and DVT[3,29,30]; although the absolute magnitude of these risks remains unquantified. Furthermore, preoperative discontinuation of blood thinners is inconvenient for the patient, may necessitate the costly monitoring of coagulation parameters, and requires coordination with the patient's primary care physician. One might conclude that the relatively minor effects of persistent bleeding and hematoma do not outweigh the major impact of MI, CVA, and DVT and this argues for continued administration of ACA and PLTI during cutaneous surgery.

Although it is generally recommended that ACA and PLTI be discontinued prior to cutaneous surgery procedures, there are no controlled studies to support the beneficial effect of withholding medication preoperatively or an increased risk of hemorrhagic complications if medication is continued. Increased hemorrhagic complications from continued administration of ACA and PLTI during the perioperative period have been documented in non-controlled studies of cardiac, dental, ocular, general, urologic, and gynecologic surgery.[31–35] By extrapolation, it has been recommended that blood thinners be stopped before dermatologic procedures although only one study supports this advice.[26]

Nine studies over the last decade have attempted to address the risks of the continued administration of ACA and PLT in cutaneous surgery.[20–28] Eight of the studies, five of which were controlled, found no benefit of withholding ACA and PLTI before any type of cutaneous surgery.[20–25,27,28] Three of these studies, however, found that INR values greater than 3.5 in warfarinized patients may be associated with an increased postoperative bleeding risk.[25,27,28] Levels of international normalized ration (INR) above 5 may result in major bleeding.[36] Only one study found that warfarin increased the risk of major postoperative bleeding complications in cutaneous surgery.[26]

Ultimately, the practice of medicine is a based on a balance between the physician's personal experience and information garnered from the medical literature. Despite recent literature that indicates that severe hemorrhagic complications are rare in the anticoagulated dermatologic surgery patient, many physicians still believe that minor bleeding complications frequently occur in patients using ACA and PLTI. Examples of minor hemorrhagic complications include increased intraoperative bleeding, increased duration of procedure, choice of a suboptimal closure, extra nursing assistance, the need for extra equipment (e.g., suction, ligating sutures), additional pain from anesthesia "wash out," added surgeon frustration, and increased wound erythema and bruising.[21,37] These minor complications may increase the difficulty of surgery even if the ultimate clinical outcome is satisfactory. Consequently, it is still a common practice among dermatologic surgeons to discontinue ACA and PLTI preoperatively despite the conclusions of recent studies.

There is evidence that the discontinuation of ACA and PLTI preoperatively may increase the risk of thrombo-embolic complications in cutaneous surgery.[3,29,30] Reported complications include stroke, transient ischemic attack, myocardial infarction, pulmonary embolus, deep vein thromboses, death, and blindness due to retinal artery occlusion.[29] The authors of the aforementioned studies all concluded that medically necessary blood thinners should be continued during cutaneous surgery because there is no documented increased risk of severe hemorrhagic complications and because any bleeding problems that may occur are negligible, easily managed, and are not comparable to the morbidity and mortality of thromboembolic events.

However, none of the studies reporting thromboembolic complications compared the incidence of adverse vascular events in patients who had blood thinners discontinued preoperatively with the incidence of thrombotic episodes in patients who continued warfarin and aspirin or in patients who did not take blood thinners before surgery. Many of the patients in these studies were elderly and at risk for adverse vascular events independent of aspirin and warfarin therapy. Thus, a direct relationship has yet to be conclusively established between the preoperative discontinuation of blood thinners and perioperative thrombotic events.[38]

The cutaneous surgeon should develop a strategy for the perioperative management of patients on ACA and PLTI based on the recent evidence in the literature of the low risk of hemorrhagic complications in cutaneous surgery patients taking blood thinners and the potential for thrombotic complications if these medicines are withheld. It would seem prudent to continue warfarin during cutaneous surgery unless strictly prohibited by the primary care physician or if the INR is not within therapeutic range (2.0–3.5). Because of the tendency of INR values to unpredictably wander from baseline, it would seem logical to check INR values before surgery. Aspirin should be continued during surgery only if prescribed out of medical necessity. In general, NSAIDS, herbal supplements, and vitamin E may be safely discontinued preoperatively (some herbal supplements and vitamin E may have an adverse affect on platelet function, as discussed later in this chapter). Many patients are not aware of the many prescription and over-the-counter medications that contain aspirin and NSAIDS (Table 4-1). It is important to obtain a thorough preoperative history of all medications so that medically unnecessary drugs can be stopped before surgery. Cyclooxygenase 2 inhibitors, which have minimal antiplatelet effects, may be a useful preoperative alternative to traditional NSAIDS in patients with chronic conditions.[8]

Inadequate Intraoperative Hemostasis

Inadequate intraoperative hemostasis is another common cause of persistent bleeding and hematoma. Hemostasis rituals must be approached in a thorough and meticulous manner to prevent hemorrhagic complications. Ferric subsulfate (Monsel's solution) and aluminum chloride may achieve hemostasis of superficial wounds by denaturing protein and causing protein precipitation.[39] Small vessels should be electrodessicated, electrofulgurated, or electrocoagulated. These techniques rely on heat to denature protein. Electrocoagulation may be a more effective hemostatic modality than electrodessication and electrofulguration for excisional surgery. It is important to examine undermined skin for bleeding vessels by having assistant retract skin edges with skin hooks. Excess electrocoagulation should be avoided because charred, necrotic tissue may increase the risk of infection. Larger arteries and veins should be electrocoagulated or clamped with a hemostat and ligated with appropriate sized absorbable sutures. A suction device is helpful in clearing the surgical field and visualizing bleeding vessels that require ligation. It may be prudent to ligate large, visible vessels lying in the wound bed even if they appear undamaged. Such vessels can be nicked during surgery but may not bleed until the vasoconstrictive effects of epinephrine in the local anesthetic resolve.

Persistent intraoperative bleeding that can't be stopped with electrosurgery or ligation may be managed with firm, direct pressure for 10 to 15 minutes with a gauze pad, elevation of the affected area if feasible, and cold compresses. Cold compresses, which decrease bleeding through local vasoconstriction, are more effective if applied to the area surrounding the wound instead of the wound itself. In addition, the wound bed and surrounding edges may be injected with an epinephrine-containing local anesthetic or an epinephrine-soaked gauze pad may be placed in the wound bed. Topical absorbable hemostatic agents that may be applied to open wounds include gelatin sponges, oxidized cellulose, thrombin, and collagen. These agents work initially by transmitting pressure to the wound. Once hemostasis is achieved, they also provide a scaffold for the organization of a stable clot.

Drains are useful to siphon off excess blood when persistent bleeding is anticipated, such as a wound with a large dead space or one that has been widely undermined. Drains allow persistent bleeding to egress from the wound bed rather than to accumulate as a hematoma. Drains should be removed within 24 hours because they may increase the risk of wound infection by serving as portals of entry for bacteria into the wound bed.

Pressure dressings, which are very important in the postoperative management of the wound that persistently bleeds, are made of multiple layers of folded gauze. Pressure dressings serve multiple purposes: they immobilize the wound and prevent the dislodgement of fragile new clots, draw blood away from the suture line before clots form and separate wound edges, protect against bacteria, and prevent traumatic injury to the wound.[1] In general,

pressure dressings can be replaced in 24 to 48 hours with a less bulky bandage. Patients should be instructed to remove pressure dressings if they become soaked because they will subsequently lose their rigidity and compressive capacity.

Less Common Causes of Bleeding and Hematoma

In addition to drug-induced coagulopathy and inadequate intraoperative hemostasis, there are many less common factors and conditions that may increase the risk of bleeding during the perioperative period. Hypertension (blood pressure greater than 150/100 mm Hg) at the time of surgery may increase the risk of bleeding and hematoma.[37] A preoperative blood pressure level should be measured to detect hypertension and the surgeon must decide whether to postpone surgery and send the patient to the primary care physician for antihypertensive medication. Patients may forget or erroneously discontinue their medication before surgery. In such a case, the patient may then take their medicine and have blood pressure remeasured 1 to 2 hours later. Surgery may proceed if the patient is becomes normotensive. Sublingual antihypertensives (e.g., nifedipine) are not recommended for the immediate management of hypertension because the patient's blood pressure may quickly drop and precipitate a stroke or cardiac event.[37] The surgeon should consider preoperative anxiety as a cause of hypertension, in which case anxiolytics (e.g., diazepam 5–10 mg) may be beneficial.

Over 50% of patients take herbal supplements and vitamins prior to and at the time of surgical procedures.[40,41] Many of these products have anticoagulant effects and may increase the risk of perioperative bleeding, particularly if taken concomitantly with ACA and PLTI, although no reported cases of bleeding have occurred in cutaneous surgery.[40] Dietary supplements that may increase the risk of perioperative bleeding are grouped according to their mechanism of anticoagulation in Table 4-3.[40] The products most implicated in perioperative bleeding problems are ginkgo biloba, garlic, ginger, ginseng, feverfew, vitamin E, and ephedra.[7] Ephedra, which does not have antiplatelet effects, may potentiate the effects of epinephrine and increase blood pressure. Less than 40% of patients disclose alternative medicine use with their physicians,[7] so it is important to specifically ask about the use of supplements before surgery during the preoperative evaluation. Because the majority of these supplements are not medically necessary, it may be prudent to discontinue these products 7 to 10 days prior to cutaneous surgery to minimize bleeding risk.

Genodermatoses that may be associated with an increased risk of bleeding include hereditary hemorrhagic telangiectasia, osteogenesis imperfecta, Down's

TABLE 4-3. Dietary supplements and effects on coagulation.

Name	Medical uses	Effects on coagulation	No. of patients
Alfalfa	Prothrombinemic purpura	Contains coumarins	0
Capsicum	Dyspepsia, arthritis	Contains coumarins, inhibits platelet aggregation	0
Celery	Arthritis, urinary infection	Contains coumarins	0
Chamomile	Dyspepsia, anxiety	Contains coumarins	0
Chinese herbal teas/green tea	Cancer prevention, gastrointestinal disorders, cognition enhancement	Inhibits platelet aggregation	11
Danshen	Cardiovascular disease	Inhibits platelet aggregation, decreases elimination of warfarin in rats	0
Dong quai	Menopausal complaints, menstrual disorders	Contains coumarins	
Fenugreek	Dyspepsia, gastritis	Contains coumarins	0
Feverfew	Migraines, arthritis, fever	Inhibits platelet aggregation	0
Fish oils	Hypercholesterolemia	Decreases platelet aggregation and platelet adhesion	5
Garlic	Atherosclerosis, hypertension, hypercholesterolemia, infection	Decreases plasma viscosity, increases clotting time, inhibits platelet aggregation	4
Ginger	Nausea, arthritis	Inhibits platelet function	2
Gingko	Cardiovascular disease	Inhibits platelet aggregation and function, decreases plasma viscosity	2
Ginseng	Stress reduction, improves vitality	Inhibits platelet aggregation, contains coumarins	2
Horseradish	Infection, inflammation	Contains coumarins	0
Huang qui	Immunostimulant	Inhibits platelet aggregation and fibrinolysis	0
Kava kava	Anxiety, stress, muscle pain	Decreases platelet aggregation	0
Licorice	Cough, peptic ulcer	Contains coumarins	0
Passionflower	Anxiety, insomnia	Contains coumarins	0
Red clover	Infections, psoriasis	Contains coumarins	0
Vitamin E	Antioxidant	Decreases platelet adhesion and aggregation	24

Source: Adopted from Collins and Dufresne.[40]

syndrome, Ehler's Danlos syndrome, and Marfan's syndrome.[42] There are no reported cases of perioperative bleeding in dermatologic surgery patients with these hereditary diseases.

Patients with congenital bleeding disorders are at risk for intraoperative and postoperative hemorrhagic complications when their coagulation defect is not at least partially corrected.[42] Von Willebrand's disease, factor VIII deficiency (hemophilia A), and factor IX deficiency (hemophilia B or Christmas disease) are the most common inherited bleeding disorders, collectively affecting about 1% of the population.[43] Bleeding may occur with minor surgery unless coagulation factor levels are 40% to 50% of normal.[44] After major surgery, which requires 100% of normal clotting activity, replacement of coagulation factors is continued 7 to 10 days.[44] Preoperative consultation with a hematologist is essential in the management of dermatologic surgery patients with inherited bleeding disorders in order to prevent perioperative hemorrhagic complications.

Other factors that may be associated with perioperative bleeding include conditions associated with increased fibrinolysis (e.g., coronary artery bypass grafts, liver transplantation, disseminated intravascular coagulation, and fibrinolytic disorders) and atrophy of the skin (e.g., increasing age and chronic steroid use).[42]

Hemorrhagic Complications

The first type of hemorrhagic complication is an ecchymosis, which is a bruise that typically occurs within the first 24 hours after surgery. Ecchymoses develop secondary to scattering of red blood cells through natural soft tissue planes as a result of the trauma from the surgical procedure, whereas a hematoma is a focal collection of blood within the wound bed (Fig. 4-1). Gravity plays a very important role in the spread of blood within tissue planes postoperatively. Consequently, eyelids are very susceptible to ecchymoses and edema, particularly after surgical procedures on the scalp, forehead, temple, and upper nose (Fig. 4-2). Likewise, surgery on the cheek or chin may result in ecchymoses on the jawline and neck. Ecchymoses, which always resolve spontaneously within a few days, may frighten and alarm the patient because of their sometimes gruesome appearance. It is important, therefore, to warn the patient immediately after surgery about the possibility of this complication. Beginning on the first postoperative day, the application of cold compresses on a regular basis to high-risk surgical sites, such as the periocular area, may help prevent or lessen the formation of ecchymoses.

The second type of hemorrhagic complication is persistent postoperative bleeding after the patient leaves the

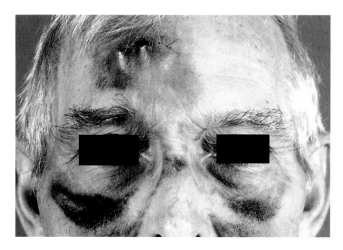

FIGURE 4-1. This patient developed a hematoma within the surgical site on his forehead and ecchymoses of the infraorbital area. A hematoma is a focal collection of blood within the wound bed, whereas ecchymoses develop as a result of the scattering of blood through tissue planes.

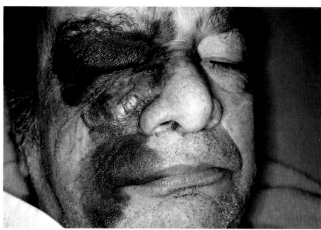

FIGURE 4-3. This patient developed a hematoma after surgery on the right medial cheek. He also has severe ecchymoses of the periorbital area, lower cheek, and upper lip.

surgical facility. Persistent postoperative bleeding is managed in a similar fashion to persistent intraoperative bleeding. First, the patient is instructed to apply firm pressure to the surgical site for 20 to 30 minutes. If possible, the affected area should also be elevated above the level of the heart. If these measures are unsuccessful, cold compresses — in addition to firm pressure — may be applied an additional 20 to 30 minutes. Cold compresses are more effective if applied to the area surrounding the wound instead of the wound itself. If bleeding persists, the patient should receive medical attention so that hemostasis may be achieved.

The third type of hemorrhagic complication is a hematoma, which is a focal collection of blood within the wound bed (Fig. 4-3). Hematomas typically go through four stages of development, each of which has therapeutic implications.[1] During the initial 48 hours, they are amorphous, gel-like masses that can easily be expressed from the wound. Between 2 and 5 days, they become adherent, rubbery clots that cannot be easily evacuated. From 7 to 14 days, hematomas are often liquefied by the fibrinolytic system. Liquified hematomas are easily aspirated from the wound. After 14 days, most hematomas undergo total resorption. Occasionally, hematomas do not liquefy and instead form organized, calcified tumors or hypertrophic scars that may persist indefinitely without intervention, such as intralesional steroids or surgical revision (Fig. 4-4).

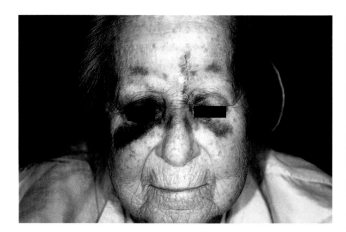

FIGURE 4-2. This patient developed periorbital ecchymoses after a surgical procedure on the forehead. Gravity plays an important role in the spread of blood within tissue planes after surgery.

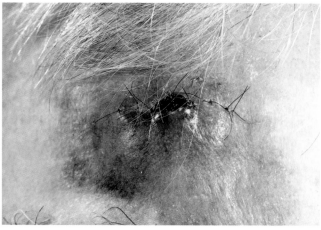

FIGURE 4-4. Organized hematoma of the temple that did not undergo resorption. Organized hematomas may form calcified tumors or hypertrophic scars that are difficult to treat.

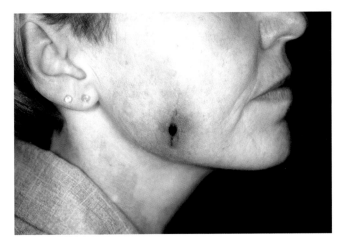

FIGURE 4-5. Small hematoma that became clinically apparent 3 days postoperatively.

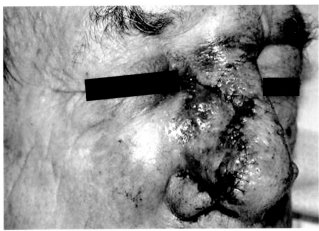

FIGURE 4-7. Acute hematoma that developed 4 hours postoperatively under a bilobed flap.

Anything that increases the risk of bleeding may lead to the development of a hematoma. Predisposing factors that have been discussed earlier in this chapter include medications (anticoagulants and platelet inhibitors), inadequate intraoperative hemostasis, hypertension, herbal supplements, certain genodermatoses, and coagulation disorders. Additional events that may precipitate a hematoma include postoperative trauma to the surgical site, excessive movement or manipulation of the surgical site, extensive undermining, a surge of bleeding after the dissipation of epinephrine in the local anesthetic, and a sudden increase in blood pressure (e.g., excessive exercise, heavy lifting, sneezing, coughing). Many of these factors may be prevented with a thorough preoperative evaluation, meticulous surgical technique, and adequate postoperative education of the patient.

There are two types of hematomas: small, indolent hematomas and large, expansile hematomas. Small hema-

tomas form insidiously and are usually noticeable 1 to 3 days postoperatively after edema subsides (Figs. 4-5, 4-6). Small hematomas are easily managed by removing one or more sutures, inserting a sterile hemostat into the wound, and expressing the clot through the suture line.

In contrast, large, expansile hematomas develop rapidly, typically within 24 hours postoperatively, and most commonly within the first 6 hours after surgery (Figs. 4-7, 4-8). Symptoms include sudden pain and the rapid appearance

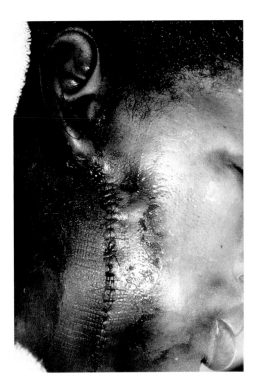

FIGURE 4-8. Acute hematoma that developed 12 hours postoperatively after keloid surgery on the cheek. (Photo courtesy of Carl Washington, MD.)

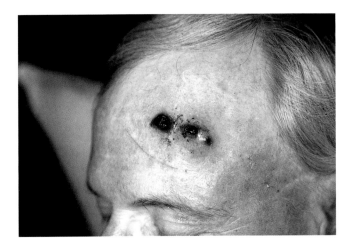

FIGURE 4-6. Small hematoma that the patient noticed when the pressure dressing was removed 48 hours after surgery.

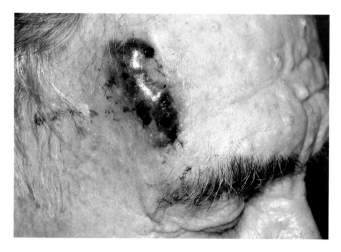

FIGURE 4-9. This expanding hematoma increased wound edge tension leading to ischemia and necrosis of the overlying skin.

of reddish-blue, tender swelling around the surgical site. Expansile hematomas constitute an acute surgical emergency and require immediate medical attention because they may impinge upon vital structures, serve as media for wound infection, and increase wound edge tension, which in turn can lead to ischemia, necrosis, and dehiscence (Fig. 4-9).[45]

The most important step in the initial management of a large, expansile hematoma is immediate relief of wound edge tension. The wound should be anesthetized and sterilely prepared. Cutaneous and subcutaneous sutures should be removed and the clot promptly evacuated. To improve visualization, the wound should be irrigated with saline. Hemostasis may then be obtained either with electrocoagulation, ligation of visible bleeding vessels, or a combination of the two. The wound generally may be resutured unless it appears infected, in which case it should be packed with iodoform gauze and the patient placed on antibiotics. If persistent oozing is anticipated, a drain may be inserted in the wound. Drains should be removed after 24 hours because they may provide a portal of entry for bacteria. Although no studies support this dogma, most physicians institute antibiotics because hematomas are thought to serve as potential media for infection.

If the hematoma is discovered several days after surgery, the surgeon must decide whether or not to open the wound and evacuate the clot. The presence or absence of infection, necrosis, or dehiscence determines if the wound should be opened or not. If any of these complications are present, the wound must be opened. The clot should be soaked with warm saline for 5 to 10 minutes and then removed with sterile forceps. Again, although no studies exist to support this advice, it is commonly recommended that antibiotics be instituted in this scenario because the clot may serve as a nidus for infection.

The wound should be allowed to heal by second intention and scar revision, if necessary, may be performed at a later date.

It is not necessary to open the wound in the absence of infection, necrosis, or dehiscence. Instead, the clot may be managed expectantly and allowed to be resorbed by the fibrinolytic system. Alternatively, the surgeon can wait until the clot liquefies and aspirate it by inserting a large-bore (16- or 18-gauge) needle into the wound. This process may be repeated if necessary. It may again be prudent to institute appropriate antibiotics.

Conclusion

The cutaneous surgeon should be capable preventing, diagnosing, and managing bleeding complications. The first step in prevention is a thorough history and physical exam focused on identifying risk factors that may predispose the patient to bleeding episodes. The second preventive step is the maintenance of meticulous intraoperative hemostasis, the use of proper pressure dressings, and providing clear postoperative instructions to the patient. Despite these precautions, bleeding problems may still occur, in which case the surgeon must be skilled in proper diagnosis and management. Fortunately, most hemorrhagic complications in cutaneous surgery are a mere nuisance to the patient and physician and, with proper management, may be successfully treated without a negative impact on the final outcome of the procedure. However, a potentially serious complication is a rapidly expanding hematoma, which may impinge on vital structures and lead to infection and increased wound edge tension with subsequent ischemia, necrosis, and dehiscence. It is incumbent upon the cutaneous surgeon manage this complication promptly and efficiently in order to provide excellent patient care.

References

1. Salasche S. Acute surgical complications: cause, prevention, and treatment. J Am Acad Dermatol 1986;15:1163–1185.
2. Salasche S, Grabski W. Complications of flaps. J Dermatol Surg Oncol 1991;17:132–140.
3. Alam M, Goldberg L. Serious adverse vascular events associated with perioperative interruption of antiplatelet and anticoagulant therapy. Dermatol Surg 2002;28:992–998.
4. Antman E. The re-emergence of anticoagulation in coronary disease. Eur Heart J Suppl 2004;6:B2–B8.
5. Amann R, Peskar B. Anti-inflammatory effects of aspirin and sodium salicylate. Eur J Pharmacol 2002;447:1–9.
6. Flower R, Moncada S, Vane J. Analgesic-antipyretics and anti-inflammatory agents: drugs employed in the treatment of gout. In: Goodman LS, Gilman AG, eds. The pharmacological basis of therapeutics. 7th ed. New York: MacMillan; 1985:690–704.

7. Chang L, Whitaker D. The impact of herbal medicines on dermatologic surgery. Dermatol Surg 2001;27:759–763.

8. Weisberg N, Becker D. Potential role of the new specific COX-2 inhibitors in dermatologic surgery. Dermatol Surg 2000;26:551–553.

9. CAPRIE Steering Committee. A randomized, blinded trial of clopidogrel versus aspirin in patients at risk of ischaemic events (CAPRIE). Lancet 1996;348:1329–1339.

10. Barnett H, Eliasziw M, Meldrum H. Drugs and surgery in the prevention of ischemic stroke. N Engl J Med 1995;332:238–248.

11. Desager J. Clinical pharmacokinetics of ticlopidine. Clin Pharmocokinet 1994;26:347–355.

12. Moake J, Funicella T. Common bleeding problems. Clin Symp 1983;35:1–32.

13. Sharis P, Cannon C, Loscalzo J. The antiplatelet effects of ticlopidine and clopidogrel. Ann Intern Med 1998;129:394–405.

14. Samlaska C, Winfield E. Pentoxifylline. J Am Acad Dermatol 1994;30:603–621.

15. Chiquette E, Amato M, Bussey H. Comparison of an anticoagulation clinic with usual medical care: anticoagulation control, patient outcomes, and health care costs. Arch Intern Med 1998;158:1641–1647.

16. Mohr J. A comparison of warfarin and aspirin for the prevention of recurrent ischemic stroke. N Engl J Med 2001;345:1444–1451.

17. Bauer K. Selective inhibition of coagulation factors: advances in antithrombotic therapy. Semin Thromb Hemost 2002;28:15–24.

18. Majerus P, Broze G, Miletich J, Tollefsen D. Anticoagulant thrombolytic, and antiplatelet drugs. In: Hardman JG, Limbird LE, eds. Goodman and Gilman's the pharmacological basis of therapeutics. 9th ed. New York: McGraw-Hill; 1996:1347–1351.

19. Horton J, Bushwick B. Warfarin therapy: evolving strategies in anticoagulation. Am Fam Physician 1999;59:1–19.

20. Goldsmith S, Leshin B, Owen J. Management of patients taking anticoagulants and platelet inhibitors prior to dermatologic surgery. J Dermatol Surg Oncol 1993;19:578–581.

21. Lawrence C, Sakuntabhai A, Tiling-Grosse S. Effect of aspirin and nonsteroidal anti-inflammatory drug therapy on bleeding complications in dermatologic surgical patients. J Am Acad Dermatol 1994;31:988–992.

22. Otley C, Fewkes J, Frank W, Olbricht S. Complications of cutaneous surgery in patients who are taking warfarin, aspirin, and nonsteroidal anti-inflammatory drugs. Arch Dermatol 1996;132:161–166.

23. Billingsley E, Maloney M. Intraoperative and postoperative bleeding problems in patients taking warfarin, aspirin, and nonsteroidal anti-inflammatory agents. Dermatol Surg 1997;23:381–385.

24. Bartlett G. Does aspirin affect the outcome of minor cutaneous surgery? Br J Plast Surg 1999;52:214–216.

25. Alcalay J. Cutaneous surgery in patients receiving warfarin therapy. Dermatol Surg 2001;27:756–758.

26. Kargi E, Babuccu O, Hosnuter M, Babuccu B, Altinyazar C. Complications of minor cutaneous surgery in patients under anticoagulant therapy. Aesthetic Plast Surg 2002;26:483–485.

27. Ah-Weng A, Natarajan S, Velangi S, Langtry J. Preoperative monitoring of warfarin in cutaneous surgery. Br J Dermatol 2003;149:386–389.

28. Syed S, Adams B, Liao W, Pipitone M, Gloster H. A prospective assessment of bleeding and INR in warfarin-anticoagulated patients having cutaneous surgery. J Am Acad Dermatol 2004;51:955–957.

29. Kovich O, Otley C. Thrombotic complications related to discontinuation of warfarin and aspirin therapy perioperatively for cutaneous operation. J Am Acad Dermatol 2003;48:233–237.

30. Schanbacher CF, Bennett R. Postoperative stroke after stopping warfarin for cutaneous surgery. Dermatol Surg 2000;26:785–789.

31. Ferraris V, Swanson E. Aspirin usage and perioperative blood loss in patients undergoing unexpected operations. Surg Gynecol Obstet 1983;156:439–442.

32. Madura J, Rookstool M, Wease G. The management of patients on chronic coumadin therapy undergoing subsequent surgical procedures. Am Surg 1194;60;542–546.

33. Amrein P, Ellman L, Harris W. Aspirin-induced prolongation of bleeding time and perioperative blood loss. JAMA 1981;245:1825–1828.

34. Hall D, Steen W, Drummond J. Anticoagulants and cataract surgery. Ophthalmic Surg 1988;19:221–222.

35. Hunter G, Barney M, Crapo R. Perioperative warfarin therapy in combined abdominal lipectomy and intraabdominal gynecological surgical procedures. Ann Plast Surg 1990;25;37–41.

36. Hirsh J, Dalen J, Anderson DR. Oral anticoagulants: mechanism of action, clinical effectiveness, and optimal therapeutic range. Chest 1998;114:444S–469S.

37. Fader D, Johnson T. Medical issues and emergencies in the dermatology office. J Am Acad Dermatol 1997;36:1–16.

38. Kimyai-Asadi A, Jih M, Goldberg L. Perioperative primary stroke: is aspirin cessation to blame? Dermatol Surg 2004;30:1526–1529.

39. Houry S, Georgeac C, Hay JM. A prospective multicenter evaluation of preoperative hemostatic screening tests. The French Association for Surgical Research. Am J Surg 1995;170:19.

40. Collins S, Dufresne R. Dietary supplements in the setting of Mohs surgery. Dermatol Surg 2002;28:447–452.

41. Norred C, Zamudio S, Palmer S. Use of complementary and alternative medicines by surgical patients. ANNA J 2000;68:13–18.

42. Peterson S, Joseph A. Inherited bleeding disorders in dermatologic surgery. Dermatol Surg 2001;27:885–889.

43. Werner E. Von Willebrand disease in children and adolescents. Pediatr Clin North Am 1996;43:683–707.

44. Kasper C, Boylen L, Ewing N, Luck J, Dietrich S. Hematologic management of hemophilia A for surgery. JAMA 1985;253:1279–1283.

45. Mulliken J, Healey N. Pathogenesis of skin flap necrosis from an underlying hematoma. Plast Reconstr Surg 1979;63:540–545.

5
Wound Infections

Gregory J. Fulchiero, Jr., and Elizabeth M. Billingsley

Wound infections are uncommon in dermatologic surgery with an overall reported incidence of 2%.[1] By definition, surgical wound infections occur within 30 days of the time of the procedure and may involve the skin, subcutaneous fat, or the muscle above the fascia. The Centers for Disease Control and Prevention (CDC) has categorized skin and subcuticular surgical site infections as *superficial*, while those involving the muscle are categorized as *deep* surgical site infections.[2] Most wound infections are thought to begin at the time of surgery whenever aseptic technique is broken, or bacteria are introduced into the wound due to inadequate preoperative cleansing or the use of contaminated instruments and suture material. However, infections may also be caused by patient-specific factors such as preoperative skin or nasal bacterial colonization and poor wound hygiene postoperatively.

Infections are classically differentiated from bacterial wound colonization by either (i) the number of bacteria identified by culture ($>10^5$ colony forming units/g of tissue)[3] or (ii) the clinical signs and symptoms that suggest infection (Table 5-1). Colonization of bacteria in a wound may be a precursor to infection, or may be temporary, as the patient's own immune system and wound bed environment promote healthy physiologic wound healing.

Most wound infections present within 4 to 10 days after the surgical procedure. The clinical appearance of wound infections is dictated by the degree of tissue insult from the inflammatory response that ensues from the inoculated bacteria. Activation of the complement cascade, secretion of cytokines and chemotactic polypeptides [interleukin (IL) 1, IL-2, IL-8, tumor necrosis factor α (TNF-α)] from neutrophils, macrophages, and keratinocytes,[4] as well as host matrix metalloproteinases, acute phase reactants, and bacteria-derived collagenases are all part of the pathophysiologic machinery leading to clinically evident wound infection.

Classification of Wounds

Surgical wounds have been classified into four main categories according to their risk for postoperative infection: clean (class I), clean–contaminated (class II), contaminated (class III), and dirty–infected (class IV).[5] Each category caries an increasingly greater incidence of postoperative wound infection (Table 5-2). This allows the surgeon to risk stratify the likelihood of developing an infection for each procedure based on the status of the surgical site and the anatomic location.

The majority of dermatologic surgery procedures results in either class I or class II wounds, and generally require no prophylactic antibiotics. Prophylactic antibiotics in class III wounds may have an uncertain benefit and should be considered by the surgeon if additional risk factors for infection are found. Antibiotics in class IV wounds are not considered prophylactic, but therapeutic, and should be continued postoperatively (Table 5-3). Class III and IV wounds may benefit from second intention healing to minimize postoperative infection.

Risk Factors for Infection

Risk factors predisposing wounds to infection have been described, and include the immune- or overall health status of the patient, diabetes, tobacco use within the past 30 days, and length of the surgical procedure (Table 5-4).[6] The rate of infection may roughly *double* for each additional hour of surgery.[6] Operative and postoperative factors that establish an environment suitable for the development of infection are relative wound edge ischemia, hematoma or seroma formation, excessive suture material, extensive electrocoagulation, and devitalized tissue.

Immunocompromised Patients

While the association between immunosuppression and wound healing has been documented, the association

TABLE 5-1. Diagnostic criteria for wound infection.

Any of the following suggest infection
  Purulent wound drainage
  Positive wound culture
  Erythema
  Induration
  Tenderness

Additional situations suggesting infection until proven otherwise
  Opening of an incision postoperatively by either the patient or surgeon, for any reason
  Infection as deemed by clinical assessment of an attending physician, with or without the results of a wound culture

TABLE 5-3. Utility of prophylactic antibiotics.

Wound classification	Prophylactic antibiotics
Class I	No role
Class II	Uncertain benefit
Class III	Possible benefit if additional risk factors are present
Class IV	Necessary; considered therapeutic and continued postoperatively

between immunosuppression and wound infection rates is less certain. It has been suggested that prophylactic antibiotics be considered for patients receiving cytotoxic drugs (chemotherapy) when either (i) granulocyte counts are below 1000/mm^3, (ii) the surgical procedure could result in significant bacterial contamination, or (iii) if the patient's immune status is inadequate to combat any bacterial insult.[7] Prophylactic antibiotics should be instituted

on an individual basis, taking into account the nature of the procedure and the immune status of the patient. Malnutrition may also be considered an immunocompromised state, with potential delayed wound healing and an increased risk of wound infection.

Chronic Corticosteroids

Chronic corticosteroid usage is also a debatable risk factor for infection. The proposed mechanisms for increased wound infections is a decrease in neutrophil chemotaxis and superoxide production,[8] as well as an increase in the time required for complete wound healing. It has been suggested that stopping corticosteroid therapy immediately prior to surgery, and for several days postoperatively, might normalize the wound healing cascade in these patients.[9] However, this is rarely done in routine excisional surgery.

Human Immunodeficiency Virus/Acquired Immunodeficiency Syndrome

The prevalence of human immunodeficiency virus (HIV)-infected patients undergoing dermatologic surgery continues to rise as the efficacy of highly active antiretroviral therapy (HAART) minimizes the morbidity and mortality from acquired immunodeficiency syndrome (AIDS).

TABLE 5-2. Classification of wound infections.

Classification	Description of wound	Infection risk
Class I Clean	Uninfected operative wound No acute inflammation Primary closure Respiratory, gastrointestinal, biliary, and urinary tracts not entered No break in aseptic technique *Example:* routine excision	<2%
Class II Clean–contaminated	Elective entry into axillae, inguinal, or mucosal regions No evidence of infection or major break in aseptic technique *Example:* axillary biopsy; healing by secondary intention	<10%
Class III Contaminated	Nonpurulent inflammation Gross spillage from gastrointestinal tract Penetrating traumatic wounds <4 hours prior Major break in aseptic technique *Example:* inflamed cyst; tumor with inflammation or ulceration	≈20%
Class IV Dirty–infected	Purulent inflammation present Devitalized or necrotic tissue Penetrating traumatic wounds >4 hours, or foreign bodies *Example:* swollen hidradenitis suppurativa nodule; furuncle	≈40%

TABLE 5-4. Wound infection risk factors.

Diabetes mellitus
Cancer
Malnutrition
Alcohol abuse
Intravenous drug abuse
Smoking within past 30 days
Vascular insufficiency
Chemotherapy
Neutropenia[a]
Immune suppression[b]
Organ transplant recipients[b]
HIV/AIDS[b]
Shaving of surgical site (≥24 hours prior to procedure)[b]

Abbreviations: AIDS, acquired immunodeficiency syndrome; HIV, human immunodeficiency virus.
[a] Granulocyte count <1000/mm^3.
[b] Relative risk factors.

Some investigators have found that HIV-infected patients may experience overall higher rates of infectious complications in general surgery.[10] Others have found no difference in the rate of wound infections nor complications in wound healing in HIV-positive patients.[11,12] In summary, neither detectable preoperative CD4+ counts nor HIV status reliably correlate with an increased rate of postoperative wound infections.

Hair Removal

Shaving of the surgical site may be considered a risk factor for infection and is generally discouraged. The microtrauma caused by a razor is thought to act as a nidus for bacterial colonization or even transient bacteremia (usually *Staphylococcus aureus*). In one study, the risk of wound infection when shaving the surgical site within 24 hours was 5.6%, compared to 0.6% if hair clipping or no hair removal was performed.[13] The infection rate exceeded 20% if shaving was performed more than 24 hours prior to surgery. Thus, if hair removal is required, gentle clipping with curved scissors at the time of operation is preferred.

Clinical Differential Diagnosis

The differential diagnosis of wound infections varies based on the clinical picture of the wound and the complaints of the patient (Table 5-5). Normal symptoms that may be mistaken for infection include incisional discomfort, pain, swelling, erythema, and tenderness in the surrounding skin (Fig. 5-1).

Hematoma and Seroma

Seroma and hematoma formation are the most frequent complications within the first 24 hours after surgery. These complications present as extensive ecchymosis or a mass, which represents a collection of fluid beneath the incision site (Figs. 5-2, 5-3). A seroma or hematoma may simply present with pain and not be clinically obvious. Extensive undermining increases the likelihood of seroma

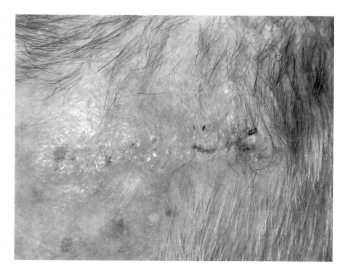

FIGURE 5-1. Normal wound healing is seen with accompanying erythema and swelling.

formation, while anticoagulation and failure to achieve meticulous hemostasis increases the risk of hematoma. Both are best managed with aspiration or evacuation as they may predispose the patient to latent wound infection or lengthen the time to full recovery. Antibiotics are often prescribed prophylacticaly when hematoma or seroma occur.

Contact Dermatitis

Allergic or irritant contact dermatitis to tape dressings, adhesive glues, or antibiotic ointments may mimic a postoperative wound infection. While irritant contact reactions may present within the first 24 hours of application, allergic contact dermatitis typically presents 24 to 72 hours after the antigenic exposure and may mimic a

TABLE 5-5. Differential diagnosis of wound infection.

Etiology	Clinical symptoms	Time course
Hematoma	Ecchymosis, hemorrhagic bullae, progressive swelling	24 to 48 hours
Seroma	Swelling, pain, erythema	12 to 72 hours
Contact dermatitis	Papules, vesicles, erythema	12 to 72 hours
Bacterial colonization	Erythema without purulence, exudate, delayed healing	Days to weeks
Spitting suture	Sterile pustule, extruded suture material, granulation	Weeks to months

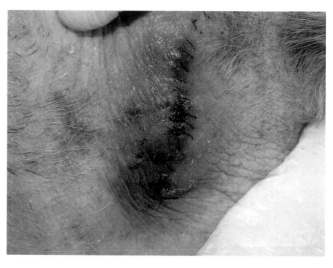

FIGURE 5-2. Extensive ecchymosis and a subcutaneous mass representing a hematoma.

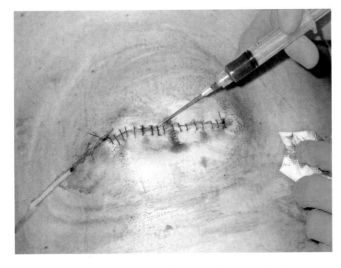

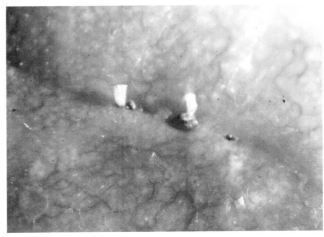

FIGURE 5-5. Obvious extruded material of a spitting suture along a healing wound.

FIGURE 5-3. Percutaneous extraction of an acute hematoma that eventually required opening of the wound to achieve hemostasis. (Courtesy of Catherine Headley, MD.)

wound infection due to its delayed presentation and progressive evolution. Contact dermatitis frequently manifests as a pruritic and geometric, well-demarcated erythema with or without papules and vesicles limited to the site of the applied antigen or irritant (Fig. 5-4).

Spitting Sutures

Spitting sutures, a common complication presenting in up to 5% of wounds with buried intradermal braided absorb-

able sutures,[14] may occur as early as several weeks, or as late as 3 to 6 months postoperatively. A painless sterile pustule or erythematous tract with frank, transepidermal elimination of suture material may be seen (Figs. 5-5, 5-6). The etiology of spitting sutures is not completely understood, but is usually related to the degree of the suture material's tissue reactivity and more superficial placement within the dermis. Monofilament absorbable sutures, which have traditionally been considered to have less overall tissue reactivity, have also been noted to cause spitting sutures.[15] The delayed onset of spitting sutures, lack of tenderness, and absence of other signs of infection, such as warmth and surrounding erythema, are clues to the diagnosis and should obviate the surgeon from starting unnecessary antibiotics.

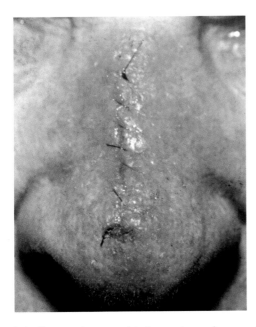

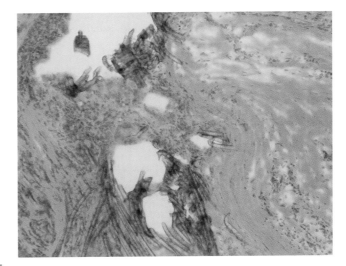

FIGURE 5-4. Geometric crusted inflammatory plaques of allergic contact dermatitis to bacitracin antibiotic ointment mimicking wound infection.

FIGURE 5-6. Foreign-body reaction seen to extruding suture material.

Wound Infection Microbiology

Most wounds are contaminated by the patient's own *endogenous* flora, which are present on the skin, mucous membranes, or gastrointestinal tract. The common pathogens on skin and mucosal surfaces are Gram-positive cocci, particularly staphylococci. Gram-negative aerobes and anaerobic bacteria frequently contaminate skin in the axillary and inquinal areas. Gram-positive organisms, such as staphylococci and streptococci, account for the vast majority of *exogenous* flora involved in wound infections.[16] Sources of these exogenous pathogens include surgical personnel and intraoperative factors, including surgical instruments, articles brought into the operative field, and the operating room air.[2,16] Culture data compiled by the CDC encompassing all surgical site infections, such as those in general and orthopedic surgery, have shown that *Staphylococcus aureus* and *Staphylococcus epidermidis* are implicated in only 20% and 14%, respectively. This is in stark contrast to the overwhelming isolates of *Staphylococcus aureus* routinely found in dermatologic surgery. Futoryan and Grande have shown in one series that over 70% of culture-positive wound infections in excisional skin surgery demonstrate *S. aureus*.[1]

Bacterial Flora

Bacterial flora, or microbiota, varies in different anatomic sites. These bacteria are divided into either (i) *resident flora* or (ii) *transient flora*. Resident flora are the most abundant number of microorganisms (10^{14} bacteria) normally found in and on healthy individuals. Transient bacterial flora are acquired through contact with people, objects, or the environment. Transient flora are not always present or are present for only a few days, weeks, or months before disappearing for various immunologic, hygienic, and environmental conditions. In spite of their smaller numbers, transient bacteria are the organisms that are largely responsible for postoperative wound infections.

Transmission

Contact transmission of transient flora into the wound may occur *indirectly* via fomites (e.g., contaminated materials such as suture or hypodermic needles) or *directly* by the surgeon or patient (e.g., a gloved or ungloved finger). Airborne transmission of bacteria often occurs as microorganisms are carried by desquamated skin cells into the wound.[17] Aerosolized water droplets and dust particles can also introduce transient flora into the surgical wound and cause infection, regardless of adherence to intraoperative aseptic techniques.

Distribution of Flora

Staphylococcus epidermidis is considered part of the normal flora, comprising over 50% of the resident staphylococci. *S. epidermidis* can be found on the skin in virtually any anatomic location but has a higher density on the extremities. While *S. epidermidis* rarely causes frank wound infections, it can be a pathogen for bioprosthetic heart valves and vascular grafts due to its ability to form a proteoglycan-rich extracellular biofilm that surrounds the bacterium and tightly binds it to the skin and inanimate surfaces. In the setting of infection, this biofilm acts as a protective barrier and prevents the bacterium from engulfment by neutrophils, making established *S. epidermidis* infections particularly difficult to treat.

Staphylococcus aureus, which is coagulase positive, is usually not among the resident flora, but can occasionally be found in intertriginous areas and increasingly in the nares. *S. aureus* also frequently colonizes the skin of patients with atopic dermatitis due to decreased production of endogenous antimicrobial peptides such as cathelicidins and β-defensins, and may predispose these patients to wound infection.[18] Although *S. aureus* is the most commonly documented pathogen in wound and routine soft tissue skin infections, it is implicated in less than 30% of the cases of bacterial endocarditis.[19] *Streptococcus viridans* is common in the oral cavity, causing oral and cutaneous wound infections, and it is routinely isolated in up to 50% of patients with diagnosed endocarditis.[19] Endocarditis as a complication in skin surgery and wound infections will be discussed in Chapter 6.

The head, neck, and upper part of the trunk have more sebaceous glands, and hence more lipophilic organisms, such as the *Propionibacterium* species. Although rarely a cause of wound infection, *P. acnes* bacteremia can occur during skin surgery and is occasionally identified on blood cultures. Exposed areas, such as the face, neck, and hands, have higher total numbers of bacteria, including more transient bacteria such as *S. aureus* and group A streptococci (Fig. 5-7). Intertriginous areas, such as the axillae and groin, can be more heavily colonized with Gram-negative rods, coryneforms, and *S. aureus*.[20]

Special Considerations

Ear Flora

The ear poses a unique challenge to the dermatologic surgeon. In one series of 530 consecutive Mohs surgery cases repaired by primary or complex closures, nearly half (46%) of the wound infections occurred on the ear.[1] Furthermore, after repair the infection rate was 28% if the ear cartilage was involved and 6% if the procedure did not involve the cartilage. Infection rates of the ear

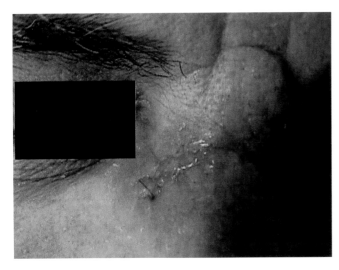

FIGURE 5-7. Wound infection of the nasal dorsum caused by *Staphylcoccus aureus.*

also correlate independently with the number of Mohs stages, and are presumably related to the cumulative duration of the surgery.

The pathogens causing wound infections of the ear are commonly staphylococci and Gram-negative rods such as

Pseudomonas aeuruginosa and, less frequently, *Serratia marcescens*. Although *P. aeruginosa* innocuously colonizes toe webspaces and complicates chronic lower extremity ulcers, it also frequently colonizes the external auditory canal and may cause cutaneous wound infections of the ear, as well as acute or delayed auricular chondritis (Fig. 5-8). *Serratia marcescens* often colonizes the urinary tract, but is an increasingly frequent cause of antibiotic-resistant ocular infections, otitis media, and wound infections of the ear.[21] Interestingly, *S. marcescens* can produce a pigment called *prodigiosin*, which ranges in color from dark red to pale pink and that may be mistaken for blood.

Gastrointestinal and Urinary Flora

Escheria coli and *Klebsiella* are Gram-negative rods found in the gastrointestinal, biliary, and urinary tracts and cause up to 8% and 3% of cutaneous wound infections, respectively.[22] These organisms, like the enterococci, frequently colonize the skin of patients in the hospital setting who have been catheterized or have had an endotracheal tube in place. They can also complicate lower extremity surgery due to patient incontinence or poor patient hygiene, especially if proper antiseptic scrubbing is not performed (Fig. 5-9).

Unlike other bacteria of the gastrointestinal tract, which are usually Gram-negative rods, enterococci are Gram-positive cocci and can be particularly difficult to treat. They can be found in up to 12% of wound infections, particularly in hospitalized or debilitated patients who have received previous courses of antibiotics. Over 90% of the cultures of enterococci are *Enterococcus faecalis*, with the remaining 10% *E. faecium*. The emerging nosocomial threat of VRE (vancomycin-resistant enterococcus) is usually found to be a resistant isolate of *E. faecium*.

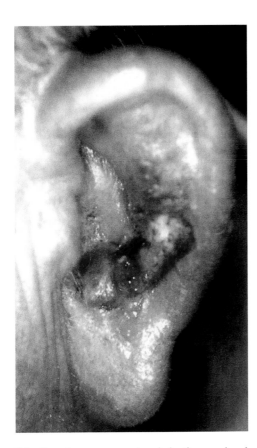

FIGURE 5-8. *Pseudomonas* causing infection and subsequent chondritis in a granulating ear wound.

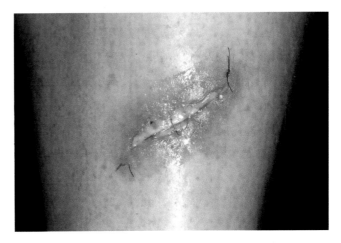

FIGURE 5-9. *E. coli* infection of an excisional leg wound.

Culture Techniques

Recent advances in the prevention and management of wound infection have focused on the level of bacterial growth rather than the mere presence of pathogenic organisms. Robson has established that a quantitative culture of 10^6 organisms per gram of tissue confirms the diagnosis of infection.[23] Though the dermatologic surgeon is more likely to swab a wound for culture than obtain a tissue sample, a quantitative assay of bacterial density can still be obtained.[24]

Quantitative Swabbing

The proper technique of quantitative swabbing involves rolling the tip of the swab in a zig-zag fashion along the length of the incision after prior debridement of dead eschar from the wound.[25] This minimizes the likelihood of impetiginized flora masking the true pathogen in a wound bed by yielding an erroneous bacterial isolate. *As a rule*, after Gram staining a wound swab on a slide, one bacterium per high-powered field is predictive of $\geq 10^5$ organisms/g of tissue.[24] Further identification of the bacteria is then carried out by culturing the swab on agar, followed by Kirby–Bauer antibiotic disk sensitivities 24 to 36 hours later.

Prevention and Management

Antisepsis and Wound Care in Preventing Wound Infection

The importance of adhering to antiseptic surgical site preparation, handwashing regimens, aseptic surgical techniques, and meticulous postoperative wound care cannot be overemphasized. Repetitive minor breaks in any of these antiseptic steps can lead to a substantial increase in the rates of wound infection for a surgeon or a surgical center at large. Once a preoperative antiseptic regimen is established in a surgical center, adherence by all members of the surgical team is critical in consistently reproducing low rates of postoperative wound infections.[26]

Surgical Site Preparation

A *systems approach* to minimizing wound infections, defined as whole body antiseptic cleansing or showering less than 24 hours prior to surgery, is recommended by the CDC.[2] This has resulted in both (i) a reduction in the observed rates of wound infection and (ii) a durable reduction in the numbers of resident and pathogenic transient flora for up to 72 hours.[27] Akin to preoperative antiseptic showering, topical application of 10% benzoyl peroxide gel to the surgical site for 7 days prior to the procedure has been shown, in one controlled study of 673 patients, to significantly reduce infection rates in seborrheic skin from 3.24% to 0.59%.[28]

Many antiseptic scrubbing solutions exist, including isopropyl alcohol, iodophors, chlorhexylenol (PCMX), and chlorhexidine gluconate. Each solution has certain disadvantages that may preclude it from being used in a particular patient or anatomic site. Alcohol, which must fully dry in order to desiccate bacteria within the surgical field, is irritating to mucous membranes and is short acting. Iodophors must remain wet and in contact with the skin for at least 2 minutes to have an antimicrobial effect by releasing bacteriocidal iodine ions. Iodophors are rapidly inactivated by blood or serum and must not be used in patients allergic to iodine or shellfish. PCMX destroys bacterial cell walls and is less effective than alcohol, iodophors, or chlorhexidine. It is inactivated by soaps, and should not be used on children because it is readily absorbed through the skin and is potentially neurotoxic. Finally, chlorhexidine is toxic to the ears and eyes and can cause an irritant conjunctivitis despite its sustained activity (hours) after application, cumulative efficacy with successive applications, and safety in pediatric patients.

A recent meta-analysis and review of the literature with an emphasis on study design by the Cochrane Database concluded that "*There is insufficient research examining the effects of preoperative skin antiseptics to allow conclusions to be drawn regarding their effects on postoperative surgical wound infections.*"[29] One finding was that there was no difference in the prevention of wound infections between isopropyl alcohol and iodine preparations. The Cochrane Database did identify a study of 371 patients undergoing clean surgery by Berry and colleagues that showed a 15.9% (28/176) infection rate with iodophors, compared with 4.1% (8/195) for chlorhexidine.[30] These results have been verified in a small study of 39 patients when a 2-minute surgical scrub with chlorhexidine was superior to both povidone–iodine and PCMX in reducing mean bacterial counts.[31]

The superior efficacy of chlorhexidine is likely due to its (i) immediate onset of action, (ii) broad spectrum of activity similar to that of povidone–iodine and PCMX (Gram-positive and -negative organisms, fungi, enveloped viruses, and *M. tuberculosis*), (iii) lack of inactivation by blood, compared to iodine, (iv) sustained activity when dry, and (v) additive antiseptic effect with repeated use.

Commercial Chlorhexidine Preparations

In accordance with the CDC recommendations,[2] the ideal surgical site scrubbing should incorporate "*a dedicated instrument . . . adapted for the purpose, (and) the applicator should be discarded once the periphery has been reached.*"

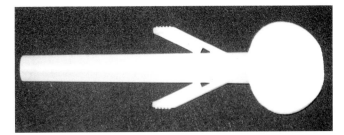

FIGURE 5-10. Disposable single-use chlorhexidine applicator with sponge.

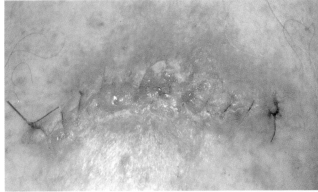

FIGURE 5-11. Extensive erythema, induration, and serosanguinous discharge suggesting infection, without frank purulence.

A sterile hemostat or towel clip on the surgical tray with a chlorhexidine-soaked gauze may adequate. However, newer commercial preparations of 2% chlorhexidine gluconate with 70% isopropyl alcohol have been developed solely for this purpose. These disposable applicators contain a breakable chamber that releases the solution, which then saturates a sterile sponge at the end of the polymer stick (Fig. 5-10). Convenient and effective in both cleansing and debridement of the surgical site, this commercial preparation is superior in reducing microbial counts than either 2% chlorhexidine or 70% isopropyl alcohol alone.[32]

Recommended Scrub Technique

After debridement of large particles or debris from the skin, the recommended preoperative scrub is 1 minute long, performed in concentric expanding circles, and left to briefly air dry. It is preferred that the surgical site be left as is, without using a gauze to remove excess cleanser. Given the above data showing its efficacy in reducing bacterial counts and postoperative wound infection rates compared to other agents, chlorhexidine is the current antiseptic of choice. A 1-minute scrub has been shown to have similar efficacy to a traditional 10-minute scrub in minimizing wound infections.[33] In general, the surgical site should be prepared with an antiseptic solution that expands far beyond the expected incision so that any surgical instruments or suture that may touch the area around the surgical site will not contaminate the wound.

Management of Established Wound Infection

When a wound infection is suspected it is imperative that an accurate assessment of pain, erythema, and tenderness be made by the surgeon. One should also inquire about the presence or absence of systemic symptoms, such as fevers, rigors, or night sweats, which may point towards occult bacteremia and require admission to the hospital for intravenous antibiotics and observation. It is normal for erythema, edema, and serosanguinous discharge to be present in healing wounds, but is much less common after

3 days postoperatively. These findings, even in the absence of frank purulence, may suggest the development of a wound infection (Figs. 5-11, 5-12).

Percutaneous sutures over the infected site may need to be removed prior to obtaining a wound culture. If the infection is diagnosed early and there is not significant fluctuance under the suture line, then it may only be necessary to remove one or two sutures. However, significant fluctuance and swelling of the infected site can increase wound edge tension and possibly lead to ischemia, necrosis, and dehiscence. In this instance, all sutures should be removed to insure adequate drainage. Local anesthesia may be used to facilitate incision, drainage, irrigation, investigation, and probing of an abscess with a swab, and packing of the wound (Figs. 5-13, 5-14, 5-15). In the setting of frank purulence, the wound should be left open and allowed to heal by second intention (Fig. 5-16). Warm compresses and gauze packing changed daily may help facilitate drainage of any residual purulent

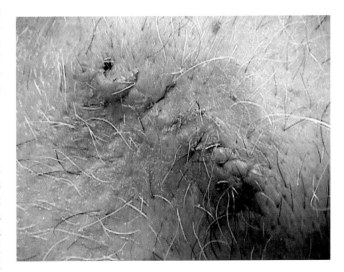

FIGURE 5-12. Erythema, induration, and yellow crust without frank purulence in this *S. aureus*–infected wound.

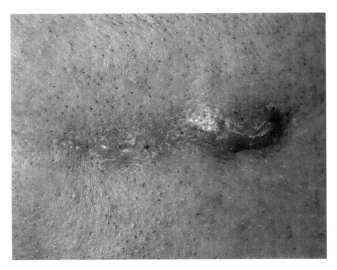

FIGURE 5-13. Wound infection abscess with little surrounding inflammation requiring incision and drainage.

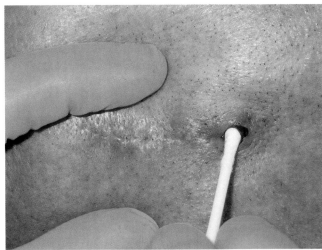

FIGURE 5-15. Abscess probed with sterile cotton swab to break any loculations prior to irrigation and packing.

debris and prevent abscess formation within the dead space of the infected wound. Scar revision, if necessary, can be performed at a later date.

Factors to consider before selecting an antibiotic are listed in Table 5-6. Empirical antibiotics should be started immediately and adjusted once culture results and antibiotic sensitivities are obtained (Table 5-7). Common empiric regimens usually involve either a first-generation cephalosporin, such as cephalexin 250 to 500 mg, or a penicillinase-resistant penicillinlike dicloxacillin, 250 to 500 mg given four times a day for 7 to 10 days. Alternatively, β-lactams/β-lactamase inhibitors, such as amoxicillin/clavulanate 500 mg every 12 hours, may be given. For penicillin allergic patients who may also have cross-reactivity to

cephalosporins, azithromycin 500 mg for the first day, followed by 250 mg for the next 4 days may be given.

A qualitative Gram stain can be performed by the laboratory prior to agar plating that may confirm the choice of empiric antibiotics within 1 hour by revealing the "appearance" of any present bacteria (e.g., Gram-positive cocci in clusters suggests *S. aureus*, Gram-positive bacilli suggests *Corynebacterium* or *Bacillus*, or Gram-negative bacilli suggests *E. coli*).

Close clinical follow-up with scheduled wound checks or phone calls, as well as specific home wound care instructions are essential. Managing the expectations of the patient by describing (i) potential scarring, (ii) the timeline of resolution, and (iii) the possible, although

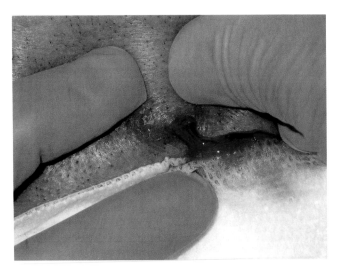

FIGURE 5-14. Wound abscess after incision with #11 blade and pressure applied to express purulent material.

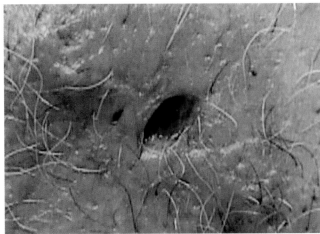

FIGURE 5-16. Wound infection with sutures removed in order to probe for a loculated abscess and allowed to heal by second intention.

TABLE 5-6. Factors in the selection of appropriate antibiotic therapy.

Intrinsic activity against the most likely pathogens (*S. aureus*,
   S. pyogenes)
Sensitivity and resistance profile of the pathogens
Propensity to promote antimicrobial resistance
Pharmacokinetics
   Absorption (bioavailability)
   Clearance (renal vs. hepatic)
   Tissue penetration (therapeutic concentrations at infection site)
Dosing convenience (1 or 2 times a day vs. 3 or 4 times a day)
Tolerability (gastrointestinal)
Formulation (tablet, suspension, taste — enhances compliance)

Source: Adapted from Hedrick J. Pediatr Drugs 2003;5(Suppl 1):35–46.

unlikely, progression of the infection, including life-threatening complications (sepsis or necrotizing fasciitis), is paramount in achieving a *good result* for both the patient and surgeon. By addressing these issues, the surgeon may also avoid potential litigation as a recent survey of the top 10 malpractice claims listed *wound infections* and *failure to communicate* as the number 8 and number 10 causes, respectively.[34]

Methicillin-Resistant *Staphylococcus aureus*

The first cases of methicillin-resistant *Staphylococcus aureus* (MRSA) were decribed in the United Kingdom in 1961, shortly after the advent of methicillin.[35] Since then increasing rates of MRSA amongst all *S. aureus* infections in the United States have risen from 2.4% in 1975 to 29% in 1991, with the overall rate of methicillin resistance for all *S. aureus* infections reported to be 43.2% in 1999–2000.[36] The dermatology community is a front-line provider in the diagnosis, treatment, and prevention of MRSA infection. A chart review examining the trends in antibiotic resistance in a large dermatology inpatient unit showed a dramatic increase in MRSA-positive superficial wounds, from 7% in 1992 to 44% in 2001.[37]

The diagnosis of MRSA should be suspected if a cutaneous wound infection persists, or progresses, during antibiotic treatment that was directed toward methicillin-sensitive *Staphylococcus aureus* (MSSA). Alternatively, one may suspect MRSA based on a patients prior medical history, such as (i) nosocomial risk factors (recent hospitalization, dialysis, or courses of antibiotics), (ii) past MRSA-positive wound infections, (iii) positive nasal cultures, or (iv) a close contact with recent MRSA colonization or infection. MRSA acquired in these settings has recently been referred to as hospital-associated MRSA (HA-MRSA) and has a different profile from MRSA acquired by overall healthy patients in the community.

Community-acquired MRSA (CA-MRSA) is another emerging threat, defined as MRSA in immunocompetent patients without recent hospitalization, antibiotic usage, or nosocomial transmission. CA-MRSA appears to affect a younger patient population compared to HA-MRSA, ranging from infants and toddlers to adolescents and

TABLE 5-7. Antibiotic options in the treatment of wound infections.

Antibiotic	Dosage	Duration	Comments
Cephalexin	250mg–500mg PO	b.i.d. to q.i.d. × 7–10 days	First-line agent *S. aureus*
Dicloxacillin	250mg–500mg PO	b.i.d. to q.i.d. × 7–10 days	First-line agent *S. aureus*
Azithromycin	250mg PO	2 tabs × 1 day, 1 tab days 2–5	First-line alternative PCN-allergic patients *S. aureus*
Amoxicillin/clavulaunate	500mg PO or 875mg PO	t.i.d. × 7–10 days or b.i.d. × 7–10 days	Second-line agent Oral surgery *S. viridans*
Ciprofloxacin	500mg PO	b.i.d. × 7–10 days	Ear or genitourinary *S. aureus, Pseudomonas*
Clindamycin	300mg PO	1 tab q.i.d. × 7–10 days	Skin or oral surgery *S. aureus, S. viridans*
Erythromycin	500mg PO	b.i.d. × 7–10 days	Second-line agent[a] Oral surgery *S. viridans*
TMP-SMX	1 DS tab PO	b.i.d. × 7–10 days	Skin or genitourinary *S. aureus, E. coli*
Vacnomycin[b]	500mg IV	q. 6 hours × 7–14 days	Skin or oral surgery MRSA, *S. viridans*

Abbreviations: MRSA, methicillin-resistant *Staphylococcus aureus*; PCN, penicillin.
[a]Increasing Gram-positive antimicrobial resistance documented.
[b]Alternative for hospitalized patients, those with MRSA wound infections, an overwhelming infection at a distant site, or those with active bacterial endocarditis.

TABLE 5-8. Morphology of methicillin-resistant *Staphylococcus aureus*/community-acquired methicillin-resistant *Staphylococcus aureus* skin infections.[38]

Diagnosis	Patients	Percentage
Abscess	32	70%
Folliculitis/furuncle	6	13%
Impetigo	4	9%
Paronychia	2	4%
Cellulitis/wound Infection	2	4%

young adults. One survey found that the average age of patients with CA-MRSA was 23 years, while those infected with HA-MRSA were 68 years old.[38] Epidemics have been seen in the university setting, where an outpatient health center found 53% of *S. aureus* culture–positive wounds in 853 patients were identified as CA-MRSA; generally manifested as abscesses and cellulitis.[39] Iyer and colleagues reported similar morphologies of CA-MRSA skin infections in 39 patients (Table 5-8), with five patients requiring admission for intravenous vancomycin.[40] Although acquired in the community, CA-MRSA is not limited to the outpatient setting, as a recent study found that 62% of hospitalized patients with staphylococcal infections had community-acquired strains.[41]

It is important to make the distinction between HA-MRSA strains and CA-MRSA strains, as they show different toxin-producing and resistance patterns (Table 5-9). As opposed to hospital-acquired MRSA infections, CA-MRSA infections (i) often occur in healthy individuals, (ii) are usually susceptible to most non–β-lactam antibiotics (ciprofloxacin, clindamycin, TMP-SMX), (iii) can be virulent and fatal, and (iv) have a type IV staphylococcal cassette chromosome (SCCmec) genetic element which carries *mecA*, the methicillin resistance gene. This is distinct from the types I, II, and III SCCmec elements that are associated with HA- MRSA infections.[39]

Management of Methicillin-Resistant Staphylococcus aureus *Wound Infection*

Vancomycin remains the drug of choice for MRSA infections in hospitalized patients, or CA-MRSA–infected patients that require hospitalization for advanced wound infections or signs of septicemia. However, HA-MRSA and CA-MRSA should be confirmed by culture because vancomycin is less rapidly bacteriocidal and less efficacious than the β-lactams (intravenous cefazolin or oral cephalexin) and the semisynthetic penicillinase-resistant penicillins (intravenous nafcillin or oral dicloxacillin) against MSSA.[42]

Outpatient management of HA-MRSA and CA-MRSA infection poses a unique challenge to the dermatologic surgeon, especially as antibiotic resistance increases and susceptibilities decrease. Due to the profile of most dermatology practices, CA-MRSA is much more likely to be encountered in wound infections. An excellent review by Jones concisely summarized the current antibiotic susceptibilities and regimens for HA-MRSA and CA-MRSA (Tables 5-9, 5-10).[38,43] Similar sensitivity profiles have been noted by dermatologists, with either trimethoprim–sulfamethoxazole or clindamycin, with or without rifampin, and linezolid having the greatest efficacy.[37,39,40,44] Linezolid belongs to a new class of synthetic antimicrobials, the oxazolidinones, and is available in either oral or intravenous forms. It has activity against *Enterococcus faecium, Enterococcus faecalis,* MSSA, MRSA, methicillin-resistant *S. epidermidis,* and many streptococcal species. Due to case reports of linezolid resistance and its high cost (approximately $1200 for a 14-day oral course), its use should be strictly limited to use in patients who fail or cannot tolerate vancomycin or other oral agents.[45]

Prevention of Hospital-Associated Methicillin-Resistant Staphylococcus aureus *and* Community-Acquired Methicillin-Resistant Staphylococcus aureus *Wound Infection*

Prevention of HA-MRSA and CA-MRSA spread and resistance is governed by three key principles: (i) use antibiotics only when necessary, (ii) use the shortest course of antibiotics necessary to cure the infection, and (iii) use the agent with the narrowest antimicrobial spectrum in order to decrease the incidence of further resistant strains. It has been shown that bathing with an antimicrobial soap (4%–10% providone–iodine, 4% chlorhexidine, or 5%–10% benzoyl peroxide),[46] in conjunction with intranasal mupirocin,[47] can effectively treat patients who are MRSA colonized.[48] Furthermore, these steps may lead to a decreased spread of MRSA to family members, other patient contacts in the community, and potential sites of colonization on the patients themselves.

TABLE 5-9. Antimicrobial susceptibility profile of community-acquired and hospital-associated methicillin-resistant Staphylococcus aureus isolates in 2000.[37,42]

Drug	CA-MRSA	HA-MRSA
Oxacillin	0%	0%
Ciprofloxacin*	79%	16%
Clindamycin*	83%	21%
Erythromycin*	44%	9%
Gentamycin*	94%	80%
Rifampin	96%	94%
Tetracycline	92%	92%
TMP-SMX	95%	90%
Vancomycin	100%	100%

Abbreviations: CA-MRSA, community-acquired methicillin-resistant *Staphylococcus aureus*; HA-MRSA, hospital-associated methicillin-resistant *Staphylococcus aureus*.
*Statistically significant difference between CA-MRSA and HA-MRSA.

TABLE 5-10. Antibiotic management of community-acquired methicillin-resistant *Staphylococcus aureus* infections in the outpatient setting.[42]

Drug	Oral dose	Comments
TMP-SMX ± rifampin	1 DS tablet q. 8–12 hours 300 mg b.i.d.	Check sulfa allergy Not for empiric therapy in suspected streptococcal infections Rifampin drug interactions
Clindamycin ± rifampin	150–300 mg q. 6 hours 300 mg b.i.d.	May induce resistance Adequate bone penetration Rifampin drug interactions
Fluoroquinolones Ciprofloxacin, or levofloxacin, or gatifloxacin, or moxifloxacin ± rifampin	500 mg q. 12 hours 500–750 mg q. 24 hours 400 mg q. 24 hours 400 mg q. 24 hours 300 mg b.i.d.	Rapid resistance is possible, addition of rifampin should be considered Absorption of quinolones impaired by antacids Rifampin drug interactions
Tetracycline, or minocycline, or doxycycline ± rifampin	500 mg q.i.d. 100 mg q. 24 hours 100 mg b.i.d. 300 mg b.i.d.	Check drug interactions Possible secondary yeast infections may occur Do not administer with dairy products Rifampin drug interactions
Linezolid	600 mg b.i.d.	Reserve for highly resistant strains; vancomycin intolerance Avoid in patients on SSRIs May cause bone marrow suppression Cost may be prohibitive

Abbreviation: SSRI, selective serotonin reuptake inhibitor.

Unusual Causes of Wound Infection

Mycobacteria

There have been increasing numbers of reports of rapidly growing mycobacterium as a cause of postoperative wound infections. These Runyon class IV organisms are part of the nontuberculoid mycobacteria and include *Mycobacterium chelonae* (formerly known as *M. abscessus*) and *M. fortuitum*. Mycobacterial organisms are fairly ubiquitous in nature and can even be found in the tapwater used to moisten wound dressings.[49] Clusters of *M. chelonae* infections have occurred in cosmetic surgery, as a result of contamination of methylene blue and gentian violet used for preoperative skin markings,[50,51] and in breast implants.[52] Additionally, several outbreaks of *M. chelonae*[53] and *M. fortuitum*[54] have occurred after outpatient liposuction and with subcuticular fat injections.[55]

Mycobacterial infections typically present days to weeks after inoculation. Clinically, they appear as violaceous or dusky papules and nodules that may ulcerate and drain a serosanguinous fluid. While most lesions are tender, longstanding infections may in fact be painless and take on the appearance of scar tissue with postinflammatory hyperpigmentation. Immunosuppressed patients and those on long-term corticosteroid therapy are more at risk for *M. chelonae* infections and the dreaded sequelae of disseminated cutaneous involvement, osteomyelitis, and occasionally fatal pulmonary infection.[56]

Treatment of mycobacterial infections usually involves the combination of surgical excision or debulking and appropriate antibiotics.[57] Intravenous amikacin is the preferred aminoglycoside for treating rapidly growing mycobacteria, with tobramycin a second choice against *M. chelonae*. First-line oral clarithromycin and azithromycin have both been used successfully and are more active than erythromycin, which no longer should be considered.[58] Some case series of *M. chelonae* infections have shown nearly 100% sensitivity to these macrolides.[56] Ciprofloxacin and levofloxacin also have activity against these organisms.[59] Occasionally, the addition of oral clofazamine and even cryotherapy might be needed to treat recalcitrant cutaneous infections.[60]

M. chelonae and *M. fortuitum* may require weeks to months of oral antibiotics, combined with surgical debridement, to completely resolve cutaneous infections. Consultation with infectious disease specialists might be indicated in some recalcitrant cases.

Candida

Candida species are ubiquitous yeastlike fungi that are the most common cause of fungal infections in humans. Isolates are frequently recovered from the hospital environment, medical personnel, and the mucous membranes of patients. *Candida* prefers to grow in a warm, moist environment with a predilection for the oropharynx, perineum, and intertriginous areas. Oropharyngeal colonization is found in 30% to 55% of healthy young adults.[61] Because *Candida* is an unusual cause of surgical site infections, management of established infections can be difficult because delays in diagnosis often occur.[62] Wounds that have an occlusive, semipermeable, or moist dressing may also be at risk for *Candida* colonization or infection, regardless of the anatomic site.

Candida albicans is the most common species (50%–60%) identified in patients, followed by other isolates, such as *C. glabrata* (20%) and *C. tropicalis* (12%). One recent analysis demonstrated that *C. albicans* was an independent predictor of mortality in surgical patients, who were more likely to be treated with various antibiotics before definitive treatment was initiated.[63] While little data exists on the incidence of *Candida* and surgical wound infections,[62] certain patient populations are clearly at risk: immunocompromised patients (granulocytopenia, transplant recipients, chemotherapy, and corticosteroids), patients on broad-spectrum antibiotics, diabetics, irradiated skin, and burn victims.

The clinical features of *Candida* wound infection may mimic those of any wound infection with erythema and frank purulence, or may be manifested only with bright red and seemingly bland erythema, with or without satellite papules and pustules. Surprisingly, *Candida* can be easily grown on most bacterial culture media, even if a fungal culture is not specifically requested. An office-based wet mount (KOH) examination demonstrating numerous hyphae and pseudohyphae may be the first step in establishing a timely diagnosis. Additionally, the Gram stain methylene blue is useful to directly demonstrate fungal cells, and may heighten the sensitivity in diagnosing *Candida* when performing a KOH examination.

The standard therapy recommended for *Candida* surgical site infections is fluconazole 400 mg as the loading dose, followed by 200 mg a day orally for at least 2 weeks of therapy after clinical signs of improvement are seen. The development of resistance to other antifungals (itraconazole and ketoconazole) has been encountered. More recalcitrant or complicated *Candida* wound infections, including candidemia, may require admission for intravenous antibiotics such as amphotericin B or caspofungin acetate.[64]

Herpes Simplex Virus

Certain surgical procedures have been known to activate herpes simplex virus (HSV); namely dermabrasion, medium-to-deep chemical peels, and ablative laser resurfacing. An estimated postoperative infection rate of 7.4% has been observed in one large series, regardless of prior HSV clinical history.[65] Because the herpes virus requires viable epidermal cells in order to proliferate, this infectious complication is usually seen 5 to 10 days after surgery.

The development of pain with or without erosions is the hallmark of postoperative HSV infection. A spectrum of symptoms ranging from mild tingling or a perioral burning sensation to severe facial pain may be described by the patient. Within hours to days after the onset of the dysthesia, vesicles and "punched out" erosions may form

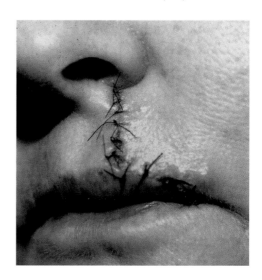

FIGURE 5-17. Grouped vesicles at the site of reactivation of herpes labialis (HSV-1) after Mohs surgery on the upper cutaneous lip.

in the deepithelialized or newly regenerated skin. Scarring is a common sequela that may or may not be prevented with prompt diagnosis and treatment.

Recent data has shown that the activation of HSV infection, and consequently postoperative infection, cannot be predicted based on a patient's history or *absence* of a cold sore.[65,66] Prophylaxis has been therefore been suggested for all patients undergoing medium-to-deep resurfacing, especially those who are immunosuppressed. Prophylaxis regimens should start the day before surgery and continued for 7 to 10 days. Valacyclovir 500 mg twice daily,[67] or famciclovir 250 to 500 mg twice daily[68] are effective regimens. Despite prophylaxis, postoperative HSV infections do develop in some patients. In the setting of HSV infection, the valacyclovir dosage should be increased to 1000 mg every 8 hours. The famciclovir dosage should also be increased to 500 mg every 8 hours. Both medications should be continued for 10 to 14 days, or until the lesions are fully healed.

For excisional surgery or Mohs procedures on the face and lip, a similar prophylactic regimen can be initiated for patients with a history of recurrent herpes labialis or simplex (Fig. 5-17). Alternatively, the patients may be given a prescription for antiviral therapy that can be started at the first signs and symptoms of a typical outbreak.

Life-Threatening Wound Infections

While most wound infections are unlikely to present within the first 24 hours after a procedure, two rare but important conditions must be considered; (i) *necrotizing fasciitis* (hemolytic streptococcal gangrene) and (ii) *clostridial cellulitis and myonecrosis* (gas gangrene).

Necrotizing Fasciitis

Necrotizing fasciitis is an infection of the underlying fascia that rapidly spreads along fascial planes. The incidence of this condition is believed to be on the rise because of a larger population of immunocompromised patients with conditions such as diabetes mellitus, cancer, alcoholism, vascular insufficiencies, organ transplants, HIV, and neutropenia.

Group A hemolytic streptococci (*S. pyogenes*) and *S. aureus* are the dominant bacterial cause of this surgical emergency which is also frequently found to be polymicrobial, containing anaerobes (*Bacteroides fragilis*) and Gram-negative organisms (*Vibrio vulnificus*). Recently, MRSA has been idenitified as a cause of several cases of necrotizing fasciitis.[69]

Hemorrhagic bullae are a classic finding in necrotizing fasciitis, which usually manifests as benign appearing cellulitis, with or without crepitus, in a febrile or septic patient. The pain described by patients is usually intense, and out of proportion with objective clinical findings. Advanced cases may be insensate as involvement of nerve fibers leads to localized anesthesia.

Patients at increased risk are frequently diabetic (20%–40% of cases) or alcoholics (35%). When necrotizing fasciitis occurs in inguinal or perineal areas it is referred to as Fournier's gangrene. Over 80% of the cases of Fournier's gangrene will occur in diabetic patients and despite aggressive treatment the mortality rate of this life-threatening condition is still 70% to 80%.[70]

Clostridial Cellulitis and Myonecrosis

Clostridial cellulitis and myonecrosis (gas gangrene), is usually caused by *Clostridium perfringens* and may clinically mimic necrotizing fasciitis with intense localized pain, fever, crepitus, and evolving septic shock. The initial stage, known as *clostridial cellulitis*, is a rapidly spreading lymphatic and fascial infection that occurs postoperatively and is readily cured with minor debridement and antibiotics. While rare, this entity is more common than nectrotizing fasciitis, and may be encountered with some frequency if properly recognized by the physician.

The later stage, referred to as *clostridial myonecrosis* or *gas gangrene*, is a highly lethal necrotizing soft tissue infection of skeletal muscle caused by one of the six known toxin- and gas-producing *Clostridium* species. They are Gram-positive, anaerobic, spore-forming bacilli that are ubiquitous in nature, and found predominantly in soil. It has been shown that up to 90% of soil-contaminated wounds demonstrate clostridial organisms, with fewer than 2% ultimately developing clostridial myonecrosis.[71] Clinical suspicion of this condition should be elevated in patients who are farmers or contractors

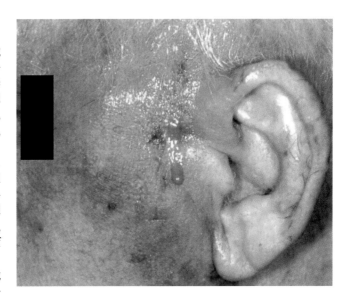

FIGURE 5-18. Bronze-colored discharge and rapid spread of tender erythema along tissue planes worrisome for clostridial cellulitis.

that may aerosolize inoculated soil into their wound or the surrounding skin.

The discharge from the incision site has a characteristic fetid, "mousy" odor and appears bronze or brown, rather than simply serosanguinous (Fig. 5-18). Clostridial myositis readily demonstrates subcutaneous air on x-ray and, like necrotizing fasciitis, is a surgical emergency requiring immediate hospitalization, wound cultures, intravenous antibiotics, and aggressive surgical debridement. If properly treated, gas gangrene still portends a poor prognosis with an overall mortality rate of 20% to 30%.

Conclusion

Meticulous surgical aseptic technique, risk stratification of patients at-risk for wound infection, and prompt identification of potential infection to direct appropriate antibiotic therapy are fundamentals paramount to achieving good results in cutaneous surgery. Establishment of uniform guidelines for addressing these issues is central to the success a surgical practice. Tracking wound infections by documenting the implicated surgical suite, personnel involved in the surgery, and the bacterial isolate are essential and easily incorporated into any surgical practice. Such documentation will help to isolate factors involved in the pathogenesis of infections for class I and class II wounds, and may prevent further events from occurring. Finally, maintaining open lines of communication for patients to report complications after surgery will assist in the timely identification and definitive treatment of surgical wound infections.

References

1. Futoryan T, Grande D. Postoperative wound infection rates in dermatologic surgery. Dermatol Surg 1995;21:509–514.

2. Mangram AJ, Horan TC, Pearson ML, et al. Guideline for prevention of surgical site infection, 1999. Hospital Infection Control Practices Advisory Committee. Infect Control Hosp Epidemiol 1999;20:250–278.

3. Krizek TJ, Robson MC. Evolution of quantitative bacteriology in wound management. Am J Surg 1975;130:579–584.

4. Barker JNWN, Mitra RS, Griffiths CEM, et al. Keratinocytes as initiators of inflammation. Lancet 1991;337:211–214.

5. Cruse PJ, Foord R. The epidemiology of wound infection. A 10-year prospective study of 62,939 wounds. Surg Clin North Am 1980;60:27–40.

6. Culver DH, Horan TC, Gaynes RP. Surgical wound infection rates by wound class, operative procedure, and patient risk index. National Nosocomial Infections Surveillance System. Am J Med 1991;16:91(3B):152S–157S.

7. Antimicrobial prophylaxis and treatment in patients with granulocyopenia. Med Lett Drugs Ther 1981;23:55–56.

8. Perner A, Nielsen SE, Rask-Madsen J. High glucose impairs superoxide production from isolated blood neutrophils. Intensive Care Med 2003;29:642–645.

9. Haas AF, Grekin RC. Antibiotic prophylaxis in dermatologic surgery. J Am Acad Dermatol 1995;32:155–179.

10. Jones S, Schechter CB, Smith C, et al. Is HIV infection a risk factor for complications of surgery? Mt Sinai J Med 2002;69:329–333.

11. Patton LL, Shugars DA, Bonito AJ. A systematic review of complication risks for HIV-positive patients undergoing invasive dental procedures. J Am Dent Assoc 2002;133:195–203.

12. Burns J, Pieper B. HIV/AIDS: impact on healing. Ostomy Wound Manage 2000;46:30–40.

13. Seropian R, Reynolds BR. Wound infections after preoperative depilatory versus razor preparation. Am J Surg 1971;121:251–254.

14. Miro D, Julia MV, Sitges-Serra A. Wound breaking strength and healing after suturing noninjured tissues. J Am Coll Surg 1995;180:659–665.

15. Coras B, Hohenleutner U, Landthaler M, et al. Comparison of two absorbable monofilament polydioxanone threads in intradermal buried sutures. Dermatol Surg 2005;31:331–333.

16. NNIS System: National Nosocomial Infections Surveillance (NNIS) report, data summary from October 1986-April 1996, issued May 1996. A report from the National Nosocomial Infections Surveillance (NNIS) System. Am J Infect Control 1996;24:380–388.

17. Davies RR. Dispersal of bacteria on desquamated skin. Lancet 1962;2:1295–1297.

18. Ong PY, Ohtake T, Brandt C, et al. Endogenous antimicrobial peptides and skin infections in atopic dermatitis. N Engl J Med 2002;347:1151–1160.

19. Bayer AS. Infective endocarditis. Clin Infect Dis 1993;17:313–320.

20. Eady EA, Coates P, Ross JI, et al. Antibiotic resistance patterns of aerobic coryneforms and furazolidone-resistant Gram-positive cocci from the skin surface of the human axilla and fourth toe cleft. J Antimicrob Chemother 2000;46:205–213.

21. Cunha BA, Koj IG. Serratia marscens: nosocomial implications. Infect Dis Pract 1999;23:49–52.

22. Podschun R, Ullmann U. Klebsiella species as nosocomial pathogens: epidemiology, taxonomy, typing methods, and pathogenicity factors. Clin Microbiol Rev 1998;11:589–603.

23. Robson MC. A failure of wound healing caused by an imbalance of bacteria. Surg Clin North Am 1997;77:637–651.

24. Robson MC, Lea CE, Dalton JB, et al. Quantitative bacteriology and delayed wound closure. Surg Forum 1968;19:501–502.

25. Levine NS, Lindberg RB, Mason AD, et al. The quantitative swab culture and smear: a quick simple method for determining the number of viable aerobic bacteria on open wounds. J Trauma 1976;16:89–94.

26. Ford DA, Koehler SH. A creative process for reinforcing aseptic technique practices. AORN J 2001;73:446–450.

27. Seal LA, Paul-Cheadle D. A systems approach to preoperative surgical patient skin preparation. Am J Infect Control 2004;32:57–62.

28. Bencini PL, Galimberti M, Signorini M. Utility of topical benzoyl peroxide for prevention of surgical skin wound infections. J Dermatol Surg Oncol 1994;20:538–540.

29. Edwards PS, Lipp A, Holmes A. Preoperative skin antiseptics for preventing surgical wound infections after clean surgery. Cochrane Database Syst Rev 2004:CD003949.

30. Berry A, Watt B, Goldacre M, Thomson J, McNair T. A comparison of the use of povidone-iodine and chlorhexidine in the prophylaxis. J Hosp Infect 1982;3:55–63.

31. Aly R, Maibach HI. Comparative antibacterial efficacy of a 2-minute surgical scrub with chlorhexidine gluconate, povidone-iodine, and chloroxylenol sponge-brushes. Am J Infect Control 1988;16:173–177.

32. Hibbard JS, Mulberry GK, Brady AR. A clinical study comparing the skin antisepsis and safety of ChloraPrep, 70% isopropyl alcohol, and 2% aqueous chlorhexidine. J Infus Nurs 2002;25:244–249.

33. Shirahatti RG, Joshi RM, Vishwanath YK. Effect of preoperative skin preparation on post-operative wound infections. J Postgrad Med 1993;39:134–136.

34. Glabman M. The top tem malpractice claims [and how to avoid them]. Hosp Health Netw 2004;78:60–66.

35. Jevons PM. "Celbenin"-resistant staphylococci. Br Med J 1961;124–125.

36. Kuehnert MJ, Hill HA, Kupronis BA, et al. Methicillin-resistant–*Staphylococcus aureus* hospitalizations, United States. Emerg Infect Dis 2005;11:868–872.

37. Valencia IC, Kirsner RS, Kerdel FA. Microbiologic evaluation of skin wounds: alarming trend toward antibiotic resistance in an inpatient dermatology service during a 10-year period. J Am Acad Dermatol 2004;50:845–849.

38. Naimi TS, LeDell KH, Como-Sabietti K, et al. Comparison of community- and health care-associated methicillin-resistant *Staphylococcus aureus* infection. JAMA 2003;290:2976–2984.

39. Cohen PR, Kurzrock R. Community-acquired methicillin-resistant *Staphylococcus aureus* skin infection: an emerging clinical problem. J Am Acad Dermatol 2004;50:277–280.

40. Iyer S, Jones DH. Community-acquired methicillin-resistant *Staphylococcus aureus* skin infection: a retrospective analysis of clinical presentation and treatment of a local outbreak. J Am Acad Dermatol 2004;50:854–858.

41. Tacconelli E, D'Agata EM, Karchmer AW. Epidemiological comparison of true methicillin-resistant and methicillin-susceptible coagulase-negative bacteremia at hospital admission. Clin Infect Dis 2003;37:644–649.

42. Quintiliani R, Kuti J. Drug therapy for methicillin-resistant *Staphylococcus aureus*. Conn Med 2001;65:23–25.

43. Jones RS. Expert advice on eradicating the MRSA threat. Pract Dermatol 2005;2:33–37.

44. Cohen PA, Grossman ME. Management of cutaneous lesions associated with an emerging epidemic: community-acquired methicillin-resistant *Staphylococcus aureus* skin infections. J Am Acad Dermatol 2004;51:132–135.

45. Anderegg TR, Sader HS, Fritsche TR, et al. Trends in linezolid susceptibility patterns: report from the 2002–2003 worldwide Zyvox Annual Appraisal of Potency and Spectrum (ZAAPS) Program. Int J Antimicrob Agents 2005;26:13–21.

46. Guilhermetti M, Hernandes ED, Fukushigue Y, et al. Effectiveness of hand-cleansing agents for removing methicillin-resistant *Staphylococcus aureus* from contaminated hands. Infect Control Hosp Epidemiol 2001;22:105–108.

47. Semret M, Miller MA. Topical mupirocin for eradication of MRSA colonization with mupirocin-resistant strains strains. Infect Control Hosp Epidemiol 2001;22:578–580.

48. Boyce JM. MRSA patients: proven methods to treat colonization and infection. J Hosp Infect 2001;48(Suppl A):S9–S14.

49. Kline S, Cameron S, Streifel A. An outbreak of bacteremias associated with Mycobacterium mucogenicum in a hospital water supply. Infect Control Hosp Epidemiol 2004;25:1042–1049.

50. Mycobacterium chelonae infections associated with face lifts — New Jersey, 2002–2003. MMWR 2004;53:192–194.

51. Safranek TJ, Jarvis WR, Carson LA, et al. Mycobacterium chelonae wound infections after plastic surgery employing contaminated gentian violet skin-marking solution. N Engl J Med 1987;317:197–201.

52. Brickman M, Parsa AA, Parsa FD. Mycobacterium chelonae infection after breast augmentation. Aesthetic Plast Surg 2005;29:116–118.

53. Meyers H, Brown-Elliot BA, Moore D, et al. An outbreak of *Mycobacterium chelonae* infection following liposuction. Clin Infect Dis 2002;34:1500–1507.

54. Murillo J, Torres J, Bofill L, et al. Skin and wound infection by rapidly growing mycobacteria: an unexpected complication of liposuction and liposculpture. The Venezuelan Collaborative Infectious and Tropical Diseases Study Group. Arch Dermatol 2000;136:1347–1352.

55. Prado AC, Castillo PF. Lay clinics and an epidemic outbreak of mycobacterium skin and soft-tissue infection. Plast Reconstr Surg 2004;113:800–801.

56. Wallace RJ Jr, Brown BA, Onyi GO. Skin, soft tissue, and bone infections due to *Mycobacterium chelonae chelonae*: importance of prior corticosteroid therapy, frequency of disseminated infections, and resistance to oral antimicrobials other than clarithromycin. J Infect Dis 1992;166:405–412.

57. Madjar DD Jr, Carvallo E, Proper SA, et al. Adjunctive surgical management of cutaneous *Mycobacterium fortuitum* infection. J Dermatol Surg Oncol 1985;11:708–712.

58. Saluja A, Peters NT, Lowe L, et al. A surgical wound infection due to *Mycobacterium chelonae* successfully treated with clarithromycin. Dermatol Surg 1997;23:539–543.

59. Gutknecht DR. Treatment of disseminated *Mycobacterium chelonae* infection with ciprofloxacin. J Am Acad Dermatol 1990;23:1179–1180.

60. Kullavanijaya P, Rattana-Apiromyakij N, Sukonthapirom-Napattalung P, et al. Disseminated *Mycobacterium chelonae* cutaneous infection: recalcitrant to combined antibiotic therapy. J Dermatol 2003;30:485–491.

61. Segal E. Candida, still number one — what do we know and where are we going from there? Mycoses 2005;48(Suppl 1):3–11.

62. Garman ME, Orengo I. Unusual infectious complications of dermatologic procedures. Dermatol Clin 2003;21:321–335.

63. Hughes MG, Chong TW, Smith RL, et al. Comparison of fungal and nonfungal infections in a broad-based surgical patient population. Surg Infect 2005;6:55–64.

64. Bille J, Marchetii O, Calandra T. Changing face of healthcare associated fungal infections. Curr Opin Infect Dis 2005;18:314–319.

65. Nanni CA, Alster TS. Complications of carbon dioxide laser resurfacing. An evaluation of 500 patients. Dermatol Surg 1998;24:315–320.

66. da Silva LM, Guimaraes AL, Victoria JM, et al. Herpes simplex virus type 1 shedding in the oral cavity of seropositive patients. Oral Dis 2005;11:13–16.

67. Beeson WH, Rachel JD. Valacyclovir prophylaxis for herpes simplex virus infection or infection recurrence following laser skin resurfacing. Dermatol Surg 2002;28:331–336.

68. Alster TS, Nanni CA. Famciclovir prophylaxis of herpes simplex virus reactivation after laser skin resurfacing. Dermatol Surg 1999;25:242–246.

69. Hsiao GH, Chang CH, Hsiao CW, et al. Necrotizing soft tissue infections. Surgical or conservative treatment? Dermatol Surg 1998;24:243–247.

70. Miller LG, Perdreau-Remington F, Rieg G, et al. Necrotizing fasciitis caused by community-associated methicillin-resistant *Staphylococcus aureus* in Los Angeles. N Engl J Med 2005;352:1445–1453.

71. Feingold DS. Gangrenous and crepitant cellulitis. J Am Acad Dermatol 1982;6:289–299.

6
Prophylaxis for Wound Infections and Endocarditis

Michelle Pipitone and Hugh M. Gloster, Jr.

There are three instances when prophylactic antibiotics are indicated: prophylaxis for prevention of a sugical site infection (SSI), prevention of endocarditis, and prevention of prosthesis infection. Postoperative SSI are a serious complication in cutaneous surgery, and although some limited guidelines exist, many physicians are unaware of the proper use of antibiotics.[1–3] Furthermore, the emergence of resistant bacteria makes the prudent use of antibiotics crucial. A thorough understanding of the various factors related to SSI prophylaxis, the Centers for Disease Control and Prevention (CDC) guidelines pertaining to SSI prophylaxis, and proper antibiotic usage is vital to the practice of cutaneous surgery and will be discussed in this chapter. Treatment of definitive SSI is discussed in Chapter 5.

In addition to SSI prophylaxis, many cutaneous surgery patients are at high risk for developing bacterial endocarditis. The dermatologic surgeon must be aware of the American Heart Association guidelines pertaining to prophylactic antibiotics in these patients. Additionally, bacteremia can cause infections of various hardware (i.e., orthopedic prostheses), which may be prevented with the use of prophylactic antibiotics.

There have been several excellent reviews[3–7] of prophylactic antibiotics in dermatologic surgery, as well as several informative online references.[7–9]

Surgical Site Infection Prophylaxis

Surgical site infection occurs when a significant inoculum of pathogenic bacteria overcome the local tissue defenses and incite a host response.[10] SSI is rare in dermatologic surgery (1%–3%),[11–15] but can cause significant morbidity and have a devastating cosmetic result. Most dermatologic procedures are conducted on clean (less than 3% infection rate) or clean–contaminated wounds (less than 10% infection rate; see Table 6-1)[6,11–15] and as such, most authorities do not recommend prophylactic antibiotics

for SSI, with the exception of certain instances discussed below. Due to the low overall incidence of wound infection in dermatologic surgery, very few patients would benefit from antibiotic prophylaxis. Furthermore, the overuse and misuse of antibiotics is prevalent in medicine, and is a major factor in the development of resistance and potentially severe antibiotic side effects (hypersensitivity, pseudomembranous colitis, etc.) There have been no randomized, controlled studies examining the use of antibiotics to prevent SSI in dermatologic surgery, so any recommendations are based on various authors' opinions or consensus groups.

Factors to Consider in Assessing the Risk of Surgical Site Infection

Although there are many published guidelines for the use of prophylactic antibiotics in SSI, minimal data exists that is specific to dermatologic procedures. According to the Center for Disease Control (CDC) guidelines, the risk of developing a SSI is largely dependant on the amount, type, and virulence of the microorganism, the condition of the surgical site pre- and postoperatively, and patient characteristics.[8,11] The following section will discuss wound, surgical, intraoperative, and patient characteristics that may place a patient at higher risk for a SSI, and recommendations of how to prevent SSI.

Preoperative Condition of the Skin

Preoperative antiseptic preparation of the surgical field (see Table 6-2), the surgeon, and surgical environment are important in preventing SSI. There is insufficient evidence to conclude which of the skin antiseptics is superior.[16] Most surgeons advocate using iodophors or chlorhexidine as skin antiseptics for longer procedures, and alcohol (70%) for procedures less than 5 minutes in length.[17] Clipping hairs immediately preoperatively instead of shaving is the recommended method of hair removal by the CDC.[8]

TABLE 6-1. Surgical wound classification and subsequent risk of infection if no antibiotics are used.

Classification	Description	Risk of surgical site infection (%)[6,11,12]	Role of prophylactic antibiotics
Clean (class I)	Uninfected operative wound No acute inflammation Closed primarily Respiratory, gastrointestinal, biliary, and urinary tracts not entered No break in aseptic technique *Example*: primary excision, noninflamed cysts	<2	No role
Clean–contaminated (class II)	Elective entry into oral/mucosal, axillary, inguinal regions, with minimal spillage Minor breaks in aseptic technique No evidence of infection *Example*: secondary intention healing wounds	<10	Benefit uncertain; individual patient characteristics must be evaluated (e.g., immunocompromised)
Contaminated (class III)	Nonpurulent inflammation present Penetrating traumatic wounds <4 hours Major break in aseptic technique *Example*: inflamed cyst, tumor with inflammation/ulceration	About 20–25	Although controversial, most sources consider antibiotic use for class III therapeutic
Dirty–infected (class IV)	Purulent inflammation present Devitalized or necrotic tissue Penetrating traumatic wounds >4 hours Foreign-body penetration *Example*: ruptured cysts, hidradenitis, tumors with purulent or necrotic material, incision and drainage of abcesses or furuncles	About 40	Antibiotics are considered therapeutic, not prophylactic; must be continued postoperatively

Source: Modified from Garner.[11]

Shaving within 24 hours of the surgery results in a risk of wound infection of 5.6% versus 0.6% if hair is clipped or if no hair removal is performed. Furthermore, if hair is shaved greater than 24 hours prior to surgery, the infection risk increases to greater than 20%.[8]

Wound Characteristics

Most dermatologic procedures can be classified into class I (clean) or class II (clean–contaminated) wounds. Surgi-

cal site categorization (Table 6-1) takes into account the preoperative skin condition and anatomic location and is a widely used method of categorizing wounds. Subsequently, studies have established the rate of infection in these classes, which is helpful in determining which patients need prophylactic antibiotics for wound infection.[6,11,12] Antibiotics are not administered for class I wounds, "clean, performed on surgically scrubbed skin" (see Table 6-1),[6,11,12] due to the low risk of infection. Primary closures should be protected with a sterile

TABLE 6-2. Antiseptics used in cutaneous surgery.

Antiseptic	Mechanism of action	G+	G-	MB	Fun	V	Onset and residual activity	Toxicity
Chlorhexidine (biguanine, Hibiclens, Hibistat)	Disrupt cell membrane	E	G	P	F	G	I; Excellent	Minimal percutaneous absorbtion, toxic to wound, ears, and eyes (ototoxicity & keratitis)
Iodine, Iodophors (iodine + surfactant; i.e., Betadine)	Oxidation/substitution by free iodine	E	G	G	G	G	I; Minimal iodophor lasts much longer than plain iodine	Iodophor less irritating than iodine, 15% allergic sensitization, inactivated by blood or serum, absorption occurs
70% ethyl alcohol	Denature proteins	E	E	G	G	G	R; None	Drying, volatile (flammable)

Source: Adapted from the 1999 CDC guidelines.[8]
Abbreviations: E, excellent; F, fair; Fun, fungi; G, good; G-, Gram-negative bacteria; G+, Gram-positive bacteria; I, intermediate acting; MB, Mycobacterium tuberculosis; P, poor; R, rapid; V, virus.

dressing for 24 to 48 hours postoperatively to prevent infection.

Prophylactic antibiotics are most controversial for class II wounds (clean–contaminated), due to the higher but still low rate of infection. This category includes dermatologic procedures involving oral–nasal areas invading mucosa, genitourinary areas, and the axilla, which are considered clean–contaminated by most authors, and contaminated (class III) wounds by others. Because of this ambiguity, many surveys of physician behavior reveal that antibiotics are used in these situations, despite guidelines to the contrary.

Infection rates for these specific areas have been documented, but need further study. The overall rate of SSI for Mohs micrographic surgery has been reported to be equivalent to clean procedures.[15,18] However, certain clinical sites and surgical procedures may increase the risk of bacteremia. One study examined Mohs micrographic surgery procedures on the ear and found an increased rate of infection (12.5%–28%), especially for wounds that reach the level of the cartilage.[15] However, data regarding infections of the ear may be complicated by the difficulty in distinguishing chondritis from definitive wound infections. Studies of head and neck surgery have attempted to establish in what clinical settings antibiotics may be useful, but results have been mixed.[19,20] One study failed to demonstrate a beneficial effect of antibiotic administration when used for otologic sinonasal reconstructive procedures that are considered clean–contaminated (exposure to mucosa lined cavities of the head and neck).[19] Another study of head and neck procedures did demonstrate the efficacy of perioperative administration of antibiotics in the prevention of SSI.[20]

Maragh and colleagues in their recommendations state that they do not use antibiotic prophylaxis for SSI for skin flaps and grafts on the scalp, neck, and body, but that they administer a single preoperative dose of antibiotics before flap and graft reconstruction on the nose and ears because of the prolonged operative times associated.[3] A postoperative course of antibiotics up to 10 days may be administered depending on a variety of environmental and patient factors. The authors list "flap or graft reconstruction on the nose and ear, high-tension closures, inflamed or infected skin close to the surgical site, multiple simultaneous procedures, below the knee full thickness procedures and hand surgery" as scenarios for potential administration of surgical site prophylaxis. Mohs procedures with large defect sizes, and/or prolonged surgeries (greater than 2 hours) are also instances when surgeons may decide to use prophylactic antibiotics. Unfortunately, there are no studies specifically evaluating infection rates in the setting of multistep repairs, such as delayed repairs and interpolation take-downs.

A prophylactic antibiotic for laser resurfacing with carbon dioxide or erbium laser and medium-to-deep chemical peels is another controversial area. These areas become colonized with bacteria, similar to a burn injury, shortly after the procedure. Also, these procedures are performed close to mucosal areas on the richly sebaceous skin of the head and neck. The overall infection rate for laser resurfacing is less than 10%, placing it in the clean–contaminated (class II) category.[8,21–26] Several authors have actually found increased infection rates with selection for pathologic organisms with the use of prophylactic antibiotics.[21,25,27] It is the accepted practice among burn surgeons not to prophylactically treat burn patients with oral antibiotics, but topical antibiotic agents are employed such as silver sulfadiazine, which has a low incidence of contact sensitivity.[28–31] Prophylactic topical antibiotic use in this setting is hotly debated among dermatologists due to the risk of contact sensitivity.[24,31,32] However, antiviral prophylaxis is widely accepted in the dermatologic community for laser resurfacing.[33–37]

Class III (contaminated) wounds, which have an infection rate of 6% to 25%, are usually due to breaks in sterile technique and obvious inflamed skin, such as an inflamed cyst. Due to the high risk of infection, antibiotics are considered empiric and are indicated for these procedures. Class IV (dirty–infected) wounds are, by definition, infected and therefore are treated with the appropriate antibiotics, which are considered therapeutic instead of prophylactic. For class III and IV wounds, the CDC promotes the use of delayed closure or leaving the wound incision open to heal by secondary intention. Furthermore, if draining a wound is necessary, the drain should be placed so that it exits from a separate incision distant from the wound, and the drain should be removed as soon as possible.[8]

Most physicians would prescribe antibiotics for incision and drainage of abscesses due to the high incidence of bacteremia (38%). However, a study examining the incidence of bacteremia after incision and drainage of cutaneous abscesses in afebrile adults revealed 0/150 blood cultures positive ($n = 50$ patients; one baseline blood culture prior to procedure, two cultures after procedure at time 1 and 10 minutes), but 64% of wound cultures revealed *Staphylococcus aureus*.[37] Further studies are needed to establish the risk of infection after incision and drainage of abscesses.

Topical Antibiotics

Topical antibiotics may decrease rates of colonization in healing wounds, thus decreasing the risk of infection. Although petrolatum is commonly applied to surgical wounds, multiple topical antibiotic ointments are available, such as bacitracin, neomycin sulfate, mupirocin, triple antibiotic ointment (neomycin–polymixin B–bacitracin), and silver sulfadiazine. These antibiotics are active against Gram-positive organisms (e.g., *S. aureus*). Neo-

TABLE 6-3. Considerations for the use of antibiotic prophylaxis for surgical site infection.

Location	Highly contaminated areas (ear, axilla, groin, mucosa)
Duration	Long excisions, Mohs micrographic surgery
Surgery type	Grafts, flaps, Mohs micrographic surgery with large defects, laser resurfacing of large areas
Skin condition	Eroded, ulcerated, infected, dermatitis
Patient characteristics	See Table 6-4.

mycin sulfate and silver sulfadiazine also provide coverage against *Pseudomonas* infections.

The use of topical antibiotics in SSI prophylaxis is controversial and no clear guidelines exist that clarify the ability of topical antibiotics to prevent wound infections in dermatologic surgery. A randomized, controlled study of 922 patients revealed no statistical difference in SSI in patients who applied bacitracin versus petrolatum to their sites.[38] Bacitracin also appeared to promote Gram-negative bacilli infections compared to petrolatum by selectively removing resident Gram-positive skin flora. There was also an increased risk of allergic contact dermatitis in those treated with bacitracin, which has been found to have a sensitivity rate of 9.2% according to the North American Contact Dermatitis Group.[39]

Comparative studies of the use of topical antibiotics versus petrolatum have failed to show a benefit in the antibiotic group for patients with uncomplicated partial-thickness outpatient burns,[40] and auricular secondary intention healing wounds,[41] both considered class II or III wounds. In fact, one study found a disproportionate number of cases of inflammatory chondritis with the prophylactic use of topical antibiotics on ear wounds.[41]

Topical antibiotics appear to have minimal benefit in the prevention of infection in cutaneous wounds. Topical antibiotics may disrupt resident skin flora and promote infections, induce allergic contact dermatitis, and increase the likelihood of the development of resistant strains of bacteria, such as methicillin-resistant *Staphylococcus aureus* (MRSA). Generally, topical antibiotic prophylaxis may have a role in the postoperative period of class III and IV wounds, in which the risk of infection is higher than class I and II wounds. Table 6-3 lists considerations for SSI antibiotic prophylaxis.

Intraincisional Antibiotics

In this technique, antibiotics are incorporated into the local anesthetic to create a local antimicrobial environment that decreases the risk of postoperative wound infection. Intraincisional clindamycin in patients undergoing Mohs micrographic surgery has been shown to be effective in preventing wound infections.[18,42] In one study, culture-positive wound infections were found in 2.4% of

patients in the control group versus 0.7% in those patients receiving anesthesia containing 408 μL/mL of clindamycin.[42] In another study, intraincisional buffered lidocaine was compared to a lidocaine/nafcillin solution in 797 patients and 908 wounds were studied. Eleven infections (2.5%) occurred in the control group versus 1 infection (0.2%) in the treated group ($p = 0.003$).[18] Intraincisional prophylaxis eliminates the risk of gastrointestinal upset, which may somewhat minimize the risks of resistance. Intraincisional clindamycin is an alternative to nafcillin in penicillin-allergic patients. Both antibiotic preparations use only several milligrams of antibiotics per patient, at a low cost of a few cents per syringe.

Surgical/Intraoperative Characteristics that Increase the Risk of Surgical Site Infection

Aside from wound characteristics, certain intraoperative events may place a patient at higher risk for SSI. The length of the procedure (a surgery greater than 2 hours may be considered a contaminated class III wound) and improper surgical technique must be considered when deciding upon prophylactic antibiotics. The rate of infection doubles after each hour of surgery.[43] Improper surgical technique includes breaks in sterile field, high-tension closures, inadequate hemostasis/hematoma formation, rough handling of tissue, excessive devitalized tissue with inefficient use of electrosurgery, inadequate obliteration of dead space, and incorrectly designed flaps and grafts with insufficient blood supply, all of which contribute to wound infection.[8]

Patient Characteristics that Increase the Risk of Surgical Site Infection

Table 6-4 summarizes the various patient characteristics that may predispose to SSI. A patient's risk of infection must be individualized. Physicians must ascertain whether the risk of not using antibiotics outweighs the potential

TABLE 6-4. Patient characteristics that may influence the risk of surgical site infection development.

Advanced age
Nutritional status/malnutrition
Diabetes mellitus
Smoking
Alcohol use
Obesity
Coexistant infections at a remote body site
Colonization with microorganisms
Altered immune response, immunosuppression
Chronic renal insufficiency
Peripheral vascular disease

Source: Adapted from the 1999 CDC guidelines and Maragh and colleagues.[3,8]

for antibiotic resistance and the rare but serious risk of severe drug reactions that can result in death.

Colonization of the nares with *S. aureus* has been shown to be associated with the development of a SSI with *S. aureus*.[17,44–46] This pathogen is carried in the nares of 20% to 30% of healthy humans.[46] A multivariate analysis demonstrated that such carriage was the most powerful independent risk factor for SSI following cardiothorasic operations.[17] The use of mupirocin to treat the nares of patients with *S. aureus* colonization is effective, but the effect of mupirocin on reducing SSI risk is yet to be determined.[44,45] Unfortunately, the incidence of staphylococcal resistance is rising due to excessive intranasal application without documentation of nasal colonization by culture.

Intranasal mupirocin should be reserved for patients who have nasal cultures positive for *S. aureus* or MRSA who are at risk for wound infection, have had a recent skin or nosocomial infection with *S. aureus* or MRSA, or are undergoing treatment for a *S. aureus* wound infection. To treat nasal colonization, mupirocin should be applied twice daily for 5 days along with total body cleansing with chlorhexidine or benzoyl peroxide.

Wound Infection Pathogens and Prophylactic Antibiotics

The CDC clearly defines infections of the skin and subcutaneous tissue as "superficial incisional" SSI.[8] According to the data of the National Nosicomial Infection Survey (NNIS) system,[9] the distribution of pathogens isolated from SSI has not changed markedly in the last decade (Table 6-5). Gram-positive organisms, particularly staphylococci and streptococci, account for the vast majority of exogenous flora involved in SSIs (Table 6-5). Sources of such pathogens include surgical/hospital personnel, surgical instruments, articles brought into the operative field, and the operating room air. Most SSIs are contaminated by the patient's endogenous flora, which

are present on the skin, mucous membranes, or hollow viscera (Table 6-6). The usual pathogens on skin and mucosal surfaces are Gram-positive cocci (notably staphylococci); however, Gram-negative aerobes and anaerobic bacteria contaminate skin in the groin/perineal areas (Table 6-6).

Antimicrobial prophylaxis refers to a very brief course of an antimicrobial agent initiated just before an operation begins, ideally 1 to 2 hours prior to surgery, to allow adequate tissue distribution and incorporation into the wound coagulum. It is not an attempt to sterilize the tissues, but rather it is critically timed to reduce the microbial burden of intraoperative contamination to a level that cannot overwhelm the host defenses. Antimicrobial prophylaxis does not address postoperative contamination. The CDC recommends that a prophylactic antibiotic should be used for all operations in which "its use has been shown to reduce SSI rates based on evidence from clinical trials [none have been done in dermatologic surgery], or ... if SSI would represent a catastrophe [in dermatologic surgery, infection and necrosis of a graft or flap, or a catastrophic cosmetic result]."[8] The CDC also recommends using an agent that is "safe, inexpensive, and bactericidal with an in vitro spectrum that covers [appropriate] organisms, given at a time prior to surgery so that the concentration of the drug is established in serum and tissues by the time the skin is incised, and maintained at a therapeutic level throughout the operation and until a few hours after the incision is closed."[8] Some physicians give a second dose administered 6 hours after surgery if the surgery is prolonged or significant breaks in aseptic technique occur. No data exists to support continued prophylaxis after 24 hours when an antibiotic regimen was initiated preoperatively.[47]

In some clinical situations, physicians decide during or after surgery that prophylactic antibiotics should be given, such as a long duration of surgery or major breaks in aseptic technique. Antibiotics should then be initiated immediately and continued for 3 to 7 days postoperatively. Table 6-6 lists the most likely pathogens and antibiotics that may provide coverage if clinically indicated. There are no formal recommendations nor are there randomized, controlled trials for wound prophylaxis.

The most frequently isolated pathogens of SSI are *S. aureus*, coagulase-negative staphylococci, *Enterococcus* species, and *Eschericha coli*[9] (Table 6-5). Antimicrobial-resistant organisms and candidal infections have also been reported, and the increase in incidence is attributed to the overuse of antimicrobial agents and an increase in immunocompromised patients.[9]

S. aureus, which can be part of the transient microbial flora colonizing the perineum (20% of normal persons) and nasal surfaces (20%–40% of normal persons), is present on diseased skin in high concentrations. The risk

TABLE 6-5. Pathogens commonly associated with wound infections and frequency of occurrence.

Pathogen	Frequency (%)
Staphylococcus aureus	20
Coagulase-negative staphylococci	14
Enterococci	12
Escherichia coli	8
Pseudomonas aeruginosa	8
Enterobacter species	7
Proteus mirabilis	3
Klebsiella pneumoniae	3
Other streptococci	3
Candida albicans	3

Source: Adapted from NNIS system.[9]

TABLE 6-6. Likely surgical site infection pathogens and potential choices for prophylactic antibiotics if clinically indicated.

Antibiotic	1 hour preoperatively	6 hours later	Comments
Cephalexin or cefadroxil[c]	1 g PO	500 mg PO	First-line agent Glabrous skin, non-oral S. aureus, streptococci pyogenes
Dicloxacillin[b]	1 g PO	500 mg PO	First-line agent Glabrous skin, non-oral S. aureus, streptococci pyogenes
Azithromycin	500 mg PO	250 mg PO[d]	First-line alternative to penicillin Glabrous skin, non-oral Penicillin-allergic patients S. aureus
Amoxicillin/clavulaunate	2 g PO	1 g PO	Oral or nasopharyngeal surgery S. viridans, oropharyngeal anerobes (peptostreptocci)
Ciprofloxacin	500 mg PO	500 mg PO[e]	Ear or genitourinary S. aureus, Pseudomonas
Clindamycin	600 mg PO	300 mg PO	Glabrous skin, oral, nasopharyngeal S. aureus, S. viridans Methicillin-resistant S. aureus (MRSA) resistance increasing
Erythromycin	1 g PO	500 mg PO	Second-line agent Oral surgery S. viridans Gram + resistance increasing
TMP-SMX	1 DS tab PO	1 DS tab PO[e]	Skin or genitourinary S. aureus, E. coli
Vacnomycin[a]	500 mg IV	250 mg IV	Skin or oral surgery MRSA, S. viridans

Source: Information on antibiotic coverage obtained from the Sanford Guide to Antimicrobial therapy, 2005, in regards to definitive therapy, not prophylaxis.[5,21] Information also adapted from Haas AF, Grekin RC. J Am Acad Dermatol 1995;32(2 Pt 1):155–176.
See text for details.
[a]Alternative for hospitalized patients, those with MRSA wound infections, an overwhelming infection at a distant site, or those with active bacterial endocarditis.
[b]Twenty-five percentor more S. aureus are resistant to penicillins and cephalosporins in some populations.
[c]Repeat dosing of cephalexin may be needed to sustain the MIC90, which is about 1 to 2 hours. If the course of antibiotics will be continued after surgery 3 to 10 days, some use the dosing of cephalexin 500 mg PO b.i.d. for surgical site infection prophylaxis, compared to 500 mg q.i.d. for definitive infection.[3]
[d]May not be necessary due to sustained tissue concentrations, give 12 hours later.
[e]If desired, second dose should be given 12 hours later.

of SSI is increased from two- to ninefold in carriers of S. aureus.[18,44–46] Streptococcus pyogenes and S. aureus are the major pathogens of SSI on glabrous skin, while on mucosal sites, Streptococcus viridans and peptostreptococcus are the primary pathogens. S. aureus and Streptococcus pyogenes are treated by the administration of penicillinase-resistant penicillins (e.g., dicloxacillin) and first-generation cephalosporins (e.g., cephalexin), with the exception of MRSA (25% or higher incidences have been documented).[48,49] Cephalosporins are active against most Gram-positive cocci, E. coli, Klebsiella, and Proteus mirabilis, but not against Pseudomonas, S. epidermidis, or MRSA. Erythromycin has fallen out of favor due to extensive resistance in some studies (up to 70%).[47] Growing clindamycin resistance in MRSA isolates has been documented.[50] However, clindamycin is active against S. aureus and is suggested as the agent of choice for penicillin-allergic patients. Dicloxacillin and nafcillin are both semisynthetic penicillinase-resistant penicillins effective against S. aureus and Streptococcus.

S. epidermidis constitutes more than 50% of the resident staphylococci and colonizes the upper parts of the body. S. epidermidis can be a common pathogen for prosthetic valve endocarditis and vascular grafts, but is not a common pathogen in wound infections. Intravenous vancomycin must be employed for MRSA, S. epidermidis, or Enterococcus.

Amoxicillin provides optimal coverage for S. viridans, but is not effective against S. aureus. Amoxicillin is the antibiotic of choice for oral mucosal procedures. Inflamed or infected axillary skin may harbor a broad array of microorganisms, so broad coverage would be necessary (i.e., amoxicillin–clavulanate, gatifloxacin, cefadroxil, and others).[45] Finally, the perineum and groin may be contaminated with Enterococcus or E. coli, although enterococci are not common wound pathogens. TMP-SMX or cephalosporins are effective against Enterococcus and E. coli because of their broad spectrum and are excellent choices when operating in the inguinal or perineal areas. TMP-SMX is not effective against Pseudomonas *aeruginosa* or anaerobic Gram-negative bacilli such as *Bacteroides fragilis*, and thus should not be considered in ear or toe webspace surgery where *Pseudomonas* may be encountered.

Infections of wounds on the ear are most commonly caused by *S. aureus*, *P. aeruginosa*, and *Serratia marcens*. Half of the infections in Mohs cases occurred on the ears in one study, with a rate of 28% if the cartilage was involved, and 6% if not involved.[15] There are four generations of quinolones with increasing Gram-positive coverage. The second generation quinolones (e.g., ciprofloxacin) have moderate *S. aureus* activity, minimal streptococcal activity, and excellent activity against *Pseudomonas*. Thus, ciprofloxacin is an excellent candidate for prophylaxis before surgery on the ear or genital region. The widespread use of quinolones for various infections has resulted in substantial *Pseudomonas* resistance, and should be discouraged.[51] Table 6-6 summarizes likely SSI pathogens and potential choices for prophylactic antibiotics.

Timing of Antibiotics

Antibiotics should be given 1 to 2 hours prior to the procedure in order to obtain adequate blood and tissue levels at the time of surgery. Most authorities believe that extending antibiotic coverage beyond 24 hours increases the risk of developing resistant strains of bacteria and drug toxicity. Some authors do give another dose of antibiotics (typically half the amount of the first dose) 6 hours after the procedure, especially if the procedure is prolonged and in a contaminated area.

Overall, many physicians reserve the use of prophylactic antibiotics in the prevention of wound infection to situations in which the clinical indication is so overwhelming that the risk of not doing so may result in a catastrophic event. It is important to refer to the most updated and recent antibiotic guidelines before prescribing prophylactic antibiotics.

Antibiotics for Endocarditis Prophylaxis

Bacteremia

Endocarditis and prosthesis infection result only if there is a significant bacteremia, which causes seeding of the endocardium or hardware with pathogens. Bacteremia, which is a common event in everyday life (Table 6-7), is considered transient because in most instances, it lasts only a few minutes. It has not been established whether various dermatologic procedures cause bacteremia, but there have been several studies attempting to quantify

TABLE 6-7. Incidence of bacteremia in procedures and daily activities.

Procedure or activity	Incidence of bacteremia (%)
Tooth extraction	60–90
Periodontal surgery	32–88
Incision of abscess	38
Tonsillectomy	28–38
Cystoscopy	17
Rigid bronchoscopy	15
Endoscopy	4–8
Cardiac catheterization	5
Sigmoidoscopy	2–9
Normal birth	0–5
Tooth brushing	24–40
Chewing food	17–24

Source: Adapted from Everett ED, Hinschmann IV. Transient bacteremia and endocarditis prophylaxis. A review. Medicine 1977;56:61–77.

the risk.[37,52–54] Furthermore, the incidence of endocarditis following a dermatologic procedure or condition is a rare but serious complication.[52,53,55–58]

Endocarditis

For endocarditis to develop, the endothelium must be damaged and a bacteremia caused by adherent organisms must occur. Although bacteremia is a frequent problem after invasive procedures, only certain bacteria cause endocarditis. Most reported cases of endocarditis are not attributable to procedures.[59] Additionally, approximately 50% of reported cases of infective endocarditis occurred in patients with no detectable cardiac abnormality. Furthermore, the use of antibiotics does not completely reduce the chance of endocarditis, as it has been reported in patients receiving prophylactic antibiotics according to the American Heart Association (AHA) recommendations.[60] In these cases infection was attributed to inadequate antimicrobial coverage. Approximately one third of endocarditis cases are caused by organisms not adequately covered by recommended regimens.[6]

Native valve infective endocarditis is most commonly caused by *Streptococcus viridans*, enterococci, other streptococci, *S. aureus*, and coagulase-negative staphylococci, which comprise more than 90% of the cases[61,62] (Table 6-8) Prosthetic valve endocarditis is most commonly caused by coagulase-negative staphylococci, streptococci (non-enterococcal), and *S. aureus*. α-Hemolytic streptococci are the most common cause of endocarditis following dental and oral procedures and upper respiratory tract procedures, and a single dose of amoxicillin is the proper prophylactic agent. Bacterial endocarditis following genitourinary and gastrointestinal tract procedures is most often caused by *Enterococcus faecalis*. Gram-negative bacilli rarely are responsible for endocar-

TABLE 6-8. Microorganisms causing infective endocaridits.

Microorganism	% native valve (nonaddicts)	% prosthetic valve early	% prosthetic valve late
Streptococci	50–70	5–10	25–30
Staphylococci	25	45–50	30–40
S. aureus	90	15–20	10–12
S. epidermidis	10	25–30	23–28
Enterococci	10	<1	5–10
Gram-negative bacilli	<1	20	10–12
Fungi	<1	10–12	5–8
Diphtheroids	<1	5–10	4–5
Culture negative	5–10	5–10	5–10

Source: From Korzeniowski OM, Kaye D. Endocarditis. In: Gorbach SL, Bartlett JA, Blacklow NR, eds. Infectious diseases. Philadelphia: Sauders; 1992:548–557.

ditis, although they may cause bacteremia. There are no randomized, controlled trials in regards to endocarditis prophylaxis. The AHA has created guideline based upon the following points:

1. The degree to which the patient's underlying condition creates a risk of endocarditis.
2. The apparent risk of bacteremia with the procedure.
3. The potential adverse effects of the prophylactic antimicrobial agent to be used.
4. The cost–benefit aspects of the recommended prophylactic regimen.[59]

American Heart Association Recommendations for Endocarditis Prophylaxis

Based upon these considerations, the AHA has stratified patients into high, moderate, or low risk based upon their cardiac defect (Table 6-9), and has listed which types of procedures are higher risk of causing bacteremia and subsequent endocarditis. The AHA has recommended that those in high- or moderate-risk categories be given prophylactic antibiotics prior to certain procedures, because compared with the general population, patients in the high-risk category are much more likely (high risk)

or more likely (moderate risk) to develop a severe endocardial infection resulting in morbidity and mortality (Tables 6-9, 6-10) In patients with mitral valve prolapse, it can be difficult to determine when endocarditis prophylaxis is needed. This common condition represents a heterogeneous population; the natural history of mitral valve prolapse ranges from extremely benign to severe mortality of morbidity.[63] The moderate-risk category includes those patients with mitral valve prolapse and leaking mitral valves, as evidenced by audible clicks and murmurs of mitral regurgitation or by Doppler-demonstrated mitral insufficiency, whom are considered to be at increased risk for endocarditis.

Procedures that Require Endocarditis Prophylaxis According to the American Heart Association Guidelines

Procedures that require prophylactic antibiotics are listed in Table 6-11 and the recommended antibiotic regimens based upon location are listed in Tables 6-12 and 6-13. However, most cases of bacterial endocarditis are not attributable to a specific invasive procedure. Prophylaxis

TABLE 6-9. Patients that require prophylactic antibiotics according to the AHA recommendations.

High-risk patients	Moderate-risk patients
Prosthetic cardiac valves	Most other congenital cardiac malformations
Previous bacterial endocarditis	Valvular dysfunction of any origin
Complex cyanotic congenital heart disease	Hypertrophic cardiomyopathy
Surgically constructed systemic to pulmonary shunts or conduits	Mitral valve prolapse with valvular regurgitation

Source: Adapted from JAMA 1997;277:1794–1801.

TABLE 6-10. Cardiac defects in the negligible risk category (no greater risk than general population and prophylactic antibiotics are not indicated).

Isolated secundum atrial septal defect
Surgical repair of ASD, VSD, or PDA without residua beyond 6 months
Previous coronary artery bypass graft surgery
MVP without valvular regurgitation
Physiological, functional, or innocent heart
Murmurs
Previous Kawasaki disease without valvular dysfunction
Previous rheumatic fever without valvular dysfunction
Cardiac pacemakers (intravascular and epicardial) & implanted defibrillators

Abbreviations: ASD, atrial septal defect; VSD, ventricular septal defect; PDA, patent ductus arteriosus; MVP, mitral valve prolapse.

TABLE 6-11. Selected procedures and American Heart Association recommendations for and against prophylactic antibiotics for endocarditis prevention.

Endocarditis prophylaxis recommended for high-risk and moderate-risk patients (selected items)	Endocarditis prophylaxis not recommended (selected items)
Dental	**Dental**
Extractions	Local anesthetic injections
Periodontal procedures	Postoperative suture removal
Prophylactic cleaning of teeth or implants where bleeding is anticipated	
Respiratory tract	**Respiratory tract**
Surgical operations that involve respiratory mucosa	Tympanostomy tube insertion
Gastrointestinal tract	**Gastrointestinal tract**
Surgical operations that involve intestinal mucosa	Endoscopy with or without gastrointestinal biopsy
Genitourinary tract	**Genitourinary tract**
Prostatic surgery	Vaginal hysterectomy[a]
Cystoscopy	Vaginal delivery[a]
Urethral dilation	
Skin	**Skin**
Procedure involving infected tissues, i.e., soft tissue infection (cellulitis) or bone and joint infections	Incision or biopsy of surgically scrubbed skin, noninfected
	Circumcision

[a]Prophylaxis optional for high-risk patients.

is recommended for procedures that are known to induce significant bacteremias with the organisms commonly associated with endocarditis and attributable to identifiable procedures. Invasive procedures performed through surgically scrubbed skin are not likely to produce such bacteremias, and as such, the AHA has addressed dermatologic procedures involving noninfected glabrous skin; "incision or biopsy of surgically scrubbed skin" is listed in the "negligible risk" category, not requiring antibiotic prophylaxis (Table 6-11).

Skin Condition and the Need for Endocarditis Prophylaxis According to the American Heart Association

Surgical Procedures Involving Infected Tissue

Antibiotic prophylaxis is needed for procedures that involve grossly infected tissue because these procedures can cause a bacteremia with the organism causing the infection. Therefore, if a procedure requires endocarditis

TABLE 6-12. Antibiotic regimines for dental/oral/respiratory tract/esophageal procedures for patients at-risk.

Standard general prophylaxis for patients at-risk	Adult: Amoxicillin 2g orally
	Children: 50mg/kg PO 1 hour before procedure
Unable to take oral medications	Adult: Ampicillin 2g IV or IM
	Children: 50mg/kg, IM or IV 30 minutes prior to procedure
Amoxicillin/ampicillin/penicillin allergic	Clindamycin
	Adults: 600mg
	Children: 20mg/kg orally 1 hour before procedure
	or
	Cephalexin[a] or Cefadroxil[a]
	Adult: 2g orally
	Children: 50mg/kg PO 1 hour before procedure
	or
	Azithromycin or clarithromycin
	Adult: 500mg orally;
	Children: 15mg/kg PO 1 hour before procedure
Amoxicillin/ampicillin/penicillin-allergic patients unable to take oral medication	Clindamycin
	Adult: 600mg
	Children: 20mg/kg IV 30 minutes before procedure
	or
	Cefazolin[a]
	Adult: 1g
	Children: 25mg/kg IM or IV 30 minutes before procedure

Source: Adapted from JAMA 1997;277:1794–1801.
[a]Cephalosporins should not be used in individuals with immediate-type hypersensitivity reactions (urticaria, angioedema, or anaphylaxis) to penicillin.

TABLE 6-13. Genitourinary/gastrointestinal (excluding esophageal) procedures and recommendations from the American Heart Association for endocarditis prophylaxis.

High-risk patients	Adults: Ampicillin 2 g IM or IV 30 minutes before procedure plus gentamycin 1.5 mg/kg (not to exceed 120 mg) IM or IV 20 minutes before procedure followed by ampicillin 1 g IM or IV or amoxicillin 1 g orally Children: Ampicillin 50 mg/kg IM or IV (not to exceed 2 g), plus gentamycin 1.5 mg/kg IM within 30 minutes of starting the procedure; 6 hours later ampicillin 25 mg/kg IM or IV or amoxicillin 25 mg/kg orally
High-risk patients allergic to ampicillin/amoxicillin	Adults: Vancomycin 1 g IV over 1–2 hours plus gentamycin 1.5 mg/kg (not to exceed 120 mg) IM[a] or IV, both to be completed 30 minutes prior to procedure Children: Vancomycin 20 mg/kg IV over 1–2 hours, plus gentamycin 1.5 mg/kg IV or IM; both to be completed within 30 minutes of starting the procedure
Moderate-risk patients	Adults: Amoxicillin 2 g orally 1 hour before procedure or ampicillin 2 g IM or IV 30 minutes before procedure Children: Amoxicillin 50 mg/kg orally 1 hour before the procedure, or ampicillin 50 mg/kg IM or IV within 20 minutes of starting procedure
Moderate-risk patients allergic to ampicillin/amoxicillin	Adults: Vancomycin 1 g IV over 1–2 hours to be completed 30 minutes prior to procedure Children: 20 mg/kg IV over 1–2 hours; infusion should be completed within 30 minutes of starting the procedure

[a]Intramuscular injections must be avoided in patients who are receiving heparin therapy. The use of warfarin is a relative contraindication to intramuscular infections.
A second dose of vancomycin or gentamycin is not recommended.
The total pediatric dose should not exceed the adult dose.

prophylaxis, the patient should be given both antibiotics appropriate for the established infection and for endocarditis prophylaxis (Table 6-14). While some organisms that cause tissue infections are unlikely to cause endocarditis, they could cause life-threatening sepsis. For nonoral soft tissue infections, or bone and joint infections, an antistaphylococcal penicillin or a first-generation cephalosporin is an appropriate choice for prophylaxis in patients who are at high and moderate risk for endocarditis. Clindamycin is an alternative in patients allergic to penicillin, and intravenous vancomycin is the drug of choice in patients who are unable to take oral antibiotics or those with known MRSA bacteremia.[59]

Special Situations

If the patient did not take the antibiotic prior to surgery, it has been established in animal models that effective

TABLE 6-14. Endocarditis prophylaxis for procedures involving infected tissues [soft tissues (cellulitis) bone and joint infections]: Recommendations from the American Heart Association.[a]

High- and moderate-risk patients	Cephalexin or dicloxacillin 2 g PO 1 hour prior to procedure or clindamycin 600 mg or Azithromycin or clarithromycin 500 mg PO 1 hour prior to procedure

[a]If the procedure or suspected organism is one that requires a different agent for endocarditis prophylaxis than listed above, both agents should be given (i.e., coverage of the microorganism causing infection and endocarditis prophylaxis agent of choice for that location or procedure). Antibiotic coverage should continue after the procedure if there is definitive infection in order to treat the infection.

prophylaxis can be achieved when the appropriate antibiotic is administered within 2 hours after the procedure and no later than 4 hours after the procedure.[64] If the patient is already on an antibiotic normally used for endocarditis prophylaxis, a drug from a different class should be selected.[59]

Dermatologic Procedures and Skin Conditions that May Warrant Endocarditis Prophylaxis

Bacteremia after Dermatologic Procedures

The prevalence of bacteremia after various dermatologic procedures, conditions, and locations has been studied and may aid in deciding when prophylactic antibiotics may be needed. The AHA comments on surgical procedures on infected tissue and normal skin, but does not address surgery on eroded or otherwise diseased skin. Similarly, dermatologic procedures and their subsequent risk of bacteremia and endocarditis have not been adequately studied, which has led to varying practices among dermatologists.[1,3,65] Despite British guidelines against prophylactic antibiotics for endocarditis for routine dermatologic procedures, even in the setting of cardiac disease, 58% of physicians prescribe antibiotics: 57% for simple excisions, 63% for secondary intention wounds, 76% for flaps, 69% for grafts, and 39% for Mohs micrographic surgery.[65]

Procedures on eroded or diseased skin are considered clean–contaminated wounds (i.e., class II lesions) and may increase the risk of endocarditis. A study comparing excision of eroded versus noneroded lesions revealed 1/35 (2.8%) patients with *S. aureus* bacteremia in the eroded group, compared to 0/15 in the noneroded group. After statistical analysis, the incidence of bacteremia for surgery on eroded lesions was 8.4%, and the authors recommended 1 to 2g of a first-generation cephalosporin or dicloxacillin to be administered 1 to 2 hours before surgery and continued for 1 to 2 doses in patients with prosthetic heart valves who undergo surgery on eroded skin.[53] Wilson and colleagues found a 2.1% incidence of bacteremia on normal subjects who had random blood cultures drawn.[66] Zack and colleagues studied blood cultures of 21 patients undergoing electrodessication and curettage or scalpel excision of either eroded or intact, noninfected skin and found all cultures negative.[67] Halpern and coworkers studied 45 patients undergoing Mohs micrographic surgery with repair, hair transplantation, dermabrasion, skin grafting, cyst and wart excision, and scar revision. Six of the neoplasms were eroded but not clinically infected. Three patients (7%) had a positive blood culture at 15 minutes postprocedure. The cultures grew *P. acnes* in two cases and *S. hominis* in one case. Neither of these organisms commonly cause endocarditis, but there have been reports of *P. acnes* causing endocarditis. The authors concluded that prophylaxis should be considered for patients with prosthetic valves.[52]

There has been a report of endocarditis occurring after a dermatologic procedure on noninfected but crusted skin.[68] Acne[69] and atopic dermatitis[70–75] have been also been associated with endocarditis. Because there is minimal data regarding the incidence of bacteremia and subsequent endocarditis from various dermatologic procedures and dermatologic conditions (i.e., inflamed skin or crusted lesions), the use of antibiotics in these situations is controversial. From the available data, the overall incidence of bacteremia seems to be low for dermatologic procedures performed on intact skin, but further studies are needed for surgery on eroded or otherwise diseased skin, as well as for surgery in highly contaminated areas (i.e., the axilla, ear, and groin).

Maragh and colleagues[3] have defined their recommendations for endocarditis prophylaxis for various dermatologic procedures and conditions of skin (Table 6-15). Their guidelines, which were based on available authoritative guidelines of the AHA and CDC and consultation with infectious disease specialists, take into account the procedure type, condition of the skin, and the patient's cardiac risk. According to their guidelines, antibiotic prophylaxis is not indicated for low-risk patients for the prevention of endocarditis (or prosthesis infection) even in the presence of eroded, inflamed, or infected skin.

TABLE 6-15. Mayo Clinic Division of Dermatologic Surgery guidelines for antibiotic prophylaxis for the prevention of endocarditis and prosthesis infection.

Procedure	Risk	Skin condition	Prophylaxis
Mohs surgery	High[a]	All	Yes
Excision, biopsy, cryotherapy, ED&C ablative laser	High	Intact skin	No[b]
		Inflamed or infected	Yes
		Eroded	No[c]
Mohs surgery, excision, biopsy, cryotherapy, ED&C, ablative laser	Low	All	No

Source: Maragh et al.[3]

[a]The authors define "high-risk" patients as those with prosthetic valves, mitral valve prolapse with regurgitation, mitral valve prolapse without regurgitation in men greater than 45 years of age (a non–American Heart Association recommendation), any valve dysfunction, cardiac malformation, hypertrophic cardiomyopathy, orthopedic prosthesis, central nervous system shunts, or shunts/fistulas with nearby inflamed or infected tissue.

[b]An exception is breach of nasal or oral mucosa. Prophylaxis is used in these locations.

[c]An exception is excision of eroded skin with prosthetic valve. Prophylaxis is used in this scenario.

Non-oral sites: Cephalexin 2g PO 30–60 minutes prior to surgery or clindamycin 600mg or azithromycin or clarithromycin 500mg PO 30–60 minutes prior to procedure.

Oral sites: Amoxicillin 2g PO 30–60 minutes prior to surgery or clindamycin 600mg or cephalexin (if non–type I allergic reaction) 2g PO or azithromycin or clarithromycin 500mg PO 30–60min prior to procedure.

However, those patients with prosthetic heart valves who undergo non-Mohs procedures on eroded skin will receive antibiotics. The recommendations state that antibiotics are indicated for the prevention of SSI in the presence of inflamed and infected skin.

In high-risk patients with intact, noninfected, noninflamed skin, Maragh and colleagues[3] do not recommend antibiotic prophylaxis to prevent endocarditis in patients undergoing sterile excision, biopsy, cryosurgery, electrodessication and curettage, or ablative laser procedures. However, in high-risk patients, antibiotics are administered for all skin lesions that are inflamed or infected, even for minor procedures such as excision, biopsy, electrodessication and curettage, laser ablation, or ablative cryotherapy.

The guidelines proposed by Maragh and colleagues[3] also recommend that all high-risk patients having Mohs surgery receive prophylaxis due to the prolonged operative time and intermittent bandaging, regardless of the condition of the skin. The increased risk of bacteremia and endocarditis that may occur is not really consistent with the overall low risk of infection for Mohs' surgery (i.e., 2% to 3%). However, it has been shown that in certain locations (i.e., the ear) that the risk of infection may be as high as 12% to 28%.[15] Maragh and colleagues also recommend that prophylactic antibiotics should be administered to patients with high risk indications undergoing procedures that breech the nasal or oral mucosa.

A study of patients undergoing surgery of the head and neck revealed that 3 of 45 patients had a transient bacteremia after the procedure, 2 patients with *P. acnes*, and 1 patient with *Staphylococcus hominis*, which yielded a 7% incidence of bacteremia. The authors of this study concluded that for noninfected skin of the head and neck, patients with prosthetic heart valves should receive prophylactic antibiotics.[52]

All guidelines and opinions should not serve as standard of care or a substitute for clinical judgment, as randomized, controlled studies are lacking. Physicians should use their own judgment in selecting an antibiotic and determining the number of doses that should be administered to patients in certain circumstances. Even with antibiotics, endocarditis may occur and warning signs include fever, night chills, weakness, myalgia, arthralgia, lethargy, or malaise in a patient who has had a procedure.

Antibiotics for Prosthesis Infection Prophylaxis

There is little data concerning the prevention of prosthetic joint infection from bacteremia in dermatologic surgery. Most of the data is related to urologic or dental procedures. The following is a quote from the American Academy of Orthopedic Surgeons bulletin, 1997:

An expert panel of dentists, orthopedic surgeons and infectious disease specialists, convened by the American Dental Association (ADA) and the American Academy of Orthopedic Surgeons (AAOS) performed a thorough review of all available data to determine the need for antibiotic prophylaxis to prevent hematogenous prosthetic joint infections in dental patients who have undergone total joint arthroplasties. The result is this report, which has been adopted by both organizations as an advisory statement. The panel's conclusion: Antibiotic prophylaxis is not indicated for dental patients with pins, plates and screws, nor is it routinely indicated for most dental patients with total joint replacements. However, it is advisable to consider premedication in a small number of patients who may be at potential increased risk of hematogenous total joint infection. [These patients include immunocompromised and immunosuppressed patients (those with inflammatory arthropathies such as rheumatoid arthritis, systemic lupus erythematosus, or disease, drug- or radiation-induced immunosuppression), or other patients (insulin-dependent diabetes, first 2 years following joint replacement, previous prosthetic joint infections, malnourishment, hemophilia).][76]

There is no data supporting the use of prophylactic antibiotics in patients with artificial joints who undergo cutaneous surgery. As stated above, patients with prosthetic joints usually do not require antimicrobial prophylaxis when undergoing gastrointestinal, genitourinary, or dental procedures. Most infections of prosthetic joints arise from contamination at the time of their insertion or from distant sites of suppurative infection,[77,78] and the most common pathogens are *S. aureus* and *S. epidermidis*. However, in some instances, an orthopedic surgeon may request that prophylactic antibiotics be administered prior to a dermatologic procedure for a patient who has undergone joint replacement or other orthopedic procedures in the recent past or if surgery is performed in an infected area. It is always prudent to contact the patient's surgeon if there is any ongoing infection at the time of surgery. Antibiotic prophylaxis should be administered to those patients who are undergoing surgery on infected or abscessed skin or if the patient has a distant wound infection.[7] Maragh and colleagues[3] combined the guidelines for endocarditis prophylaxis and hardware infection prophylaxis in their antibiotic recommendations (Table 6-15).

Conclusion

In conclusion, prophylactic antibiotics may be used in various clinical situations in dermatologic surgery. Surgical site infection prevention, endocarditis prevention, and prosthesis infection prevention are the three main instances when antibiotics are used for prophylaxis. The risks of allergic reactions and the growing problem of antibiotic resistance must be considered before antibiotics are initiated. Consultation with specialists in cardiology, orthopedic surgery, and infectious diseases may be necessary. The dermatologic surgeon must be aware of the patient's comorbidities, such as any distant cutaneous infections, immunosuppression, status of prosthetic valves, other heart diseases or orthopedic hardware, allergies to antibiotics, and colonization of microflora if MRSA is a problem in the community. (See Table 6-16 for suggestions to the dermatologic surgeon and a preoperative questionnaire for patients.) Proper surgical scrub and surgical technique, as well as elimination of possible contamination of the surgical site, are necessary to prevent surgical site infections. Finally, the dermatologic surgeon should be aware of the warning signs and symptoms of wound infection, endocarditis, and hardware infection and act promptly to evaluate and treat the patient appropriately.

TABLE 6-16. Suggested questionnaire for the dermatologic physician and surgery patient.

In regards to surgical site infection prophylaxis
Wound issues
What is the surgical wound classification (Table 6-2); that is, is the surgical site contaminated or infected prior to surgery? Is the surgical site a high-risk, contaminated location?
Patient issues
Does the patient have any of the conditions listed in Table 6-3; that is, is the patient methicillin-resistant *Staphylococcus aureus* (MRSA) positive?
In regards to endocarditis prophylaxis
Patient issues
Does the patient have a condition listed by the American Heart Association as high or moderate risk for endocarditis (Table 6-9)?
Wound issues
Is the surgical site infected (or eroded), which may place the patient at higher risk of endocarditis?
In regards to other hardware infection prophylaxis
Wound issues
Is the surgical site infected, which may place the patient at higher risk of hardware infection?
Patient issues
Does the patient have any underlying conditions that may predispose to hardware infection (see text)?

Sample questionnaire

Do you have any allergies to antibiotics? If so, what happened when you took them?
Do you take antibiotics prior to dental procedures? If so, why?
Do you have a history of any of the following:
  a. Diabetes mellitus?
  b. Smoking?
  c. Alcohol use?
  d. Obesity?
  e. Current infection? Are you taking antibiotics or antiviral medications?
  f. Herpes simplex virus on your lips (i.e., cold sores)? If so how often, and are you taking medication for it?
  g. Colonization with microorganisms — do you know if you carry staphylococcus bacteria on your skin (i.e., MRSA)?
  h. Altered immune response (immunosuppression) — are you a transplant recipient, or do you take medications that decrease your ability to fight infection?
Do you have any of the following diseases, conditions, or medical devices?
  a. Chronic renal insufficiency?
  b. Peripheral vascular disease?
  c. Prosthetic cardiac valves?
  d. Previous bacterial endocarditis?
  e. Complex cyanotic congenital heart disease?
  f. Congenital cardiac malformations?
  g. Valvular dysfunction of any origin?
  h. Hypertrophic cardiomyopathy?
  i. Mitral valve prolapse with valvular regurgitation?
  j. Prosthetic joint or other hardware?
  k. Defibrillator or pacemaker? (Not important for antibiotic prophylaxis, but important preoperative assessment)
  l. Surgically constructed systemic pulmonary shunts or conduits?
  m. Synthetic shunts or grafts?

References

1. Scheinfeld N, Struach S, Ross B. Antibiotic prophylaxis guideline awareness and antibiotic prophylaxis use among New York State dermatologic surgeons. Dermatol Surg 2002;28:841–844.
2. George PM. Dermatoligsts and antibiotic prphylaxis: a survey. J Am Acad Dermatol 1995;33:418–421.
3. Maragh SL, et al. Antibiotic prophylaxis in dermatologic surgery: updated guidelines. Dermatol Surg 2005;31:83–93.
4. Rabb DC, Lesher JL Jr. Antibiotic prohylaxis in cutaneous surgery. Dermatol Surg 1995;33:418–421.
5. Messingham MJ, Arpey CJ. Update on the use of antibiotics in cutaneous surgery. Dermatol Surg 2005;31:1068–1078.
6. Hass AF, Grekin RC. Antibiotic prophylaxis in dermatologic surgery. J Am Acad Dermatol 1995;32:155–176.
7. Billingsley E. The role of antibiotics in cutaneous surgery. Available at: http://www.emedicine.com/derm/topic821.htm. Accessed October 2006.
8. Centers for Disease Control and Prevention. Guideline for prevention of surgical site infection, 1999. Available at: http://www.cdc.gov. Accessed October 2006.
9. National Nosocomial Infection Survey (NNIS). Report, October 2004. Available at: http://www.cdc.gov/ncidod/dhqp/nnis_pubs.html. Accessed October 2006.
10. Salache SJ. Acute surgical complications: cause, prevention, and treatment. J Am Acad Dermatol 1986;15:1163–1185.
11. Garner JS. CDC guideline for prevention of surgical wound infections, 1985. Supercedes guideline for prevention of

surgical wound infections published in 1982. (Originally published in November 1985). Revised. Infect Control 1986; 7(3):193–200.

12. Hirschmann JV. Antimicrobial prophylaxis in dermatology. Semin Cutan Med Surg 200;19:2–9.

13. Altemeier WA, et al. American College of Surgeons manual on control of infection in surgical patients. Philadelphia: Lippincott; 1994:133–139.

14. Cruse PJ, Foord R. The epidemiology of wound infection. A 10-year prospective study of 62,939 wounds. Surg Clin North Am 1980;60:27–40.

15. Futoryan T, Grande D. Postoperative wound infection rates in dermatologic surgery. Dermatol Surg 1995;21:509–514.

16. Edwards PS, Lipp A, Holmes A. Preoperative skin antiseptics for preventing surgical wound infections after clean surgery. Cochrane Database Syst Rev 2004:CD003949.

17. Kluytmans JA, et al. Nasal carriage of *S. aureus* as a major risk factor for wound infections after cardiac surgery. J Infect Dis 1995;171:216–219.

18. Griego RD, Zitelli JA. Intra-incisional prophylactic antibiotics for dermatologic surgery. Arch Dermatol 1998;134:688–692.

19. Johnson JT, Wagner RL. Infection following uncontaminated head and neck surgery. Arch Otolaryngol Head Neck Surg 1987;113:368–369.

20. Weber RS, Callender DL. Antibiotic prophylaxis in clean contaminated head and neck oncologic surgery. Ann Otol Rhinol Laryngol 1992;101:16–20.

21. Alster TS. Against antibiotic prophylaxis for cutaneous laser resurfacing. Dermatol Surg 2000;26:697–698.

22. Friedman PM, Geronemus RG. Antibiotic prophylaxis in laser resurfacing patients. Dermatol Surg 2000;26:695–697.

23. Gaspar Z, Vinciullo C, Elliott T. Antibiotic prophylaxis for full-face laser resurfacing: is it necessary? Arch Dermatol 2001;137:313–315.

24. Manuskiatti W, Fitzpatrick RE, Goldman MP, Krejci-Papa N. Prophylactic antibiotics in patients undergoing laser resurfacing of the skin. J Am Acad Dermatol 1999;40:77–84.

25. Walia S, Alster TS. Cutaneous CO2 laser resurfacing infection rate with and without prophylactic antibiotics. Dermatol Surg 1999;25:857–861.

26. Sriprachya-Anunt S, Fitzpatrick RE, Goldman MP, Smith SR. Infections complicating pulsed corbon dioxide laser resurfacing for photoaged facial skin. Dermatol Surg 1997;23:527–535.

27. Ugburo AO, Atoyebi OA, Oyeneyin JO, Sowemimo GO. An evaluation of the role of systemic antibiotic prophylaxis in the control of burn wound infection at the Lagos University Teaching Hospital. Burns 2004;30:43–48.

28. Hoffmann S. Siver sulfadiazine: an antibacterial agent for topical use in burns. A review of the literature. Scand J Plast Reconstr Surg 1984;18:119–126.

29. Monafo WW, West MA. Current treatment recommendations for topical burn therapy. Drugs 1990;40:364–273.

30. Shirani KZ, Vaughan GM, Mason AD Jr, Pruitt BA Jr. Update on current therapeutic approaches in burns. Shock 1996;5:4–16.

31. Waldorf HA, Kauvar AN, Geronemus RG. Skin resurfacing of fine to deep rhytides using a char-free carbon dioxide laser in 47 patients. Dermatol Surg 1995;21:940–946.

32. Weinstein C, Ramirez OM, Pozner JN. Postoperative care following CO2 laser resurfacing: avoiding pitfalls. Plast Reconstr Surg 1997;100:1855–1866.

33. Beeson WH, Rachel JD. Valacyclovir prophylaxis for herpes simplex virus infection or infection recurrence following laser skin resurfacing. Dermatol Surg 2002;28:331–336.

34. Gilbert S, McBurney E. Use of valacyclovir for herpes simplex virus 1 prophylaxis after facial resurfacing: a randomized clinical trial of dosing regimens. Dermatol Surg 2000;26:50–54.

35. Gilbert S. Improving the outcome of facial resurfacing-prevention of herpes simplex virus type 1 reactivation. J Antimicrob Chemother 2001:47(Suppl T1):29–34.

36. Perkins SW, Sklarew EC. Prevention of facial herpetic infections after chemical peel and dermabrasion: new treatment strategies in the prophylaxis of patients undergoing procedures of the perioral area. Plast Reconstr Surg 1996;98:427–433.

37. Bobrow BJ, Pollack CV Jr, Gamble S, Seligson RA. Incision and drainage of cutaneous abscesses is not associated with bacteremia in afebrile adults. Ann Emerg Med 1997;29:404–408.

38. Smack DP, Harrington AC, Dunn C, et al. Infection and allergy incidence in ambulatory surgery patients using white petrolatum vs bacitracin ointment. A randomized controlled trial. JAMA 1996;276:972–977.

39. Marks JG, Belsito DV, DeLeo VA, et al. North American Contact Dermatitis Group patch test results for the detection of delayed-type hypersensitivity to topical allergens. J Am Acad Dermatol 1998;38:911–918.

40. Heinrich JJ, Brand DA, Cuono CB. The role of topical treatment as a determinant of infection in outpatient burns. J Burn Care Rehabil 1998;9:253–257.

41. Campbell RM, Perlis CS, Fisher E, Gloster HM Jr. Gentamicin ointment versus petrolatum for management of auricular wounds. Dermatol Surg 2005;31:664–669.

42. Huether MJ, Griego RD, Brodland DG, Zitelli JA. Clindamycin for intraincisional antibiotic prophylaxis in dermatologic surgery. Arch Dermatol 2002;138:1145–1148.

43. Culver DH, Horan TC, Gaynes RP. Surgical wound infection rates by wound class, operative procedure, and patient risk index. National Nosocomial Infections Surveillance System. Am J Med 1991;16:91(3B):152S–157S.

44. Perl TM, Golub JE. New approaches to reduce *Staphlococcus aureus* nosocomial infection rates: treating *S. aureus* nasal carriage. Ann Pharmacother 1998;32:S7–S16.

45. Perl TM, Cullen JJ, Wensel RP, et al. Intranasal mupriocin to prevent postoperative *S. aureus* infections. N Engl J Med 2002;346:1871–1877.

46. Wenzel RP, Perl TM. The significance of nasal carriage of *Staphylococcus aureus* and the incidence of post-operative wound infection. J Hosp Infect 1995;31:13–24.

47. Babcock MD, Grekin RC. Antibiotic use in dermatologic surgery. Dermatol Clin 2003:21:337–348.

48. Gilbert D, et al. Sanford guide to antimicrobial therapy. Antimicrobial Therapy, Inc; 2005:37.

49. Johns Hopkins Point of Care information technology. Surgical Site Injections. May 23, 2007. Available at: http://hopkins-abxguide.org.

50. Braun L, Craft D, Williams R, Tuamokumo F, Ottolini M. Increasing clindamycin resistance among methicillin-resistant *Staphylococcus aureus* in 57 northeast United States military treatment facilities. Pediatr Infect Dis J 2005; 24:622–626.

51. Cao B, Wang H, Sun H, Zhu Y, Chen M. Risk factors for multlidrug-resistant *Pseudomonas aeruginosa* nosocomial infection. J Hosp Infect 2004;57:209–216.

52. Halpern AC, Leyden JJ, Dzubow LM, McGinley KJ. The incidence of bacteremia in skin surgery of the head and neck. J Am Acad Dermatol 1988;19:112–116.

53. Sabetta JB, Zitelli JA. The incidence of bacteremia during skin surgery. Arch Dermatol 1987;123:213–215.

54. Maurice PD, Parker S, Azadian BS, Cream JJ. Minor skin surgery. Are prophylactic antibiotics ever needed for curettage? Acta Derm Venereol 1991;71:267–268.

55. Griffin MR, Wilson WR, Edwards WD, et al. Infective endocarditis: Olmsted County, Minnesota, 1950 through 1981. JAMA 1985;254:1199–1202.

56. Spelman DW, Weinmann A, Spicer WJ. Endocarditis following skin procedures. J Infect 1993;26:185–189.

57. Carmichael AJ, Flanagan PG, Holt PJ, Duerden BI. The occurrence of bacteraemia with skin surgery. Br J Dermatol 1996;134:120–122.

58. Zack L, Remlinger K, Thompson K, Massa MC. The incidence of bacteremia after skin surgery. J Infect Dis 1989;159: 148–150.

59. Dajani AS, Taubert KA, Wilson W, et al. Prevention of bacterial endocarditis. Recommendations by the American Heart Association. JAMA 1997;277:1794–1801.

60. Durack DT, Kaplan EL, Bisno AL. Apparent failures of endocarditis prophylaxis: analysis of 52 cases submitted to a national registry. JAMA 1983;250:2318–2322.

61. Cotrufo M, Carozza A, Romano G, De Feo M, Della Corte A. Infective endocarditis of native cardiac valves: 22 years'surgical experience. J Heart Valve Dis 2001;10:478–485.

62. Mandell GL, Bennett JE, Dolin R, eds. Non-injection drug abusers. In: Principles and practice of infectious diseases. 4th ed. New York: Churchill Livingstone; 1995:753.

63. Avierinos JF, Gersh BJ, Melton LJ 3rd, et al. Natural history of asymptomatic mitral valve prolapse in the community. Circulation 2002;106:1355–1361.

64. Berney P, Fancioli P. Successful prophylaxis of experimental streptoccal endocarditis with single-dose amoxicillin administered after bacterial challenge. J Infect Disease 1990;161: 281–285.

65. Affleck AG, Birnie AJ, Gee TM, Gee BC. Antibiotic prophylaxis in patients with valvular heart defects undergoing dermatological surgery remains a confusing issue despite apparently clear guidelines. Clin Exp Dermatol 2005;30: 487–489.

66. Wilson WR, Van Scoy RE, Washington JA. Incidence of bacteremia in adults without infection. J Clin Microbiol 1975;2:94–95.

67. Zack L, Remlinger K, Thompson K, et al. The incidence of bacteremia after skin surgery. J Infect Dis 1989;159:148–150.

68. Zahariadis G, Ross H. A crusty cause of prosthetic valve endocarditis. Can J Cardiol 1999;15:693–695.

69. Vanagt WY, Daenen WJ, Delhaas T. Propionibacterium acnes endocarditis on an annuloplasty ring in an adolescent boy. Heart 2004;90:e56.

70. Harada M, Nishi Y, Tamura S, et al. Infective endocarditis with a huge mitral vegetation related to atopic dermatitis and high serum level of infection-related antiphospholipid antibody; a case report. J Cardiol 2003;42:135–140.

71. Conway DS, Taylor AD, Burrell CJ. Atopic eczema and staphylococcal endocarditis: time to recognize an association? Hosp Med 2000;61:356–357.

72. Onoda K, Mizutan H, Komada T, et al. Atopic dermatitis as a risk factor for acute native valve endocarditis. J Heart Valve Dis 2000;9:469–471.

73. Kobayashi H, Sugiuchi R, Tabata N, et al. Guess what! Acute infectious endocarditis with Janeway lesions in a patient with atopic dermatitis. Eur J Dermatol 1999;9:239–240.

74. Grabczynska SA, Cerio R. Infective endocarditis associated with atopic eczema. Br J Dermatol 1999;140:1193–1194.

75. Pike MG, Warner JO. Atopic dermatitis complicated by acute bacterial endocarditis. Acta Paediatr Scand 1989;78: 463–464.

76. Americal Dental Association/American Academy of Orthopaedic Surgeons Expert Panel. Antibiotic prophylaxis for dental patients with total joint replacements. AAOS Bull; July 1997. Available at: http://www.aaos.org.

77. Hirschmann JV. Antimicrobial prophylaxis in dermatology. Semin Cutan Med Surg 2000;19:2–9.

78. Segreti J, Levin S. The role of prophylactic antibiotics in the prevention of prosthetic device infections. Infect Dis Clin North Am 1989;3:357–370.

7
Dehiscence and Necrosis

Ross M. Campbell and Raymond G. Dufresne, Jr.

Wound healing is comprised of a complex cycle of inflammation, proliferation, and remodeling. Vast numbers of cellular growth factors, cytokines, and cell types are involved. Recent research has provided new information that may enable clinicians to improve wound healing in the future. Although there is currently a wealth of knowledge about the science of wound healing, the incidence of acute wound failure has not decreased significantly in the last 75 years.[1]

Normal Wound Healing

Wound healing may be divided into four phases: hemostasis, inflammation, fibroproliferation or scar formation, and scar remodeling. Vasoconstriction, which is initiated by platelet plug formation, occurs during the first 5 to 10 minutes of wound healing. Platelets and clotting factors, which are activated by exposed collagen and basement membrane, begin the hemostatic response to injury. Prostaglandin (PG) F2a, thromboxane, and catecholamines mediate the transient vasoconstriction. Fibrin is produced as a result of the clotting cascade and provides the framework for the inflammatory responses that follow. Platelets release platelet-derived growth factor (PDGF) and transforming growth factor β (TGF-β), which initiate chemotaxis and proliferation of inflammatory cells in the fibrin matrix.[2]

The inflammatory stage of wound healing begins immediately after tissue injury. After hemostasis is obtained, vasodilation and increased endothelial cell permeability occur via histamine, PGE2, PGI2, and vascular endothelial cell growth factor (VEGF), which increase local blood flow and the influx of inflammatory cells. The polymorphonuclear leukocyte (PMN) is the first inflammatory cell type to invade the wound, attaining large numbers by 24 hours. PMNs begin the process of clearing the wound of devitalized tissue, clots, bacteria, extravasated serum proteins, and foreign material introduced at the time of injury. Macrophages follow the PMNs into the wounded tissue and proliferate over days 2 and 3 to assist in the removal of waste materials by phagocytosis. Macrophages are the source of numerous growth factors and cytokines, which induce fibroblast and endothelial cell proliferation and the production of the extracellular matrix. The extracellular matrix is the foundation for the proliferative phase of wound healing.[3]

Collagen synthesis is the hallmark of the fibroproliferative phase of wound healing and beginning of renewed structural integrity. Fibroblasts proliferate in response to growth factors released by macrophages to produce procollagen which, through enzymatic processes, forms an extensive cablelike network that provides increased tensile strength to the wound.[4] Neovascularization is induced by growth factors released by macrophages that regulate the growth and proliferation of endothelial cells to form new capillaries.

Collagen production continues for 2 to 3 weeks after wounding, at which point it reaches equilibrium and the remodeling phase of wound healing begins. Collagen generation continues, as does collagen degradation by collagenases, ultimately producing a more organized network of collagen fibers with more intermolecular bonds.[5] More type III collagen is produced initially, but after remodeling the ratio of type I : type III returns to 4 : 1, the normal adult ratio of collagen in the skin. The tensile strength of wounds is estimated to be 3% to 5% of nonwounded skin at 2 weeks, 15% at 3 weeks, and 35% at 4 weeks. Collagen organization in scars never achieves the degree of order that is found in normal, unwounded skin, but does reach approximately 70% of unwounded skin strength after 6 months.

Epithelialization occurs during the first 24 hours after tissue injury and provides no strength to a healing wound. Basal keratinocytes migrate from the wound margins to cover the wound tissue in 18 to 24 hours. The migration of basal keratinocytes may be impaired by bacteria, serous exudate (protein), or necrotic tissue. Impaired epithelialization leads to a prolonged inflammatory phase of healing that may contribute to unsatisfactory healing.

Wound healing is an elaborate system of clearing devitalized tissue, initiating new growth, and rebuilding tissue integrity. Many physiologic processes can impede wound healing and are important to address because they are also causes of wound failure, or dehiscence. Oxygen (O_2) is vital for the actively proliferating and metabolically stimulated cells involved in wound healing.[6] Oxygenation of new tissue is the primary determinant of wound healing. Suboptimal tissue O_2 levels have been clinically correlated with increased surgical complication rates. The initial wound bed is avascular with P_{O_2} levels approaching 0 mm Hg. Angiogenesis quickly brings the delivery of greatly needed oxygenated blood. PMNs require P_{O_2} levels of 25 mm Hg to produce superoxide radicals needed for bactericidal activity. Collagen synthesis is also dependent on tissue oxygen tension. Factors such as atherosclerosis, small vessel disease as seen in diabetes mellitus, local scarring and fibrosis, smoking-related arteriopathy, or even hypovolemia reduce the tissue O_2 levels to surrounding skin and impede wound healing.[7]

Edema impedes wound healing by impairing the delivery of essential nutrients and oxygenation. Whether due to inflammation, venous stasis, or other causes of edema, the increased extravascular and extracellular fluid causes a greater distance to form between cells and the delivery of oxygen. In cases of chronic edema, a persistent leakage of protein leads to a pericapillary cuffing, which further impedes oxygen delivery.

Necrotic tissue, blood, and exudate also impede wound healing. Large amounts of necrotic tissue are a barrier to healing, but even small amounts of debris will prolong inflammation and delay healing. Hematomas or seromas are physical barriers to wound healing, but also lead to tissue asphyxia by compressing vessels and cellular destruction by inducing cytotoxic free radicals. Devitalized tissue is also a breeding ground for bacterial colonization that may inhibit healing or potentially lead to more serious infectious complications.

Dehiscence

Wound dehiscence occurs when the wound edges fail to heal in apposition (Fig. 7-1A,B). This may be secondary to a multitude of factors including systemic causes associated with the patient's preoperative health condition, local factors of the wound environment, or surgical and/ or postoperative management error.

Many underlying health conditions may lead to impaired wound healing, thereby increasing the risk of wound dehiscence.[8-10] Hypoalbuminemia, vitamin C deficiency, and zinc deficiency, which can adversely affect collagen synthesis and thus decrease wound strength, are often indications of poor nutritional states. Medical conditions

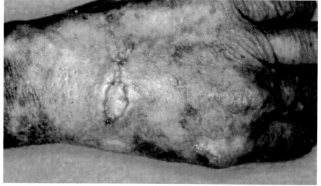

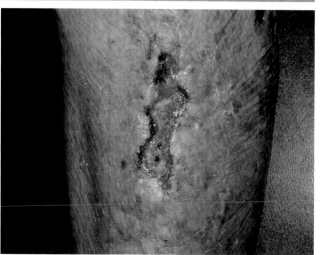

FIGURE 7-1. (A) Dehiscence of a sutured wound on the dorsal hand. (B) Dehiscence of a sutured wound on the shin of an elderly woman.

that may have a negative impact on wound healing include obesity, diabetes mellitus, uremia, hypertension, peripheral vascular disease, immunosuppression, thyroid disease, liver disease, Cushing disease, and congestive heart failure. Underlying malignancy or systemic infection may also impede wound healing because much of the patient's nutritional and inflammatory resources are already directed at these diseases. Patient age greater than 65 years and prolonged sun exposure often lead to thinning of the skin, which can increase the risk of wound failure.

Environmental stressors may increase the risk of dehiscence. The use of tobacco-containing products, especially smoking, has been shown to impair wound healing by decreased oxygenation of tissue and tissue perfusion. Excess physical activity after surgery and trauma to the surgical site may impair wound integrity. Certain anatomic sites, such as the back, chest, deltoids, and sebaceous areas of the face, are often sites of high tension and are prone to dehiscence.

Many medications may have adverse effects on wound healing. The negative effect of corticosteroids on wound healing is well known and must be considered when undergoing surgical procedure on any patient with a significant history of systemic steroid treatment (>30 mg/day).[11] Penicillamine, cyclosporine, metronidazole, and other cytotoxic chemotherapeutic agents have been demonstrated to impair wound healing.[12] Anticoagulants, antiplatelet medications, nonsteroidal anti-inflammatory medications, and aspirin may increase the risk of intraoperative and postoperative bleeding or hematoma and thus impair wound healing.

Local factors may directly impede wound healing and wound margin approximation. As mentioned previously, edema, blood products, and devitalized tissue are physical barriers to tissue healing. High bacterial levels and wound infection are also powerful impediments to wound healing. The use of proper sterile technique is important in the prevention of wound infection.

Perhaps the most preventable cause of wound dehiscence is poor surgical technique. Inadequate undermining may lead to excessive wound edge tension. The sheer mechanical force across the wound can inhibit the approximation of the wound margins and lead to wound failure. Surgeons may try to overcompensate for the tense closures by tying excessively tight sutures that only increase tissue strangulation and wound failure.[13] Excessive use of the cautery not only devitalizes tissue, but also creates an inflammatory response that impedes wound healing.[14] Hematomas and seromas may also result in dehiscence by increasing wound edge tension. Care must be taken intraoperatively to identify and properly ligate vessels and lymphatics to reduce the risk of hematoma or seroma formation.

Postoperatively, a common cause of wound dehiscence is removal of cutaneous sutures before adequate collagen production has occurred to provide adequate tensile strength to the wound. This is especially true in wounds that have not had sufficient buried dermal sutures placed to increase tensile strength. The tensile strength of wounds is estimated to be 3% to 5% of nonwounded skin at 2 weeks. Thus, the importance of buried dermal sutures in preventing dehiscence cannot be overemphasized. It has been recommended that cutaneous sutures placed on the face be removed in 5 to 7 days to reduce the amount of scarring at suture sites. Wounds sutured on the extremities and trunk may be left from 10 to 14 days, with sutures placed over areas of movement and tension allowed to remain closer to 2 weeks duration. Many of the risk factors for dehiscence are listed in Table 7-1.

TABLE 7-1. Risk factors for wound dehiscence.

Systemic
Age >65 years old
Nutrition (zinc, vitamin C, protein deficiency)
Obesity
Uremia
Cushing disease
Thyroid disease
Liver disease
Congestive heart failure
Pulmonary hypertension
Ascites
Hyperalimentation
Systemic infection
Malignancy
Peripheral vascular disease
Anemia
Edema
Diabetes

Surgical complications
Crush injury
Electrocautery
Hematoma
Infection
Tension

Medications
Anticoagulants
Aspirin
Colchicines
Systemic corticosteroids
Penicillamine
Cyclosporine
Metronidazole
B-Aminoproprionitrile
Cytotoxic/chemotherapeutic medications

Location
Chest
Back
Extremities
Sebaceous regions of face

Other
Smoking
Radiation
Physical activity
Trauma

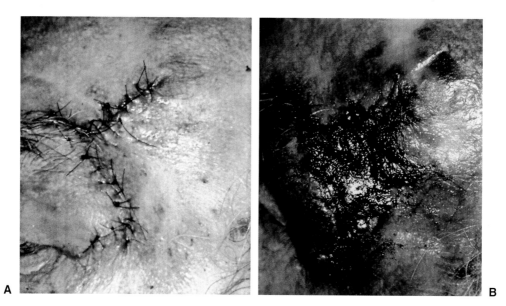

FIGURE 7-2. (A) Advancement flap demonstrating immediate postoperative pallor. (B) Flap necrosis 2 weeks postoperatively.

Wound Necrosis

Tissue necrosis occurs secondary to tissue ischemia (Fig. 7-2A,B). Necrosis differs from dehiscence in that the underlying pathology of necrosis is always the lack of adequate oxygenation of the healing wound tissue resulting in cell death, whereas dehiscence is a result of impaired healing, but not necessarily cell death. Any cause of decreased oxygenated blood flow to the involved tissue may contribute to tissue necrosis.

The primary cause of necrosis is excessive tension at the wound edges, either from insufficient undermining, poor surgical design, or expanding hematomas or seromas. Expanding hematomas or seromas may compress vessels that are bringing much-needed oxygenation and nutrients to the healing wound leading to tissue necrosis.[15] In addition, hematomas may lead to flap necrosis by a free radical–induced cytotoxic mechanism.[16,17] Patients on antiplatelet and/or anticoagulant medications near or at the time of surgery may be at increased risk of hematoma formation.

Necrosis may occur as a result of the surgical procedure itself if wound edges are sutured too tightly or if excessive cautery is performed in order to obtain hemostasis of the wound bed. Overzealous electrocautery may produce charred, necrotic, and devitalized tissue. It is difficult for neovascularization to occur in charred tissue.

Another common cause of tissue necrosis is poor flap design in the reconstruction of surgical defects. Blood supply may be decreased in flaps by compromised pedicles, excessive edema, venous congestion, hematomas, or

excessive superficial undermining, which can damage critical vessels in the subdermal plexus high in the subcutaneous fat. Flaps that exceed the 4:1 length-to-base ratio are at higher risk of necrosis secondary to poor circulation to the flap margins, particularly at the distal tip of the flap (Fig. 7-3). Skin grafts are also susceptible to tissue necrosis as a result of poor vascular supply at the base of the graft or lack of appropriate attachment to the base, allowing for movement, hematoma, or seroma formation (Fig. 7-4). Many of the risk factors for wound necrosis are the same as for wound dehiscence (Table 7-1), particularly the use of tobacco products, which decrease tissue perfusion and enhance vasoconstriction.

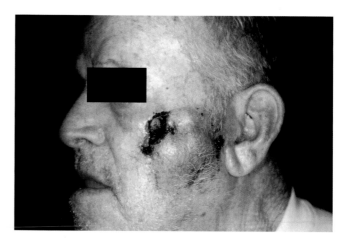

FIGURE 7-3. Tip necrosis of a rotation flap that exhibits venous congestion and edema.

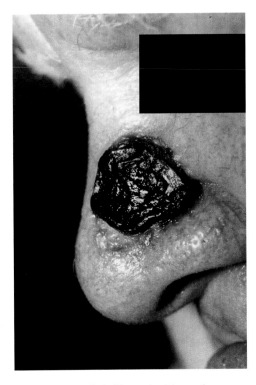

FIGURE 7-4. Necrotic skin graft.

Management

Dehiscence

Evaluation and monitoring of a surgical wound for signs of dehiscence are important for early detection. Wounds must be inspected for evidence of epithelialization, which should take place over the first 24 to 48 hours, to insure that the wound has not separated. Redness, heat, purulent exudate, edema, or pain are signs of infection and, if suspected, cultures should be obtained and empiric antibiotic therapy initiated, with further therapy dictated by culture results. The incision should have evidence of a palpable healing ridge by postoperative day 5. Absence of a ridge by postoperative day 9 signals delayed healing and a significant risk for wound dehiscence. Most dehiscences occur between postoperative days 5 and 8.[18]

In general, dehisced wounds that are clean, such as those due to premature suture removal or trauma, may be resutured. In addition, dehisced wounds from which uncomplicated hematomas can be completely evacuated may also be resutured depending on the site. Devitalized tissue should be removed before resuturing, but the surgeon should not "freshen" the wound margins by active debridement because this will remove fibroblasts that have migrated to the wound margins and are producing collagen for wound healing.[10] Alternatively, steri-strips may be considered in some cases for management of linear dehiscence and are beneficial in that the wound

is left partially open for drainage and no local anesthesia or debridement is required.[19]

Dehiscence associated with complicated hematomas or infection should be managed like other acute open wounds and allowed to heal by second intention with attention given to appropriate topical therapy, providing nutritional and circulatory support, and reducing comorbidities that interfere with healing. Gentle cleansing with warm water will assist with debridement of necrotic tissue. Topical antibiotics are sometimes appropriate to reduce bacterial burden in wounds that have a higher suspicion of infection or of becoming infected. In most cases, petrolatum alone will provide an optimum environment for granulation tissue formation and epithelial migration.

In wounds with little necrotic tissue and exudate, a layer of petrolatum followed by damp gauze may be applied to the wound and covered with a transparent adhesive dressing (e.g., Tegaderm™; 3 M Corporation, St. Paul, MN). This is a simple dressing that requires changing only 1 to 2 times a week and provides an optimum environment for wound healing by keeping the wound moist. It provides an effective bacterial barrier, a moist environment, and can absorb small volumes of exudate to allow wound healing.

Wounds that appear to have evidence of a high bioburden will need an additional layer to their dressings. In these wounds, an antimicrobial silver dressing (e.g., Silvercel™; Johnson & Johnson Medical, New Brunswick, NJ) in contact with the wound can be used in combination with dry gauze to increase absorption of exudates. Both silver dressing and dry gauze are then covered with foam dressing. These dressings may only need to be changed 2 to 3 times a week, but increased exudate may require more frequent changes. As the wound exudate decreases, partial closure of the wound may be considered in selected cases.[18]

Chronic, nonhealing wounds are particularly problematic, especially on the extremities and in patients with poor circulation. In these patients, wound care can be administered as described above, but the surgeon should warn patients that these wounds might take an extended period to time to heal. The addition of hyperbaric oxygen chambers or vacuum-assisted wound healing devices may be beneficial in some difficult cases.

Necrosis

Tissue necrosis may be defined as tissue cell death. The depth of necrosis depends on the degree of vascular compromise. Regardless of the level of tissue death, an eschar forms which eventually separates from the wound bed and may result in the formation of a scar. Treatment of tissue necrosis is conservative (Fig. 7-5A,B). The necrotic area should be allowed to fully demarcate before

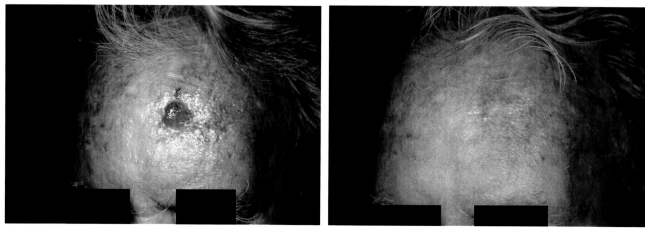

A   B

FIGURE 7-5. (A) Ulcer after scar separation at the site of flap necrosis 3 weeks postoperatively. (B) Complete healing after conservative wound care with a good cosmetic result 8 weeks postoperatively.

debridement to prevent unnecessary damage to viable tissue beneath the eschar. Once the eschar begins to separate from the wound bed, careful, sharp debridement may be undertaken with care to excise only necrotic tissue. After debridement, the wound bed should be treated as an open wound and allowed to heal by second intention and cared for as described in the management of dehisced wounds. Necrotic wounds are especially prone to infection and systemic antibiotics should be considered.

Prevention

The prevention of wound dehiscence and necrosis is fundamental to successful surgical outcomes. Unfortunately, many of the risk factors for these two complications cannot be avoided or overcome in the short time between the initial surgical consultation and the intended procedure. However, patients with identifiable risk factors for wound failure should be evaluated carefully in the immediate postoperative period before suture removal, with attention given to signs of proper wound healing.

Smoking has been identified as an important risk factor for wound failure, infection, and necrosis. Some of the effects of nicotine are reversible and can be decreased if the patient will stop smoking for as little as 2 days before surgery and 1 week after surgery. Recommendations in the literature for perioperative cessation of smoking range from 1 day to 4 weeks preoperatively and from 5 days to 4 weeks postoperatively, with a preponderance of recent recommendations advising the latter of these time periods.[20,21]

Proper surgical technique will help prevent tissue necrosis and wound dehiscence. Adequate undermining and placement of buried dermal sutures should alleviate wound edge tension. Tissue should be handled gently and the use of skin hooks may decrease the amount of acci-

dental crushing of tissue with forceps. If forceps are utilized, forceps with 1×2 teeth are preferable to forceps with smooth jaws or serrated platforms. Careful hemostasis will reduce the risk of hematoma formation, but care must be taken to not unnecessarily overcauterize viable tissue. Large vessels should be ligated with suture to prevent hematoma formation. The surgeon should consider postoperative edema when choosing a suturing technique and the type of suture to close the wound. Suture with high elasticity, such as prolene or nylon, will allow some expansion of the wound with edema and decrease strangulation of tissue. Running as opposed to interrupted sutures also allow for expansion of the wound with edema and may decrease risk of tissue necrosis.

Good postoperative management of surgical wounds may help reduce the incidence of wound failure. Adequate pain control is important because the pain response can cause vasoconstriction that may be detrimental to neovascularization and the influx of nutrients and oxygen to the healing wound bed. Management with ice packs and elevation may be helpful in the initial 24 hours postoperatively to decrease edema. However, warmth to the affected area after 24 hours may also increase circulation, especially on extremities, which is beneficial to wound healing. In patients with low oxygenation (e.g., chronic obstructive pulmonary disease or COPD), supplemental oxygenation may be helpful for initial wound healing stages. Tight glucose control is needed in diabetic patients to optimize wound healing. The use of taping, adhesive strips, polyurethane adhesive dressings, and slings may be effective reminders to limit activity of the affected areas.

The recommendations of the Centers for Disease Control and Prevention (CDC) for postoperative wound care state that a sterile dressing should be placed for the first 24 to 48 hours postoperatively. The status of showering after surgery is classified as "unresolved" by the CDC, although generally permitted after 48 hours.[22] Petrolatum, which is known to increase reepithelization time and thereby decrease scarring, promotes the natural flora, which has been shown to be beneficial to wound healing. Although the use of topical antibiotics for postoperative wound management is common, studies have not demonstrated a consistent decrease in the incidence of postoperative wound infection.[23,24] Many topical antibiotics are known to cause contact dermatitis in some patients. Several studies have shown no difference in infection rates between surgical wounds treated with petrolatum verses topical antibiotics.[25,26]

Wound dehiscence and necrosis are feared complications of cutaneous surgery. The surgeon can reduce the risk of these complications by careful evaluation and history taking to identify risk factors in patients, good surgical technique, and appropriate postoperative management of patients at increased risk for wound failure.

References

1. Wassermann RJ, Polo M, Smith PD, et al. Differential production of apoptosis modulating proteins in patients with hypertrophic burn scar. J Surg Res 1998;75:74–79.
2. Dubay DA, Franz MG. Acute wound healing: the biology of acute wound failure. Surg Clin North Am 2003;83:463–481.
3. Fine NA, Mustoe TA. Wound Healing. In: Greenfield LJ, Mulholland MW, Oldham KT, Zelenock GB, Lillemow KD, eds. Surgery: scientific principles and practice. 3rd ed. Philadelphia: Lippincott Williams & Wilkins; 2001:69–87.
4. Morgan CJ, Pledger WJ. Fibroblast proliferation. In: Cohen IH, Diegelmann RF, Lindblad WJ, eds. Wound healing: biochemical and clinical aspects. Philadelphia: Saunders; 1991:63–76.
5. Madden JW, Peacock EE. Studies on the biology of collagen during wound healing: I. Rate of collagen synthesis and deposition in cutaneous wounds of the rat. Surgery 1968; 64:288.
6. LaVan FB, Hunt TK. Oxygen and wound healing. Clin Plast Surg 1990;17:463.
7. Jonsson K, Jensen JA, Goodson WH 3rd, et al. Tissue oxygenation, anemia, and perfusion in relation to wound healing in surgical patients. Ann Surg 1991;214:6.
8. Dufresne RG. Surgical complication: prevention, recognition, and treatment. In: Ratz JL, ed. Textbook of dermatologic surgery. Philadelphia: Lippincott-Raven; 1998:59–63.
9. Koyama H, Isshiki N, Noda R, Nishimura R. Long-term survival of a split-thickness skin graft on a large seroma. Plast Reconstr Surg 1987;79:110–113.
10. Salasche SJ. Acute surgical complications: cause, prevention, and treatment. J Am Acad Dermatol 1986;15:1163–1185.
11. Levenson SM, Demetriou AA. Metabolic factors. In: Cohen IH, Diegelmann RF, Lindblad WJ, eds. Wound healing: biochemical and clinical aspects. Philadelphia: Saunders; 1991:248–273.
12. Lawrence C. Drug management in skin surgery. Drugs 1996;52:805–817.
13. Hogstrom H, Haglund U, Zederfeldt B. Tension leads to increased neutrophil accumulation and decreased laparotomy wound strength. Surgery 1990;107:215–219.
14. Rappaport WD, Hunter GC, Allen R, et al. Effect of electrocautery on wound healing in midline laparatomy incisions. Am J Surg 1991;160:618–620.
15. Riou JP, Cohen JR, Johnson H. Factors influencing wound dehiscence. Am J Surg 1992;163:324–330.
16. Angel MF, Narayanan, Swartz WM, et al. The etiologic role of free radicals in hematoma-induced flap necrosis. Plastic Reconstr Surg 1986;77:795–803.
17. Diaz DD, Freeman SB, Wilson JF, Parker GS. Hematoma-induced flap necrosis and free radical scavengers. Arch Otolaryngol Head Neck Surg 1992;118:516–518.
18. Doughty DB. Preventing and managing surgical wound dehiscence. Home Health Nurse 2004;22:364–367.
19. Khachemoune A, Krejci-Papa N, Finn DT, Rogers GS. Dehisced clean wound: resuture it or steri-stip it? Dermatol Surg 2004;30:431–432.
20. Krueger JK, Rohrich RJ. Clearing the smoke: the scientific rationale for tobacco abstention with plastic surgery. Plast Reconstr Surg 2001;108:1063–1073.
21. Wong LS, Martins-Green M. Firsthand cigarette smoke alters fibroblast migration and survival: implications for impaired healing. Wound Repair Regen 2004;12:471–484.
22. Mangram AJ, Horan TC, Pearson ML, Silver LC, Jarvis WR. Guideline for prevention of surgical site infection, 1999. Hospital Infection Control Practices Advisory Committee. Infect Control Hosp Epidemiol 1999;20:250–257.
23. Dire DJ, Coppola M, Dwyer DA, Lorette JJ, Karr JL. Prospective evaluation of topical antibiotics for preventing infections in uncomplicated soft-tissue wounds repaired in the ED. Acad Emerg Med 1995;2:4–10.
24. Mackway-Jones K. Towards evidence based emergency medicine: best BETs from Manchester Royal Infirmary. Emerg Med J 2002;19:550–557.
25. Smack DP, Harrington AC, Dunn C, et al. Infection and allergy incidence in ambulatory surgery patients using white petrolatum vs bacitracin ointment. A randomized controlled trial. JAMA 1996;276:972–977.
26. Campbell RM, Perlis CS, Fisher E, Gloster HM. Gentamycin ointment versus petrolatum for management of auricular wounds. Dermatol Surg 2005;31:664–669.

Section II
Chronic Surgical Complications

8
Hypertrophic Scars and Keloids

A. Paul Kelly

The development of hypertrophic scars (HS) and keloids are two dreaded complications of cutaneous surgery. Keloids, though medically benign, are often psychologically and socially problematic. Hypertrophic scars are elevated, thickened, and are often red, pruritic, or painful. Hypertrophic scars usually stay within the confines of the precipitating trauma, while keloids invade surrounding clinically normal skin. Keloids may also be pruritic and painful. Hypertrophic scars usually develop rapidly after cutaneous trauma, whereas keloids develop slowly but continue to enlarge for months to years. In most instances, HS regress with therapy in contrast to keloids, which often recur during therapy or when therapy is discontinued. The differences and similarities of keloids and HS are listed in Table 8-1.

The medical literature regarding HS and keloids is often confusing because many lesions which are keloids have wrongfully been called HS and vice versa. Some patients have both kinds of scars as a result of the same traumatic incident. Furthermore, clinical studies often lump the two disorders together, thus leading to dissemination of incorrect information, especially when evaluating therapeutic response.

Prevention of keloids is extremely important and nonessential surgery should be withheld from known keloid formers. Numerous treatments for HS and keloids have been utilized but lack completely satisfactory outcomes and sometimes cause significant side effects. There is no one therapeutic modality that is uniformly successful for keloids and HS and polytherapy is usually superior to monotherapy. This chapter will review the efficacy of the current therapeutic modalities available for the treatment of keloids and HS.

Keloids and HS are thought to be produced by an overgrowth of fibrous tissue secondary to a variety of causes such as wound edge tension, foreign-body reactions, infections, hormonal factors, genetic predisposition, a deficiency in metalloproteinases, or in most cases, trauma [e.g., burns (Fig. 8-1), lacerations (Fig. 8-2), surgical incisions (Figs. 8-3, 8-4), ear piercing (Fig. 8-5), vaccinations (Fig. 8-6), acne (Fig. 8-7), and insect bites]. Most keloids develop within 1 year of the precipitating trauma. There are, however, a small percentage of patients who develop keloids spontaneously with no known antecedent trauma. These types of lesions occur most often in patients with a family history of keloids and are usually located on the mid-chest area. Except for burn patients, most keloids occur in the second or third decade, although they may develop from infancy to old age. Early indications for abnormal scarring include erythema that persists and increases after 1 month, and the appearance of erythema 1 to 2 months postoperatively, particularly if associated with pruritus and pain. Early keloid formation may begin with a change of color from red to purple.

There are many strategies the physician may use to prevent the occurrence of keloids. First, nonessential cosmetic surgery should be withheld from known keloid formers (those with only earlobe keloids should not be considered keloid formers). Third, keloid formers who develop acne or varicella should be treated early and aggressively. Second, surgery on the mid-chest, an area notorious for keloid and hypertrophic scar formation, should be avoided if possible. Fourth, incisions should be as small as possible and should not cross highly mobile sites such as joint spaces and should follow relaxed skin tension lines whenever possible. Fifth, postoperative sites should be closed under minimal tension. Sixth, avoid surgery on keloid-prone areas (e.g., central chest, jawline, anterior neck, upper back, and deltoid area) should be avoided in patients with a family history of keloid formation. Seventh, delaying suture removal should be considered to avoid dehiscence. Eighth, wound infections, which may stimulate keloid formation, should be promptly treated with appropriate antibiotics. Ninth, buried sutures should be avoided if possible and long acting absorbable sutures, which tend to be less reactive, should be utilized if subcutaneous sutures

TABLE 8-1. Keloids compared to hypertrophic scars.

Property	Keloid	Hypertrophic scars
Stays in confines of injury	No	Yes
Precipitated by trauma	Not always	Yes
Area of occurrence	Area of little motion	Area of motion
Growth	For extended period	Regress in time
Symptomatic	Usually	Usually
Response to treatment	Poor	Good
Sodium (osmotic pressure)	Normal	Decreased
Magnesium (metabolic activity)	Increased	Decreased
Calcium (reflects collagen metabolism)	Increased	Decreased
Mucinous ground substance	Abundant	Scanty
Fibroblasts	Few	Numerous
Foreign-body reactions	None	Frequent
Luxol fast blue collagen stain	Reddish	Blue
Mast cells	Increased	Increased
Pathogenesis	Unknown	Unknown
Contains myofibroblasts	No	Yes
Alanine transaminase	Increased	Normal

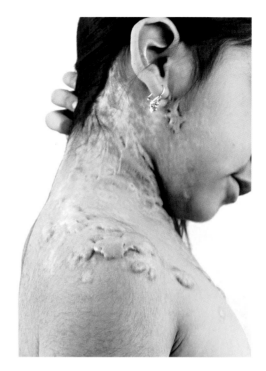

FIGURE 8-1. Patient with scarring secondary to a burn. She has hypertrophic scars on her neck and keloids on her shoulder.

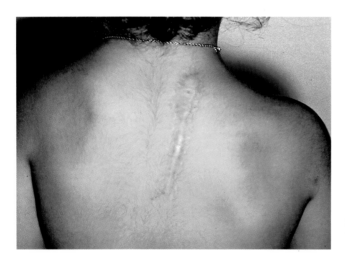

FIGURE 8-2. Hypertrophic scar on a patient's back secondary to a laceration.

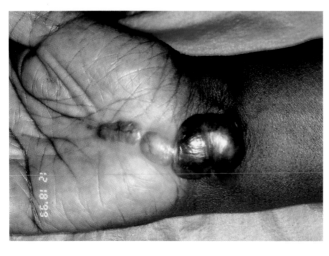

FIGURE 8-3. Keloids on right wrist secondary to surgery for carpal tunnel syndrome.

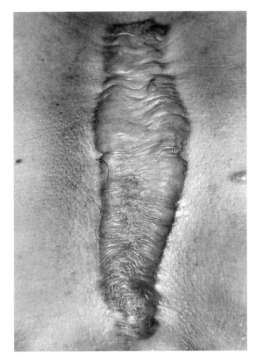

FIGURE 8-4. Vertical keloid on mid-chest area secondary to cardiac bypass surgery.

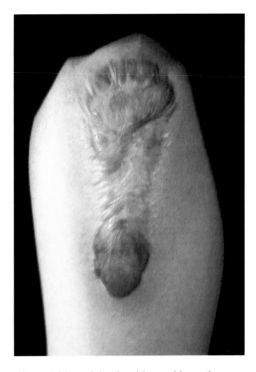

FIGURE 8-6. Keloid on right shoulder and lateral arm secondary to vaccination.

are necessary. Finally, all potential sources of persistent inflammation should be excised, including epithelial cysts, sinus tracts, trapped hair follicles, or foreign bodies.

Intralesional Steroids

Intralesional steroids (ILS) have been the cornerstone for managing keloids and HS for many years, both as primary and adjunctive therapy. As primary treatment, ILS may reduce scar elevation, thickness, pruritus, and pain in both keloids and HS. When used adjunctively, ILS may be combined with excision, silicone, pulse dye laser, or other modalities. Injections must be placed into the scar and not subcutaneously to decrease the risk of tissue atrophy.[1] Initially, the scar may be very difficult to inject.

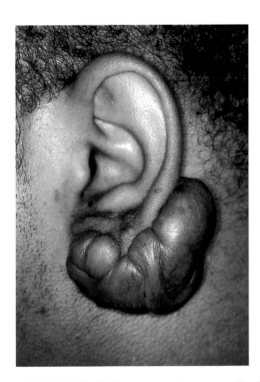

FIGURE 8-5. Keloid of left ear secondary to ear piercing.

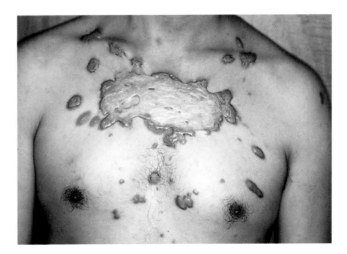

FIGURE 8-7. Keloids on chest secondary to acne.

However, with repeated injections the scar will soften and resistance to injection will decrease.

Intralesional steroids are best injected with a 27- to 30-gauge needle on a narrow-bore syringe (e.g., an insulin syringe). Larger bore needles often become plugged, especially if the keloid is hard. Multiple horizontal tracts are made with the needle and steroid is deposited into the tract. The needle hole may be plugged with tape or tissue adhesive to prevent steroid from leaking out of the injection site. A blanched appearance to the scar is the endpoint of each session. Blanching may be difficult to visualize in dark skin. The injections should be given every 2 to 4 weeks until the keloid or HS flattens. The amount injected varies according to physician preference but typically ranges from 10 to 40mg/mL. Intralesional triamcinolone acetonide (TAC), 10 to 40mg/mL, every 2 to 3 weeks followed by the daily (18–20 hours) application of flurandrenolide (Cordran®) tape or Curad Scar Therapy is usually successful in causing HS to regress.

The author prefers a maximum of 1mL of 40mg/mL of TAC. Adrenal suppression has never occurred at this dose in the author's hands. Each time the patient returns for injection the keloid(s) should be checked for a partial or complete erythematous border which, if present, indicates that the keloid is active and enlarging. Border activity is amenable to V beam or pulsed dye laser.

Intralesional corticosteroids may be unsuccessful due to utilization of an inadequate concentration of TAC (less than 10mg/mL), injection of an insufficient amount of material, or injection within the subcutaneous fat or deep dermis instead of the papillary dermis.

There is no single therapeutic modality that successfully treats keloids. Adjunctive TAC 10 to 20mg/mL may be administered intradermally at the time of surgical excision and continued postoperatively every 4 weeks.[2] Berman and Bieley reported that surgical excision as a monotherapy was fraught with a greater than 50% recurrence rate.[3] In the same study, excisional surgery with intralesional TAC had a recurrence rate of almost as high as surgical monotherapy.

Prior to keloid excision, corticosteroid can be mixed with local anesthetic, usually as a half-and-half mixture of 1% lidocaine with epinephrine and TAC 40mg/mL. This technique seems to have an inhibitory effect on keloid reformation. However, there may be a theoretical increased risk of dehiscence if corticosteroids are mixed with local anesthetic preoperatively due to adverse effects of the steroid on wound healing. Dehiscence may be avoided by leaving sutures in place an extra 7 days and by refraining from injecting the surgical site with corticosteroids for at least 2 weeks after suture removal. Fortunately, dehiscence has not been reported with intraoperative ILS.[4]

All patients receiving ILS injections should be forewarned that 3mg/mL of TAC or greater concentration may cause the injected area to become hypopigmented and remain so for 6 to 12 months. Other adverse effects of intralesional steroids include atrophy, telangiectasias, and steroid precipitation (dermal yellowish deposits).

The pain associated with the injection can be lessened by applying cool compresses or a topical anesthetic with occlusion on the keloid an hour prior to surgery. If the injection is still too painful for the patient, the area of clinically normal skin surrounding the keloid may be injected with local anesthetic, which will allow the keloid to be anesthetized enough for the patient to tolerate the intralesional corticosteroid injections. Finally, freezing the keloid with liquid nitrogen for 10 to 15 seconds, then waiting a minute or two, will induce edema and make corticosteroid injections into the keloid much easier and less painful.

Pressure Therapy

Pressure therapy may be used alone or in concert with other therapies in the treatment of HS and keloids. In pressure therapy, a compression garment or device is used to apply constant pressure to the scar. Often 15 to 45mmHg of pressure is sufficient.[5] Pressure therapy must be maintained for nearly 24 hours and is most effective for early scars. Compression should be applied for several (4–6) months for best results. An indicator of progress is reduction of erythema. Following keloid excision, pressure may be combined with silicone gel sheets to prevent recurrences.[6,7] Pressure therapy is often hot and uncomfortable, which reduces patient compliance.

Silicone

Silicone gel sheets (SGS) are effective in increasing scar pliability and reducing thickness, elevation, pain, and pruritus of both HS and keloids,[8,9] although generally HS tend to respond to SGS better than keloids. The therapeutic benefits of SGS are not derived from silicone, but from scar occlusion and hydration, which inhibit fibroblast proliferation.[10] Improvement of scars occurs in 70% to 90% of patients.[11] Silicone gel sheets, which must be applied to the scar at least 12 hours, may be combined with other therapeutic modalities (e.g., ILS and compression). Silicone gel sheets may also be used prophylactically to prevent HS or keloids after surgery in high-risk areas.[11] The greatest virtue of SGS is its low side-effect profile.

Cryotherapy

Cryotherapy with liquid nitrogen may also be employed as a monotherapeutic agent. Cryotherapy induces edema, microcirculatory disturbances, stasis, thrombosis, anoxia, and tissue necrosis in scar tissue. A freeze time of 30 to 40 seconds followed by a 1 minute rest with 1 to 3 freeze–thaw cycles at 3- to 4-week intervals for 5 to 10 sessions has been successful in reducing scar elevation and thickness.[12,13] However, the morbidity (i.e., blistering, swelling, ulceration, drainage, and pain), especially for large lesions, is not well tolerated by most patients. Again, patients should be forewarned because freezing more than 25 seconds may produce hypopigmentation that could persist 12 to 18 months or permanently.

Radiation Therapy

Radiation therapy (RT), which inhibits fibroblasts and may have effects on cutaneous vasculature, may be used as a monotherapy or combined with surgery to prevent keloids from recurring after surgical excision. As monotherapy, RT has a recurrence rate of 50% to 100% and is no better than excision alone.[14] RT is most effective in the treatment of early, thin keloids. Mature, thicker keloids often require surgery prior to RT. Although RT may not completely cure a keloid, it may eliminate the frequent pain, pruritus, and tenderness that accompany these lesions.

Radiation therapy is effective as an adjunct to excision.[15,16] Radiation therapy may be delivered as an external beam, interstitial implants, or high-dose brachytherapy. External beam radiation therapy is more successful in preventing recurrence when given within an hour or two after surgery. The usual doses are 300 rads (3 Gy) every other day for 5 days, or 500 rads (5 Gy) every other day for 3 days. A combination of pre- and postoperative irradiation has no greater efficacy than postoperative irradiation alone. In one study, high-dose brachytherapy was administered at a dose of 1200 Gy, which was delivered in four equal fractions over the first 24 hours after surgery.[16] The recurrence rate was limited to 4.7%. Cosmetic results were also good to excellent.

Side effects of RT include atrophy, alopecia, and acute and chronic radiation dermatitis. Although most studies utilizing RT to treat keloids report no carcinogenic risk,[17] the potential long-term risk for radiation-induced malignancies precludes the use of RT as primary therapy for keloids, particularly in young patients.

Lasers

The efficacy of lasers in treating keloids is still unclear. Argon, carbon dioxide, and Nd:YAG lasers decrease fibroblast activity in vitro but have yielded variable, inconsistent results when treating patients in vivo. Recurrence rates with these lasers have been high, probably due to nonspecific thermal injury to surrounding tissue.

The Q-switched, frequency-doubled 532 nm Nd:YAG laser is absorbed by hemoglobin (leading to destruction of the vascularity of the scar) and melanocytes (leading to reduction of the pigmentation of the scar).[18] Treatment with this laser resulted in statistically significant improvement in pigmented, hypertrophic scars in a small study.[18]

The 585 nm or 595 nm pulse dye laser (PDL) may improve erythema, thickness, and pliability of HS and keloids.[16,19] The PDL, which is absorbed by oxygenated hemoglobin, causes thermal injury to the scar's microvasculature, which leads to thrombosis and ischemia, ultimately resulting in reduced collagen and collagen remodeling.[20] Erythematous HS (e.g., early sternotomy scars) and keloids are, therefore, most likely to respond to PDL therapy.[20]

The most common side effects of the 585 nm PDL are posttreatment purpura, which usually subsides after 7 to 10 days, and pigmentary alterations, which are more commonly seen in skin of color.[21] The PDL may cause blistering and worsening of the scars appearance if used at excessive fluences. Consequently, minimal purpuric or subpurpuric endpoints are recommended.

The PDL may be used in combination with ILS. In one study, PDL followed by TAC 10 mg/mL improved lesion height, erythema, pruritus, and pain in 7 of 14 patients.[22] The author also believed the PDL created edema in the lesion that facilitated steroid injection.

Interferon Therapy

Injectable interferon (IFN) reduces scar formation by increasing collagenase activity and inhibiting fibroblast production of collagen and glycosaminoglycans.[23] Injected IFN α-2b, when used as monotherapy, reduced the size of existing keloids by 50%.[24] When combined with excision, IFN reduces the recurrence of keloids. Berman and Flores reported an 18.7% recurrence rate (vs. 51.1% in excision alone and 58.5% with excision with TAC) when interferon α-2b injections were given immediately after surgical excision of keloids.[23] One million units were injected intradermally into each linear centimeter of the surgical site (up to 5 million units) per day immediately after surgery and 1 to 2 weeks postoperatively. In the same study, there was a 51% recurrence rate with surgery alone and a 58% recurrence rate with surgery and TAC.

Interferon has also been used with modest success in combination with the carbon dioxide laser in the treatment of keloids.[25] One study reported no recurrences in 16 patients on the ear and 10 recurrences in 14 patients on the trunk with 3 years follow-up.[25]

Patients should be given acetaminophen preoperatively to prevent interferon-induced flulike symptoms such as fever, myalgias, headache, and arthralgias. Another limiting factor for using INF is its high cost.

Imiquimod

Topical imiquimod 5% cream (Aldara™; 3M Pharmaceuticals, Minneapolis, MN) induces local production of interferons at the site of application within 2 hours. Application to open wounds does not appear to inhibit healing. In a small pilot study involving 12 earlobe keloids and 1 back keloid, therapy was begun immediately after surgery with continued application daily for 8 weeks.[26] Although the back keloid recurred, no recurrences were noted after 6 months in all earlobe patients. In another small study of 12 patients, topical imiquimod prevented keloid recurrence in 10 patients with 6 months follow-up.[27] Patients with large surgical sites, postoperative site(s) closed with tension, or flaps or grafts should not start imiquimod cream for 4 to 6 weeks after surgery to avoid possible dehiscence.

Irritation, inflammation, burning, and pain may occur during treatment with imiquimod and rest periods during therapy may be required. Patients should also be monitored for signs of secondary bacterial infection such as increasing pain, erythema, purulence, and odor.

5-Flurouracil

Intralesional 5-flurouracil (5FU) decreases fibroblast proliferation and the production of collagen leading to an increase in scar pliability and reduction in scar elevation, thickness, pain, pruritus, and redness. The use of intralesional 5FU (alone or in combination with TAC) for HS has been effective, although results with keloids have been less favorable.[28,29] 5FU has been touted by some clinicians as effective monotherapy for small keloids.[28]

In 1999, Fitzpatrick reported his 9-year experience with 1000 patients.[28] In this study, 0.05 mL of a 50 mg/mL solution of 5FU was injected every 1 cm to a total dose of 2 to 50 mg per session once weekly. The best results were obtained in early lesions that were erythematous, symptomatic, and indurated. Old, stable lesions responded poorly.

Manuskiatti and Fitzpatrick utilized multiple modalities (ILS alone, ILS and 5FU, 5FU alone, PDL alone) and obtained comparable results.[29] In a study by Kontochristopoulos and colleagues, 17 of 20 patients with keloids showed more than 50% improvement.[30] All 20 of their patients reported pain and hyperpigmentation of the injection site and 6/20 patients experienced tissue sloughing. Recurrence was noted in 9 of 19 patients within 1 year. Side effects, which include pain, ulceration, and hyperpigmentation, are usually temporary.[31,32] Neither skin atrophy nor telangiectasias have been noted in scars following treatment with IL 5FU.[28]

The addition of TAC [0.1 mL of TAC (10 mg/mL)] to 5FU [0.9 mL of 5FU (50 mg/mL)] in a 9:1 ratio in the same syringe may improve efficacy and reduce pain.[29] The mixture is initially injected into the keloid(s) three times a week the first week and then weekly. Up to 5 sessions may be necessary before benefits are obtained. The frequency may then be decreased based on response.

Other Medical Therapies

Intralesinal Bleomycin

Intralesional bleomycin may be useful in the treatment of small keloids and HS. Espana and colleagues treated 13 patients with keloids and HS by applying bleomycin (1.5 IU/mL) to the surface of the lesion, which was subsequently punctured (after instituting local anesthesia) repeatedly with a 25-gauge needle.[33] Patients received two to five treatments at 1- to 4-month intervals. Three of seven keloids flattened completely and some partially resolved. There were two recurrences at 10 months and 12 months.

Verapamil

Verapamil is a calcium channel blocker that decreases collagen production and enhances collagenase synthesis, thus reducing fibrous tissue formation. In one small study, verapamil 2.5 mg/mL was injected into hypertrophic burn scars in 5 patients.[34] Three of five scars became softer, flatter, and less erythematous. In another study, verapamil 2.5 mg/mL (0.5–2 mL each visit) was injected monthly into 45 earlobe keloids resulting in an 85% cure rate with a mean follow-up of 28 months.[35] D'Andrea and colleagues compared postoperative intralesional verapamil (1.25–5 mg) and SGS (22 patients) to SGS alone (22 patients) and obtained an 18% cure rate for the latter with 18 months follow-up.[36]

Tacrolimus

Tacrolimus, an immunomodulator, is an immunosuppressive agent that inhibits T-cell activation. Keloidal fibroblasts overexpress gli-1 oncogene, a possible cause of cellular transformation.[37,38] Tacrolimus is thought to inhibit gli-1 signal transduction.[39] Resolution of a keloid was noted in a patient treated with topical tacrolimus for atopic dermatitis.[37]

Others

Case reports of other medical therapies exist in the literature. Further studies of these modalities with larger numbers of patients will be necessary before valid conclusions can be made about their efficacy in the treatement of keloids and HS. These agents include zinc tape,[40] pentoxifylline,[41,42] colchicine,[43] methotrexate,[44] and D-penicillamine.[45]

Keloids and hypertrophic scars pose a tremendous challenge to the physician performing cutaneous surgery. Patients should be prepared for a lengthy treatment plan. Given the myriad possible medications and/or surgical techniques, none of which are uniformly successful therapeutic modalities, it will be necessary to continue to search for a true gold standard of therapy with a low recurrence rate.

References

1. Ketchum LD, Smith J, Robinson DW, Masters FW. The treatment of hypertrophic scar, keloid scar and scar contracture by triamcinolone acetonide. Plast Recostr Surg 1996;38:209–218.
2. Kelly PA. Medical and surgical therapies for keloids. Dermatol Ther 2004;17:212–218.
3. Berman B, Bieley HC. Adjunct therapies to surgical management of keloids. Dermatol Surg 1966;22:126–130.
4. Giovannini UM. Treatment of scars by steroid injections. Wound Repair Regen 2002;17:212–218.
5. Kerckhove EV, Stappaerts K, Fieuws S, et al. The assessment of erythema and thickness on burn related scars during pressure garment therapy as a preventive measure for hypertrophic scarring. Burns 2005;6:Epub ahead of print.
6. Chang CH, Song JY, Park JH, Seo SW. The efficacy of magnetic disks for the treatment of earlobe hypertrophic scar. Ann Plast Surg 2005;54:566–569.
7. Russell R, Horlock N, Gault D. Zimmer splintage: as simple effective treatment for keloids following ear piercing. Br J Plast Surg 2001;54:509–510.
8. Kerckhove EV, Stappaerts K, Boeckx W, et al. Silicones in the rehabilitation of burns: a review and overview. Burns 2001;27:205–214.
9. Hamanova H, Broz L. Topigel in the treatment of hypertrophic scars after burn injuries. Acta Chir Plast 2002;44:18–22.
10. Borgognoni L. Biological effects of silicone gel sheeting. Wound Repair Regen 2002;10:118–121.
11. Gold MH. A controlled clinical trial of topical silicone gel sheeting in the treatment of hypertrophic scars and keloids. J Am Acad Dermatol 1994;30:506–507.
12. Rusciani L, Rosse G, Bono R. Use of cryotherapy in the treatment of keloids. J Dermatol Surg Oncol 1993;19:529–534.
13. Ceilley RI, Barin RW. The combined use of cryosurgery and intralesional injections of suspension of fluorinated adrenocorticosteroids for reducing keloids and hypertrophic scars. J Dermatol Surg Oncol 1979;5;54.
14. Borok TL, Bray N, Sinclair I, et al. Role of ionizing irradiation for 343 keloids. Int J Radiat Oncol Biol Phys 1998;15:836–870.
15. Garg MK, Weiss P, Sharma AK, et al. Adjuvant high dose rate brachytherapy (Ir-192) in the management of keloids which have recurred after surgical excision and external beam radiation. Radiother Oncol 2004;73:233–236.
16. Guix B, Henriquez I, Andres A, et al. Treatment of keloids by high-dose rate brachytherapy: a seven year study. Int J Radiat Oncol Biol Phys 2001;50:167–172.
17. Botwood N, Lewanski C, Lowdell C. The risks of treating keloids with radiotherapy. Br J Radiol 1999;72:1222–1224.
18. Bowes LE, Nouri K, Berman B, et al. Treatment of pigmented hypertrophic scars with the 585 nm pulsed dye laser and the 532 nm frequency-doubled Nd:YAG laser in the Q-switched and variable pulse modes: a comparative study. Dermatol Surg 2002;28:714–719.
19. Clavere P, Bedane C, Bonnetblanc JM, Bonnafoux-Clavere A, Rousseau J. Postoperative interstitial radiotherapy of keloids by iridium 192: a retrospective study of 46 treated scars. Dermatology 1997;195:349–352.
20. Alster TS, Williams CM. Treatment of keloid sternotomy scars with 5858 nm flashlamp-pumped pulsed-dye laser. Lancet 1995;345:1198–1200.
21. Goldman MP, Fitzpatrick RE. Laser treatment of scars. Dermatol Surg 1995;21:685–687.
22. Connel PG, Harland CC. Treatment of keloid scars with pulsed dye laser and intralesional steroid. J Cutan Laser Ther 2000;2:147–150.
23. Berman B, Flores F. Recurrence rates of excised keloids treated with post operative triamcinolone acetonide injections or interferon alpha-2b injections. J Am Acad Dermatol 1997;37:755–757.
24. Berman B, Duncan MR. Short-term keloid treatment in vivo with human interferon alfa-2b results in a selective and persistent normalization of keloidal fibroblast collagen, glycosaminoglycan, and collagenase production in vitro. J Am Acad Dermatol 1989;21:694–702.
25. Conejo-Mir JS, Corbi R, Linares M. Carbon dioxide laser ablation associated with interferon alfa-2b injections reduces the recurrence of keloids. J Am Acad Dermatol 1998;39:1039.
26. Berman B, Kaufman J. Rolet study of the effect of postoperative imiquimod 5% cream on the recurrence rate of excised keloids. J Am Acad Dermatol 2002;47(Suppl):S209–S211.
27. Berman B, Villa A. Imiquimod 5% cream for keloid management. Dermatol Surg 2003;29:1050–1051.
28. Fitzpatrick RE. Treatment of inflamed hypertrophic scars using intralesional 5FU. Dermatol Surg 1999;25:224–232.
29. Manuskiatti W, Fitzpatrick RE. Treatment response of keloidal and hypertrophic sternotomy scars: comparison among intralesional corticosteroid, 5-fluorouracil, and 585 nm flashlamp-pumped pulsed-eye laser treatments. Arch Dermatol 2002;138:1149–1155.
30. Kontochristopoulos G, Stefanaki C, Panagiotopoulos A, et al. Intralesional 5-flurouracil in the treatment of keloids: an open clinical and histopathologic study. J Am Acad Dermatol 2005;52:474–479.
31. Apikian M, Goodman G. Intralesional 5-fluorouracil in the treatment of keloid scars. Australas J Dermatol 2004;45:140–143.
32. Nanda S, Reddy BSN. Intralesional 5-fluorouracil as a treatment modality for keloids. Dermatol Surg 2004;30:54–57.
33. Espana A, Solano T, Quintanilla E. Bleomycin in the treatment of hypertrophic scars by multiple needle punctures. Dermatol Surg 2001;27:23–27.

34. Lee RC, Doong H, Jellema AF. The response of burn scars to intralesional verapamil. Report of five cases. Arch Surg 1994;129:107–111.

35. Lawrence WT. Treatment of earlobe keloids with surgery plus adjuvant intralesional verapamil and pressure earrings. Ann Plast Surg 1996;37:167–169.

36. D'Andrea F, Brongo S, Ferraro G, et al. Prevention and treatment of keloids with intralesional verapamil. Dermatology 2002;204:60–62.

37. Kim A, DiCarlo J, Cohen C, et al. Are keloids really "gliloids"? High-level expression of gli-1 oncogene in keloids. J Am Acad Dermatol 2001;45:707–711.

38. Ladin DA, Hou Z, Patel D, et al. p53 and apoptosis alterations in keloids and keloid fibroblasts. Wound Repair Regen 1998;6:28–37.

39. Louro ID, McKie-Bell P, Gosnell H, et al. The zinc finger protein GLI induces cellular sensitivity to the mTOR inhibitor rapamycin. Cell Growth Differ 1999;10:503–516.

40. Soderberg T, Hallmans G, Bartholdson L. Treatment of keloids and hypertrophic scars with adhesive zinc tape. Scand J Plast Reconstr Surg 1982;16:261–266.

41. Wong TW, Lee JY, Sheutt M, Chao SC. Relief of pain and itch associated with keloids on treatment with oxpentifylline. Br J Dermatol 1999;140;771–772.

42. Berman B, Duncan MR. Pentoxyfylline inhibits the proliferation of human fibroblasts derived from keloid, scleroderma, morphea skin and their production of collagen, glycosaminoglycans and fibronectin. Br J Dermatolol 1990;123:339–346.

43. Lawrence WT. In search of the optimal treatment of keloids: report of a series and review of the literature. Ann Plast Surg 1991;27:164–178.

44. Onwukwe MF. Treating keloids by surgery and methotrexate. Arch Dermatol 1980;116:158.

45. Mayou BJ. D-penicillamine in the treatment of keloids. Br J Dermatol 1981;105:87–89.

9
Free Margin Distortion

Sumaira Z. Aasi and David Leffell

Surgical complications are a function of host factors, surgical skill, and other considerations that are sometimes obscure. Complications are unavoidable even in the best hands and adverse events should always be anticipated. To minimize future adverse events, a skilled surgeon should know how to manage complications and learn from mistakes. Understanding the consequences of the various options in wound reconstruction and management is essential to minimize the incidence of adverse events. In addition, a thorough discussion of the procedure, risks, benefits, and possible complications with the patient will minimize unnecessary misunderstanding or anger should the reconstruction have a suboptimal outcome. In this regard, it is important to inform the patient that more than one procedure may be required to achieve the best result. Otherwise, the patient may presume that the initial surgery has produced the best and only possible result, which is often not the case. It is critical for the surgeon to have a sense of the patient's expectations in order to anticipate the problematic patient and explain the probable outcome in advance. The patient must be prepared so that surgical outcome matches patient's expectations.

To achieve good results there is no substitute for proper planning and scrupulous surgical technique. Designing flaps that minimize donor site deformity, avoiding free margin distortion, and placing incision lines within cosmetic units and natural skin relaxation lines are the core principles of good reconstruction. Handling tissue gently, decreasing wound tension, obtaining good wound edge approximation, and eversion are as necessary as a carefully developed design.[1] Fortunately, the cutaneous anatomy of the face and factors such as the inevitable aging process, skin laxity, gravity, and time permit a wide range of options for reconstruction of surgical defects. Almost imperceptible scars can often be achieved by hiding incisions in the natural junctions and creases of the face.

However, areas of the face with free margins present special challenges to the reconstructive surgeon. The eyes, nose, and lips, each with its own functional and aesthetic importance, are sometimes less forgiving. These three structures often convey innate personality traits, inadvertent emotion, and nonverbal communication. The free margins of these structures, by definition, offer little resistance to the tension created by the surgical movement of nearby tissue. Any abnormality in the natural contours of these critical structures of the face focuses attention to the disruption or distortion. Often, however, the distortion not only leads to an unacceptable cosmetic result, but may also have functional consequences.

Free Margins: Perioperative Considerations

To design the reconstruction, one should view a defect on the face with the patient sitting in the upright position, which allows appreciation of the natural effects of gravity. Have the patient perform facial movements to clarify the relaxed skin tension lines and reservoirs of available tissue. While the reconstruction is being executed, it is important throughout the surgical procedure to remove the surgical drapes and view the patient from different positions (with eyes open and looking up, at the mouth and lips from above and below) to evoke any possible distortion. Most surgical procedures are performed while the patient is in a supine position, so the surgeon should be aware that there may be some distortion occurring which is not readily appreciable in that position. In addition, understanding effects of local swelling intraoperatively and explaining this to the patient is valuable when reconstructing near free margins. An example of transient eyelid retraction secondary to anesthetic and

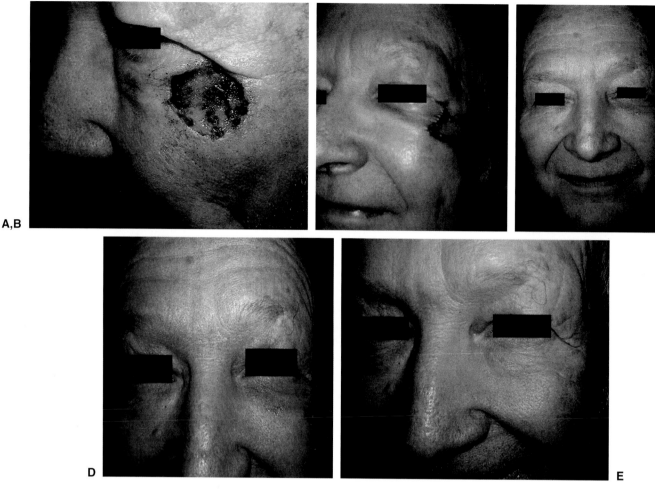

FIGURE 9-1. (A) Defect of the lateral infraorbital area. (B) A rhombic transposition flap is performed during which intraoperative swelling and eyelid retraction is appreciated. (C, D) Eyelid retraction is no longer present when the patient returns in a few days for suture removal. (E) Postoperative results in 3 months.

intraoperative swelling is illustrated in Figure 9-1. Though this may be concerning to the novice surgeon and the patient, the area of distortion resolves as the swelling recedes within a few days. The eyelid is in its normal position when the patient returns for suture removal in a week.

Factors Affecting Free Margin Healing

It is axiomatic in the biology of wound healing that a scar continues to heal, mature, and improve in appearance over 1 to 3 years. Free margin distortion may correct itself over time in certain situations, especially where gravity itself plays a role in creating change in the structure of the face. Nasal tip ptosis in the elderly patients or the return of a distorted eyebrow with time and gravity are examples (Fig. 9-2).

Scar remodeling also varies depending on the location of the scar and individual patient disposition. Occasionally, however, it is clear that the distortion will not change significantly and, in that case, the revision can be performed earlier.

Second Intention Healing

In certain situations, nature can provide a better cosmetic and functional result than surgical reconstruction. Surgeons often underestimate the benefits of second intention healing, which represents a viable option for select defects. The main concern with second intention healing is the amount of wound contraction that may occur. Wound contraction is greater with second intention healing than with linear closures, flaps, or grafts. The presence of reticular dermis is important in inhibiting wound contraction. While wounds repaired with full-thickness grafts contract very little, split-thickness skin grafts with

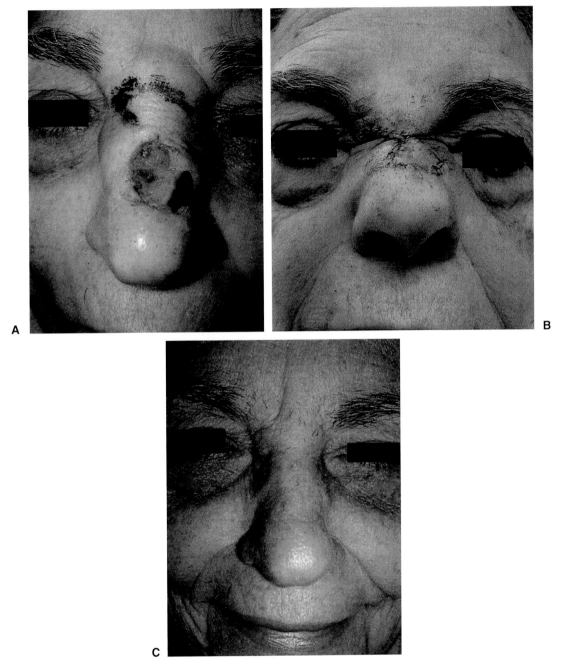

FIGURE 9-2. (A) A rhombic transposition flap is designed to reconstruct a wound on the nasal bridge. (B) Execution of the flap leads to elevation of nasal alae and upturning of the nasal tip. (C) Within 2 months, the nasal alae and tip have returned to a normal position.

very little reticular dermis will contract approximately 40%. Superficial wounds that extend only into the papillary dermis contract very little in second intention healing, while full-thickness wounds devoid of reticular dermis may contract significantly.[2]

Location of the wound is the most important factor that predicts the cosmetic and functional result after second intention healing. Wounds located in concave areas heal with excellent cosmetic results, wounds on flat surfaces usually heal with satisfactory results, and wounds on convex surfaces often heal with a noticeable scar.[3] Because of the greater degree of contraction that occurs with second intention healing, one must be acutely aware of this effect when choosing this option near free margins. In this scenario, it is not only the depth of the wound, but also its proximity to the free margin that has an

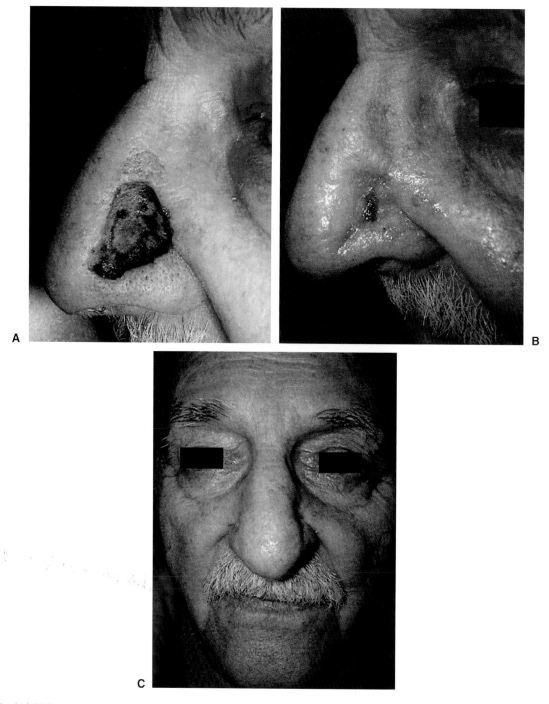

FIGURE 9-3. (A) This patient had a postoperative wound on the nasal ala that is several millimeters from the alar rim. (B) Results with second intention healing. (C) Due to the rigid and sebaceous nasal skin as well as the wound location being several millimeters from the alar rim, second intention healing does not lead to significant distortion of the alar rim.

impact on the final result or any expected distortion (Fig. 9-3). In certain cases, it is advisable to monitor the site of a highly aggressive tumor before final, aesthetically appealing reconstruction with adjacent tissue transfer is performed. In this case, it may be advantageous to temporarily reconstruct the defect with a full-thickness skin graft to prevent wound contraction and distortion of the free margin that will otherwise be more challenging to correct later (Fig. 9-4). Split-thickness skin grafts, on the other hand, will not significantly prevent wound contraction. In addition, guiding sutures can be placed across opposite wound edges to ensure that natural wound contraction occurs in a direction controlled by the sutures.[4]

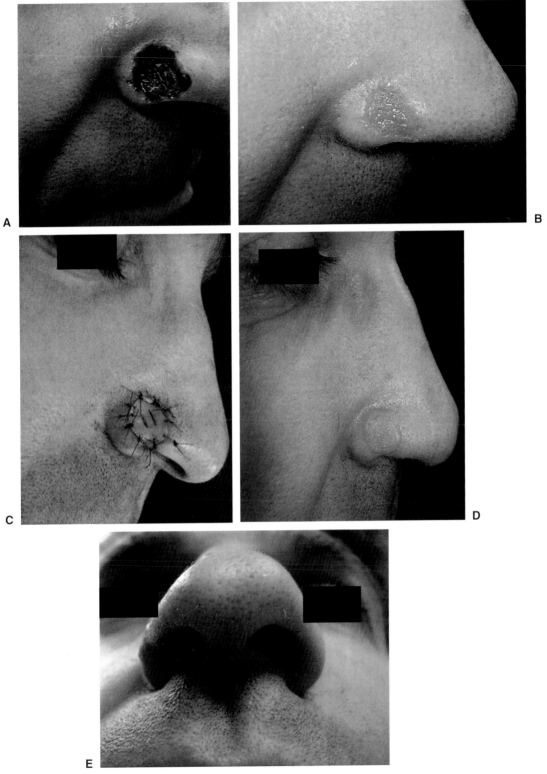

FIGURE 9-4. (A) This patient had a highly aggressive cancer on his nose treated with Mohs micrographic surgery. In contrast to the example in Figure 9-3, this wound is much closer to the alar rim. (B) Within a few days, slight notching of the alar rim is already appreciated. (C) A full-thickness skin graft was placed temporarily to minimize further distortion while the patient was monitored for tumor recurrence awaiting eventual definitive reconstruction. (D, E) There is no further alar distortion.

Revision Techniques for Free Margin Distortion

Fusiform Ellipse

Various surgical methods may be used to correct free margin distortion. One simple technique is fusiform elliptical excision of a scar that distorts a free edge, with an attempt at reapproximation of the edges in the direction of relaxed skin tension lines (Fig. 9-5). This can be attempted when there is sufficient tissue present (e.g., the lip), but may not be appropriate for a small structure such as the nasal ala. Serial excisions can also be used when the scar is exceptionally wide.

Z-Plasty

The Z-plasty is a very common and reliable method of scar revision. Its fundamental unit, a triangular double transposition flap, has the ability to lengthen a contracted scar, change the direction of the scar for better alignment with relaxed skin tension lines, and interrupt a straight line scar for better camouflage.[5–7] In terms of free margin distortion, the Z-plasty is particularly useful in lengthening and changing the direction of the scar without requiring the excision of more tissue, which is at a premium near free margins. The change in the direction of the scar frees the contracture, allowing the return of a distorted free margin to its normal position. The design of the Z-plasty comprises the central limb of the Z, which is often the original scar line being redirected, and the two arms of the Z that come off the central limb at various angles. The central limb along with its two arms creates two equilateral triangles that will transpose over each other (Fig. 9-6). Through this movement, the central limb (or original scar) is rotated variably depending on the angles of the Z-plasty. The classic 60° angle Z-plasty rotates the central limb 90°.

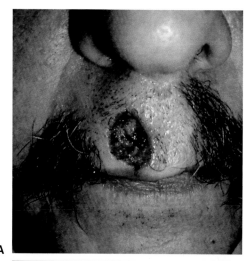

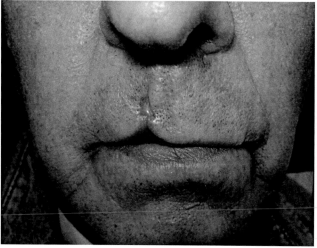

FIGURE 9-5. (A) Defect on cutaneous lip. (B) At patient's request, wound was allowed to heal in by second intent, but as expected eclabium occurred. (C) Scar excised and repaired in a linear fashion.

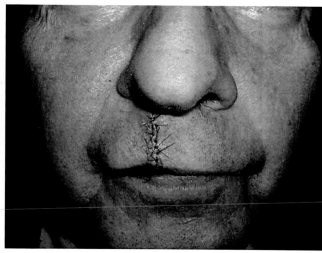

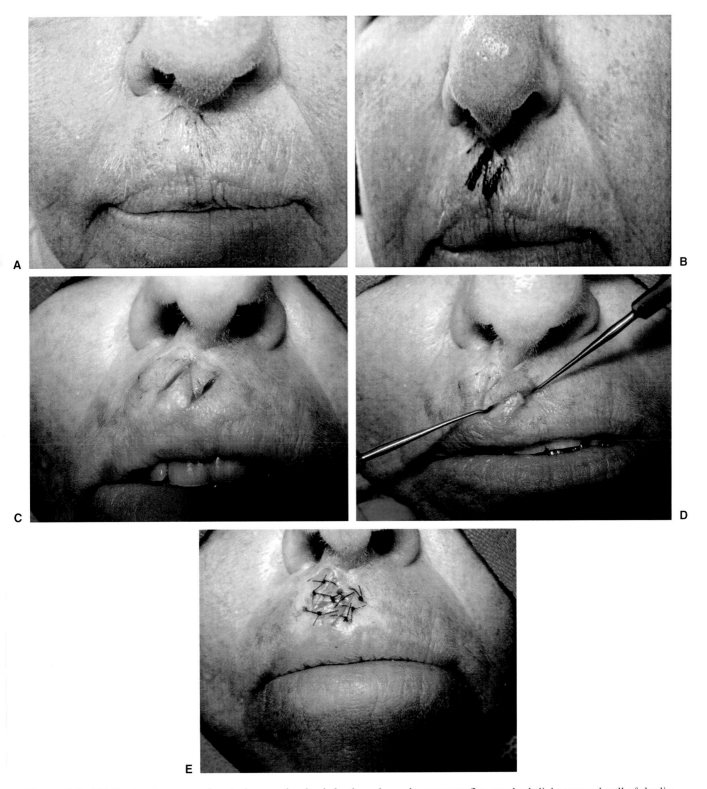

FIGURE 9-6. (A) Contracture secondary to herpes simplex infection of an advancement flap resulted slight upward pull of the lip. (B) Z-plasty designed. (C) Flap incised. (D) Two triangles of the Z-plasty transposed. (E) Flaps sutured in place.

Two-Staged Flap Reconstruction

Two-staged flaps, such as a meliolabial interpolation flap, can also be used to repair defects of the alar rim. The skin in the area of the meliolabial fold often matches the color and texture of nasal skin. This ample and sebaceous tissue can be used to contour the ala,[9] sometimes with significant inherent support without the need for an underlying free cartilage graft. One of the advantages of this flap is that it can restore a partial- or full-thickness defect. Figure 9-8 demonstrates the use of a meliolabial interpolation flap to repair the nasal ala. In this case, the wound was allowed to heal by second intention so that part of the scar tissue could be turned down as a hinge flap to form the internal nasal lining. A cartilage graft was taken from the antihelix for tissue support and placed over the hinge flap. The medial and lateral edges of the alar defect were undermined to create pockets into which the cartilage graft was inset. A pattern of the contralateral ala was drawn on the donor cheek skin above the meliolabial sulcus, keeping in mind how the flap will be rotated. The flap was then incised, sutured in place, and a primary linear closure was performed below the base of the pedicle at the meliolabial sulcus. The patient returned in 3 weeks for pedicle division and closure of the remaining portion of the proximal meliolabial fold. The distal flap was defatted aggressively and contoured to resemble the contralateral ala.

Single-Stage Nasolabial Transposition Flap

Single-stage nasolabial transposition flap can be used in certain cases to reconstruct alar defects when patients may not be able to tolerate a two-staged procedure (Fig. 9-9). This flap also relies on the reservoir of tissue available on the medial cheek and meliolabial fold. Here, a superiorly located Burrow's triangle is removed and the medial aspect of the flap is created by an incision along the nasal facial sulcus extending inferiorly to the meliolabial sulcus. The width and length of the flap is dependent upon the defect size of the wound to be reconstructed. The flap and surrounding area of the nasal sidewall are widely undermined. A buried suspension suture can placed from the deep aspect of the flap to the periosteum of the periform aperture to help recreate the nasofacial sulcus.[12] In this case, the distal tip of the flap was thinned and turned on itself to provide a lining for the inside of the nostril.

Hinged Turnover Flap

A smaller anteromedial full-thickness alar defect can be reconstructed with a hinged turnover flap (Fig. 9-10).[13] The flap is developed from the skin immediately superior to the notch. This skin of the nasal sidewall helps to create both the inner nasal lining and the outer surface of the ala. The flap is incised and raised at the level of the subcutaneous fat. It is delicately freed inferiorly until a few millimeters of subcutaneous attachment remains at the superior border of the defect. Depending on how much structural support may be required, a free cartilage graft can be inserted into pockets of the lateral and medial edges of the alar defect. The flap is then draped onto itself and sutured in place. The superior aspect of the secondary defect on the nasal sidewall is closed in a primary linear fashion.

Z-Plasty for Ecnasion

Second intention healing is often utilized for defects limited to or involving the alar crease because reconstruction with most types of flaps leads to blunting of the alar crease. However, depending on the depth of the wound and the individual characteristics of the nose (size, shape, and rigidity), the inevitable contraction with second intention healing may also lead to a variable amount of ecnasion. The patient shown in Figure 9-11 had an aggressive basal cell carcinoma in the alar crease which was initially allowed to heal by second intention. A very slight, but noticeable ecnasion developed with wound contraction. A Z-plasty was performed in the alar crease which returned symmetry to the nasal alae.

Eyelid

The most important function of the eyelids is to protect the globe and provide a consistent moist environment for the cornea. When the eye is fully opened the upper lid margin covers approximately 1 mm of the superior cornea and the lower lid rests at the limbal junction between the cornea and the sclera.[14] The lacrimal puncta or tear ducts are openings at the medial aspects of both upper and lower eyelids. Tears drain through these openings and in order to lubricate the eyes appropriately, the puncta must be opposing the surface of the globe. Even minor displacement of the punctum causes epiphora and can lead to significant discomfort. The constantly dry eye may eventually develop corneal damage or keratopathy. *Ectropion* is defined as an outward rotation of the eyelid margin and should be distinguished from upper or lower eyelid retraction, in which the lid margin is superiorly or inferiorly displaced with respect to its natural resting position against the cornea, without eyelid eversion. In both cases, displacement of the eyelid from its normal position results and can be functionally problematic for patients.

Because the eyelid skin is so thin, any procedure that causes vertical tension is transmitted to the eyelid margin, even if the margin itself is not involved in the surgery. Unlike other free margins where the skin or underlying

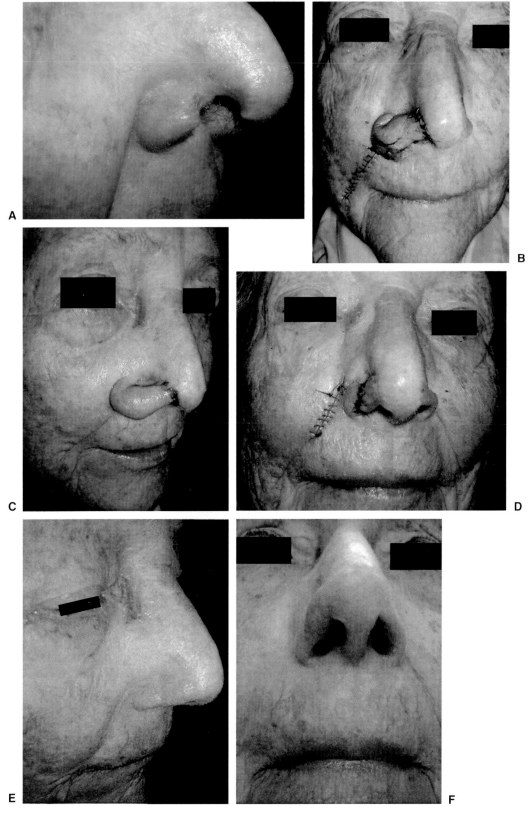

FIGURE 9-8. (A) Alar defect post–tumor extirpation. The wound was initially allowed to heal by second intention. (B) A meliolabial interpolation flap is sutured over a free cartilage graft overlying a turned down hinge flap created by the scar tissue. (C) The patient returns at 3 weeks for pedicle division. (D) The pedicle is divided, its proximal portion is discarded, and the defect at the meliolabial fold is closed primarily. The distal portion of the flap at the ala is aggressively thinned and contoured to match the contralateral ala. (E) Postoperative results: lateral view. (F) Swimmer's view.

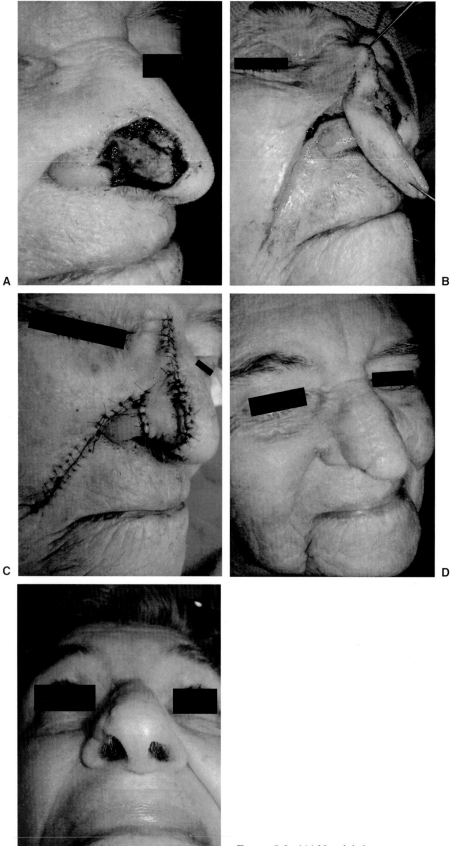

FIGURE 9-9. (A) Nasal defect post–tumor extirpation. (B) The nasolabial flap is incised and draped over the defect. (C) Flap sutured into place. (D) Postoperative result: lateral view. (E) Swimmer's view.

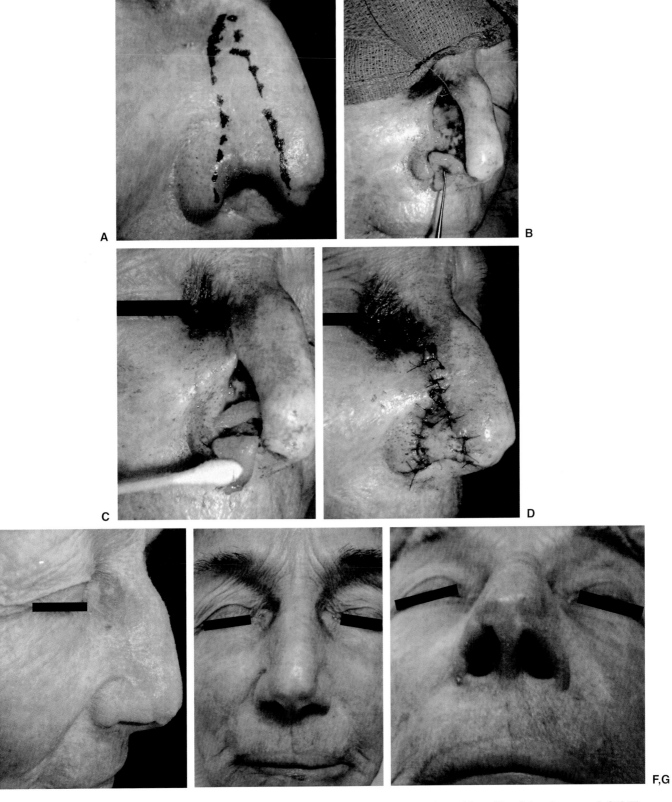

FIGURE 9-10. (A) Alar rim defect with flap design. (B) The flap is incised and freed from the underlying nasal sidewall. (C) A free cartilage graft is obtained from the antihelix and inserted into pockets created on either side of the alar wound. (D) Flap sutured into place. (E) Postoperative results: lateral view. (F) Frontal view. (G) Swimmer's view.

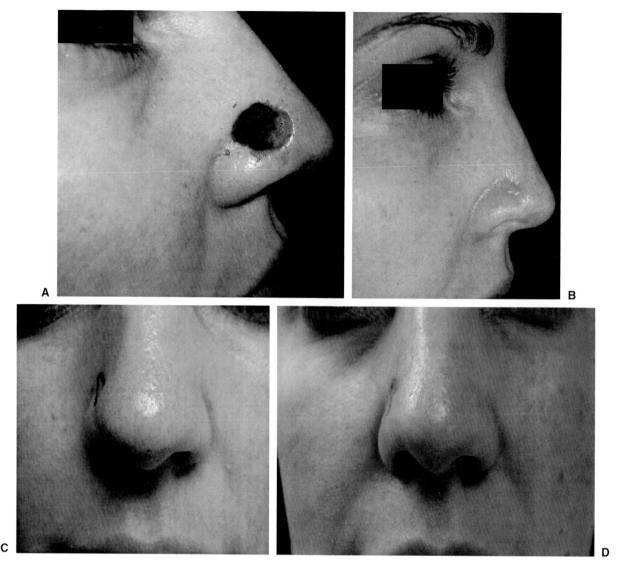

FIGURE 9-11. (A) Alar crease defect post–Mohs micrographic surgery. (B) Wound healed by second intent. (C) Slight upward pull of the right ala. (D) Z-plasty performed with normalization of the ala.

tissue is more rigid or supported, gradual postoperative scar contraction in this area can also lead to significant traction on the eyelid. The lower eyelid may sometimes be pulled down when a broad sheet of scar develops between the skin and the tissues below. This unfortunate consequence has occurred after blepharoplasty when very little skin was removed but dissection was carried down between the skin and underlying musculature. Even heavy cauterization can accentuate late wound base contraction at the expense of the eyelid.[15] Consequently, it is critical that most repairs in the periorbital area generate tension in the horizontal vector.

Avoiding vertical tension is a basic principle of eyelid surgery. One should perform flaps with a horizontal tension because the flaps' horizontal tension provides a measure of countertraction. A valuable repair for infraorbital defects that demonstrates this principle is the cheek advancement flap (Fig. 9-12). It is critical to design the flap close to the orbital rim and keep the incision lines in cosmetic units. In addition, the flap should extend upwardly at the infraorbital and lateral cheek area to compensate for height loss resulting from pivotal restraint, a limitation that occurs as the flap is rotated and advanced.[16] In addition, suspension or tacking sutures are helpful when performing repairs of this type, which involve movement of large tissue adjacent to a free margin. Suspension sutures divert tension of wound closure and decrease secondary motion to reduce distor-

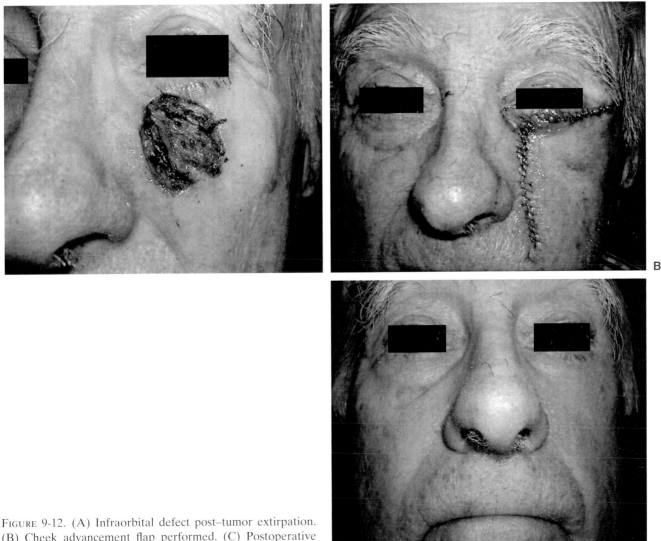

FIGURE 9-12. (A) Infraorbital defect post–tumor extirpation. (B) Cheek advancement flap performed. (C) Postoperative result.

tion of free margins secondary to wound contraction.[17] When placing suspension sutures, one must take the needle through the undersurface of the advancing tissue and ideally suture it to deep fascia or periosteum. If a flap crosses the junction of cosmetic units, the suspension suture is placed at the site anticipated to overlie the junction. It is important to make sure the suture is placed so that it parallels the blood supply and the surgeon should be aware of vessels and nerves that lie deep. For large defects, a series of suspension sutures can be placed.

Ectropion of the upper eyelid does not usually occur because gravity does not stretch the upper eyelid in the same way that the lower eyelid is affected by the weight of the midfacial structures. The lower eyelid is supported and suspended by the lateral and medial canthal tendons, the capsulopalpebral fascia, the tarsus, and the orbicularis oculi muscle. Canthal tendons tend to become lax with age and there is atrophy and degeneration of the orbicularis oris muscle with time. Thus, ectropion is more common with the lower eyelid. If the lid margin can be pulled more than 8 mm away from the globe, significant canthal tendon laxity is present. Another way to check for lower lid laxity is with the *snap test*. With the patient in the sitting position, the lower lid is grasped and pulled away from the globe. When released, it should snap back immediately. A positive snap-back test, in which the lid does not return to its normal position after distraction without a blink, is a sign of poor orbicularis tone.[14] Intraoperatively, the potential for ectropion development may also be estimated by pulling the defect together with skin hooks or toothed forceps and asking the patient to look up with the mouth open. This places maximum stress on the lower lid. With the patient in this position, if the eyelid is opposing the margin of the iris, ectropion is an unlikely outcome.

Small lesions that are mainly limited to the lid margin heal well by second intention as the remaining orbicularis oculi muscle acts as a sling to pull up the defect. However, due to thinness of the eyelid skin and its lack of significant underlying tissue or structural support, wounds involving the superficial cutaneous surface of the infraorbital eyelid may heal with ectropion. This may be prevented by full-thickness excision of the margin, including an appropriate amount of conjunctiva, so that the hammocklike contraction of both skin and conjunctiva returns the lid margin to a near normal contour.[2] Full-thickness excisions of the lid margin should be oriented vertically with careful reapproximation of the tarsal plate and the lid margin. Upper eyelid full-thickness repair does not require the suture strength of lower eyelid repair. Gravity tends to close the upper eyelid defect and thus reduces wound tension, whereas gravity tends to open the lower eyelid defect and thus increases wound tension. One must be careful not to expose the conjunctival side to suture material as this can lead to corneal abrasion.

In a patient with poor lower lid tone and significant laxity, correction of loss of tissue will not necessarily prevent an ectropion. Often, one has to repair the preexisting horizontal laxity by tightening the lateral canthal tendon.[14] A horizontal skin incision is made extending 10 mm laterally from the lateral canthus. A lateral canthotomy is made with lysis and release of the inferior crus of the lateral canthal tendon. Dissection is carried down to the periosteum of the lateral orbital rim. The lateral tarsus and canthal tendon are freed of their inferior attachments and positioned laterally towards the lateral orbital rim to determine the amount of redundancy. The point at which the lower lid overlaps with the lateral aspect of the upper lid is marked, and the skin, orbicularis, lid margin, and conjunctival epithelium are removed up to this point. The tarsal strip is sutured to the periosteum of the internal aspect of the lateral orbital rim. A suture is placed to reconstruct the canthal angle and the skin is closed with interrupted sutures.

Full-Thickness Skin Grafts

Full-thickness skin grafts can be used to reconstruct a defect on the eyelid when it cannot be closed by direct approximation or by local flaps (Fig. 9-13). The best donor site for grafts for lower eyelid defects is often the excess skin found in elderly patients in the upper eyelid. If eyelid skin is not available, preauricular or postauricular skin is

the next best choice because it provides the best match. Other possibilities are supraclavicular, inner arm, or inner thigh skin. The graft should be 50% to 100% larger than the relaxed defect to anticipate for tissue contraction once the donor skin is excised. The patient shown in Figure 9-13 had severe actinic damage with multiple coalescing basal cell carcinomas. His left eye is nonfunctioning, thus every effort was made to decrease the use of an adjacent skin flap which might contain subclinical tumors. A skin graft was performed to prevent ectropion using donor skin from the supraclavicular area. Initially, the graft appeared thickened and raised at the edges because it was cautiously oversized but within 6 months it improved in appearance. No dermabrasion was necessary.

On occasion even oversizing the full-thickness skin graft is not sufficient to prevent an ectropion, especially if the eyelid has significant baseline laxity, as is often the case in elderly patients. The patient shown in Figure 9-14 had baseline ectropion and canthal laxity. Mohs micrographic surgery was performed on an infiltrative basal cell carcinoma resulting in a large defect in the infraorbital area. Initially, a full-thickness graft was used to reconstruct the wound but postoperatively, the ectropion worsened with time. She then underwent tightening of her canthal tendon with improvement of the ectropion.

Surgical defects of the medial canthus heal well by second intention if the wound lies equally above and below the medial canthal tendon. Asymmetrically placed defects might result in an upward or downward displacement of the medial canthus, creating a webbed appearance. This can be corrected with redirecting the scar using a Z-plasty.

Lip

The lips have no bony or cartilaginous infrastructure and thus are also an area of the face where free margins can be easily distorted. The vermilion border, because it sharply demarcates the lip and forms a continuous line, is often the focus of attention in the perioral area. Restoration of the vermilion border is essential because even minute defects in reapproximation are quite conspicuous. A 2- to 3-mm pale convexity, known as the white roll, parallels the vermilion–cutaneous junction of both the upper and lower lip. The white roll is formed by a local bulging of the underlying orbicularis oris muscle and is difficult to reconstruct if damaged. Any slight malpositioning of this junction results in a distressing cosmetic deformity. Similarly, the philtrum must be maintained as a midline structure because even a slight deviation is apparent. The crests and groove of the philtrum appear to be formed and maintained by a specialized condensation of dermal collagen supported by a rich elastic tissue

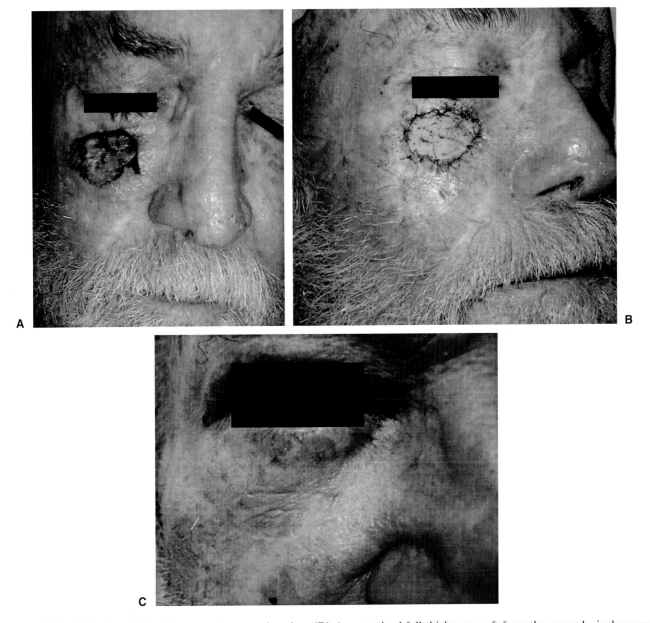

FIGURE 9-13. (A) Infraorbital defect post–tumor extirpation. (B) An oversized full-thickness graft from the supraclavicular area is used to reconstruct the defect. (C) Postoperative results at approximately 6 months with no evidence of ectropion.

component. With aging and loss of elasticity, the philtrum becomes less prominent. Laterally, the margin of the lower lip is less distinct and variable.

Surgical wounds located on the cutaneous lip or at the junction of the cutaneous lip with the mucosal lip are especially at risk for eclabium if not reconstructed appropriately. In one study, 12 of 13 patients had good-to-excellent cosmetic results and experienced neither functional impairment nor complications after surgery with second intention healing.[18] However, it was noted in the study that second intention healing should be considered for mostly superficial defects, which may be broad

and extend no deeper than the superficial portion of the orbicularis oris muscle. If, however, the defect involves the vermilion–cutaneous junction, especially on the superior lip, second intention healing may result in distortion of the vermilion border. The greater the involvement of the cutaneous lip, the greater the risk of lip distortion because the lips have no bony attachment, making vermilion border more susceptible to displacement during normal wound contracture. Deep defects involving significant portions of the orbicularis oris muscle that are allowed to heal secondarily may result in wound contracture with a subsequent depressed scar, eclabium

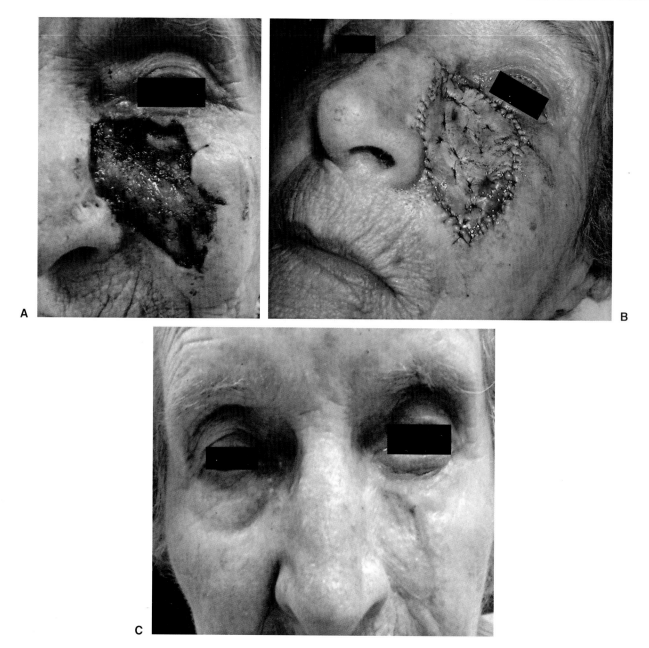

FIGURE 9-14. (A) Defect post–Mohs micrographic surgery for an infiltrative basal cell carcinoma. (B) Oversized full-thickness skin graft is performed but the patient still developed an ectropion. (C) Post–canthal tightening.

formation, and an incompetent oral aperture which may have functional consequences in speaking or being able to eat without drooling and preserving oral continence.

Revision of Eclabium

Z-Plasty

The patient shown in Figure 9-6 underwent reconstruction with an advancement flap after Mohs micrographic surgery for a basal carcinoma on the right upper lip. Postoperatively, the healing was complicated by herpes simplex infection and resulted in significant scar contracture and distortion of the vermilion border with slightly upward pull of the patient's right side of the lip. A Z-plasty was designed so that the majority of the resultant scar lines would parallel the relaxed skin tension lines and the scar is redirected to correct the upward pull on the lip.

Linear Repair

The patient shown in Figure 9-5 had a basal cell cancer removed from the upper lip. He deferred a reconstructive

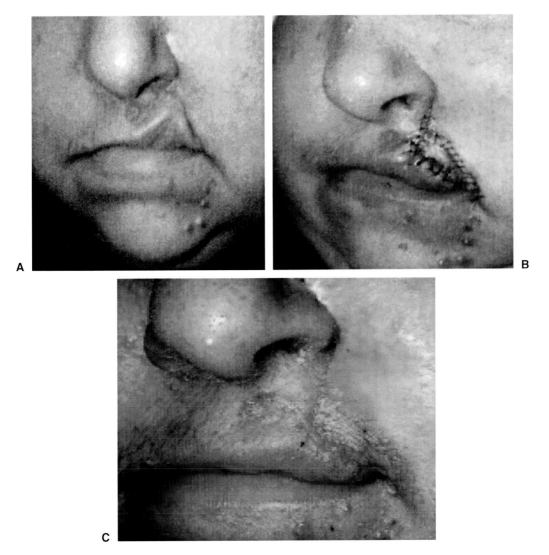

FIGURE 9-15. (A) Patient with basal cell nevus syndrome who developed eclabium. (B) A laterally based island pedicle flap is used to correct the eclabium. (C) Patient at suture removal.

procedure on the day of surgery because he felt that this area would not be visible because he normally wore a mustache. Subsequently however, the patient decided to shave in the area and the eclabium was disfiguring. There was sufficient tissue laxity so an excision of the scar and a simple linear repair was planned. The vermilion border was marked prior to local anesthetic injection and carefully reapproximated.

V to Y Repair

The patient shown in Figure 9-15 has basal cell nevus syndrome. Because of surrounding basal cell carcinomas in the adjacent skin, the wound on her upper lip was allowed to heal by second intention after tumor extirpation with Mohs micrographic surgery. This resulted in eclabium. She had an adjacent basal cell carcinoma on the upper lip medially, thus a Z-plasty was not ideal to correct the eclabium. A laterally based V to Y (or island pedicle closure) was performed and corrected the disfigurement.

Conclusion

Defects of the free margins of the lip, eyelid, and ala require special attention. Aberrancy in these areas can be both visually prominent and functionally problematic. A range of reconstructive methods are available to resurface defects in these areas, but the patient must be aware of the complexity of restoring normal anatomic and functional relationships as well as the possibility of multiple procedures in order to obtain the optimum result. Careful preparation of the patient enhances acceptance of final results.

References

1. Davidson TM. Subcutaneous suture placement. Laryngoscope 1987;97:501–504.
2. Zitelli JA. Wound healing by first and second intention. In: Roenigk RR, Roenigk HH, eds. Dermatologic surgery principles and practice. 2nd ed. New York: Marcel Dekker; 1996.
3. Zitelli JA. Wound healing by secondary intention. J Am Acad Dermatol 1983;9:407–415.
4. Albright SD. Surgical gems: placement of guiding sutures to counteract undesirable retraction of tissues in and around functionally and cosmetically important structures. J Dermatol Surg Oncol 1981;7:446–449.
5. Borges AF, Alexander JE. Relaxed skin tension lines, Z-plasties on scars, and fusiform excision of lesions. Br J Plastic Surg 1962;15:242–254.
6. Hove CR, Williams EF, Rodgers BJ. Z-plasty: a concise review. Facial Plastic Surg 2001;17:289–293.
7. Frodel JL, Wang TD. Z-Plasty. In: Baker SR, Swanson NA, eds. Local flaps in facial reconstruction. St. Louis: Mosby; 1995:131–149.
8. Wolfe D, Davidson TM. Scar revision. Arch Otolaryngol Head Neck Surg 1991;117:200–204.
9. Salasche S, Bernstein G, Senkarik M. Surgical anatomy of the skin. Norwalk, CT: Appleton & Lange; 1988.
10. Menick FJ. Reconstruction of the nose. In: Baker SR, Swanson NA, eds. Local flaps in facial reconstruction. St Louis: Mosby; 1995:305–344.
11. Adams C, Ratner D. Composite and free cartilage grafting. Dermatol Clin 2005;23:129–140.
12. Zitelli JA. The nasolabial flap as a single-stage procedure. Arch Dermatol 1990;126:1445–1448.
13. Lee KK, Gorman AK, Swanson NA. Hinged turnover flap: a one-stage reconstruction of a full thickness nasal ala defect. Dermatol Surg 2004;30:479–481.
14. Vallabhanath P, Carter SR. Ectropion and entropion. Curr Opin Ophthalmol 2000;11:345–351.
15. Harris GJ, Perez N. Anchored flaps in post-Mohs reconstruction of the lower eyelid, cheek, and lateral canthus. Ophthal Plast Reconstr Surg 2003;19:5–13.
16. Dzubow LM. The dynamics of flap movement: effect of pivotal restraint on flap rotation and transposition. J Dermatol Surg Oncol 1987;13:1348–1353.
17. Robinson JK. Suspension sutures aid facial reconstruction. Dermatol Surg 1999;25:189–194.
18. Gloster HM. The use of second-intention healing for partial thickness Mohs defects involving the vermilion and/or mucosal surfaces of the lip. J Am Acad Dermatol 2002;47:893–897.

10
Scar Revision and Camouflage

Tri H. Nguyen

Despite meticulous planning and technique, suboptimal scars will occur even in the hands of the best surgeons. Skills in scar revision, therefore, are essential to any surgeon's armamentarium. Preoperatively, patients should be informed that secondary revisions and several stages are always possible, if not probable, with complex reconstructions. An accurate assessment of the scar is a critical first step. In doing so, one should realize that what is wrong to the surgeon may not mirror what is wrong to the patient. Although patient preferences are of utmost importance, they must be balanced with objective findings and what is realistically achievable. Patients must understand that revision procedures are always more difficult and carry no guarantee. This chapter will focus on the range of options for scar revision and its application to surgically induced wounds. Traumatic, inflammatory, and burn scar revisions will not be addressed, although the concepts that will be discussed in this chapter are broadly applicable to scar revision surgery despite the initiating event.

Scar Evaluation

No two scars are alike and, therefore, therapy is highly individualized. In critically analyzing a scar, one must refrain from criticizing, especially if it is another physician's work. A positive outlook is necessary for all involved. Issues that should be considered in evaluating scars are listed in Table 10-1. Following these initial questions, the scar is objectively classified and revision options are considered (Table 10-2).

An ideal scar is one that is barely visible, less than 1 mm in width, flush with adjacent skin, does not cause dysfunction, and is similar in contour, texture, color, and softness to its surroundings. Ideal scars fall within areas of shadow, lie within existing creases or folds, follow relaxed skin tension lines (RSTL), and are either contained within or are between subunit junctions. Well-camouflaged scars are also discontinuous visually. Camouflage patterns, for example, employ broken lines and colors for conceal-

ment. Scar length is generally irrelevant as long as the scar follows the above ideals.

Given these ideals, a decision must be made on whether the existing scar is salvageable. Some scars will benefit from nonsurgical options while other scars may only be improved by a reexcision. An imperfect scar requires investigation to preempt avoidable factors. Was the initial design appropriate? Were there flaws in the closure technique? Was the wound healing compromised (poor wound care, smoking, excessive activity, infection, trauma)? Distal wounds (extremities) and highly mobile locations (joints) will heal more slowly and scar expectations should be adjusted accordingly. In some settings (Table 10-1), scars may never be optimal.

Nonsurgical Options for Scar Revision

The myriad nonsurgical options for scar therapy are listed in Table 10-3. These may be combined with one another and with surgical options for complementary benefits.

Observation

Among nonsurgical options, time and observation often produce the best results for early scar changes. Swelling, firmness, and redness usually diminish within weeks (swelling) to months (firmness and redness) as scar remodeling occurs.

Firmness and erythema are common with flaps or widely undermined tissue and should progressively improve. However, early warning signs for abnormal scarring should be noted and include erythema that persists and deepens after 4 weeks or the sudden appearance of induration and redness 1 to 2 months postoperatively, especially if accompanied by pruritus or pain. A transition from deep red to purple may herald early keloid formation. These findings should prompt closer follow-up and intervention. Wounds at risk (Table 10-1) for hypertrophic scar (HS) or keloid scar (KS) should be observed

TABLE 10-1. Issues in scar revision.

What do you wish to improve about your scar?	Always emphasize what may be "improved" upon. Listen to the patient, especially the nonverbal communication.
What stage of healing is the scar?	Noticeable scar features often resolve with continued healing and time (i.e., elevation, redness, firmness, paresthesia) and intervention that is too early may be counterproductive.
Is the scar healing normally?	Unusually poor or delayed healing should be investigated further for variables affecting wound healing. Poor wound healing is inevitable in some clinical settings. **Extrinsic factors** Poor wound care, excess activity, infection, trauma, smoking, manipulation. **Intrinsic factors** Extremity locations, advanced diabetes, irradiated skin, malnutrition, some chemotherapies, genetic diseases (Ehlers–Danlos, Marfan's syndrome, epidermolysis bullosa).
Is the site at high risk for hypertrophic scarring or keloid?	Risk factors include high wound tension, highly mobile sites (over joints or extremities), and location (jawline, neck, back, central chest, shoulders, earlobe).
Is the scar causing functional compromise?	Dysfunctional scars distort free margins (alar rim elevation, ectropion, eclabium) and/or reduce function (restrict breathing, tearing, chronic conjunctivitis). Functional needs override cosmetic restoration.
Do the subjective and the objective match?	Do the perspectives of the patient and surgeon match? A consensus of what needs correction and in what priority is essential.
Does the scar need to be excised?	Nonsurgical options should be attempted first if possible.
Can the primary surgeon perform the revisions?	Knowing one's limitations is part of good surgical judgment.
Does the patient require a second opinion?	This may be required to establish consensus and or for assistance in revision techniques.

more closely. This author follows these high-risk wounds at 1- to 2-month intervals postoperatively, observing for changes in color, symptoms, or elevation.

Scar Massage

Massage therapy is an often recommended but understudied intervention for scar modification. The results from scar massage are confounded by varied techniques, duration, compliance, and endpoints. Objectively, scar massage ameliorates pain and itching.[1–3] Subjectively, scar massage engages the patient actively in the healing process. Improperly performed, massage may also be counterproductive. Massage should consist of a deep kneading motion with lubricant (petrolatum) rather than frictional rubbing. The latter may traumatize the scar and stimulate hypertrophy.

Pressure Therapy

Pressure therapy differs from scar massage in that a minimum required pressure is constantly applied to the scar, usually via a compression garment or device. It is commonly prescribed in burn units for the prevention and reduction of contracted and hypertrophic burn scars.[4] Efficacy is best for early scars (initial 3 months). The compression is maintained for nearly 24 hours, which may be intolerable to some patients. Results may be noted as

early as 1 month but therapy should be prolonged (1 year or more) for best results. Reduction in erythema is an effective indicator of progress and as little as 15 mm Hg pressure may be sufficient.[5] Pressure devices may be combined with silicone gel sheeting following keloid excision to prevent recurrences, especially on the earlobe.[6,7]

Silicone

Since the 1980s, silicone gel sheets (SGS) have been effective in the prevention and treatment of hypertrophic and keloid scars. The silicone component is not essential as the therapeutic benefits are exerted from scar hydration and occlusion, which reduce scar thickness, pain and itching, and increase scar pliability.[8,9] Variable improvement may be seen in 70% to 90% of treated patients.[10] On a cellular level, hydration reduces fibroblast proliferation and collagen formation.[11] A change in static electricity induced by SGS is hypothesized by some authors to modulate scar formation.[12] SGS conform readily without adhesives and must remain for at least 12 hours for effect. Other than local skin irritation and maceration, silicone products are well tolerated. For high-risk wounds, SGS may be used preventively and applied after surgery. Recurrence of KS may also be prevented with SGS following excision.[10] For existing HS or KS, SGS may be combined with intralesional steroids, compression, or other options for therapy.

TABLE 10-2. Scar analysis and therapy.

Scar	Features	Revision options
Length	Scar length is not as critical as contour, texture, width, color, and proper orientation. Scar revision techniques often lengthen existing scars in exchange for better scar camouflage and altered direction	Not applicable
Contour	**Elevated** Above skin but otherwise skin colored, asymptomatic. May be due to excess tension, imprecise approximation or suturing, inadequate undermining. Step-off or overhanging edges Trapdoor bulging Persistent eversion Standing cone	Time and scar massage Silicone occlusion Intralesional steroids Scalpel sculpting Dermabrasion Reexcision Dog-ear correction
	Hypertrophic scar (HS) Elevated, thickened, often red, pruritic, or painful. Scar is confined to incision line.	See keloid options
	Keloid scar (KS) Thickened scar overgrowth that extends beyond original incision. May be symptomatic (pruritic, painful).	Time and scar massage Pressure therapy Silicone occlusion Intralesional steroids Intralesional interferon Intralesional 5-fluorouracil (5FU) Pulse dye laser Topical imiquimod Cryosurgery Reexcision ± broken line techniques Radiotherapy ± excision
	Indented Depressed concavity due to underlying tissue loss or tethering. *Example*: Thin graft mismatch with thicker periphery Indented scars are not necessarily atrophic.	Tissue augmentation to elevate depressed scar Resurfacing to plane elevated edges and reduce contour mismatch (scalpel sculpting, laser, dermabrasion) Subcision Reexcision
	Atrophic (spread) Widened scar width with cutaneous thinning. Often due to wound separation from inadequate suture support and or excessive tension. Atrophic scars may be flat or slightly depressed.	Reexcision with tissue plication for tissue support Broken line techniques
	Contracted Type of elevated scar that is tented or webbed. May have hypertrophic component. Often overlying mobile joints or between convex and concave junctions.	Similar to keloid. Broken-line techniques, especially Z-plasty to reorient scar directions
Texture	Scar is of different surface consistency to surrounding skin (i.e., smooth skin graft within sebaceous surroundings)	Resurfacing techniques Excision of remaining subunit and repair with like tissue
Color	Color should match surrounding skin. Less optimal colors include ranges of white, red, brown, and purple.	Resurfacing techniques to blend hypopigmentation Pulse dye laser for erythema Cosmetics
Width	Ideal scar is<1 mm in width. Wider scars may be seen with atrophic/spread or indented scars.	Identifying cause of spread is essential to prevention with revision (technique vs.excess tension vs. postoperative complications, etc.) Reexcision
Orientation	Scars not hidden or parallel to relaxed skin tension lines (RSTL)	• Reexcision + broken line techniques

TABLE 10-3. Nonsurgical Options for Scar Revision.

Options	Features	References
Massage	**Benefits** Improves pain, itching Involves patient actively **Side effects** Improperly performed, massage may traumatize scar and worsen healing	2, 3
Pressure	**Benefits** Reduces scar elevation, thickness, redness, pain, pruritus Prevents or reduces hypertrophic burn scars Effective in preventing recurrences from keloid excisions **Side effects** Discomfort from chronic pressure, occlusive irritation	4–7
Silicone dressings	**Benefits** Mechanism of action related to occlusion and hydration reduces scar elevation, thickness, pain, pruritus Increases scar pliability Silicone products (not inclusive): Novagel™ (Alimed, Dedham, MA), Cica-Care* (Smith & Nephew, Largo, FL), Silon® (BioMed, Allentown, PA) **Side effects** Irritation, maceration	8–12
Interferon (IFN)	**Benefits** Reduces scar elevation, thickness, pain, pruritus Prevents keloid scar recurrence when combined with excision **Side effects** Pain, inflammation, irritation, impetiginization Systemic flulike symptoms *Intralesional* 1. IFNα-2b (Intron®A, 10 million IU/1mL; Schering Corp., Kenilworth, NJ). Excision with immediate 1 million units (MU) intradermally for each 1 linear cm of scar (up to 5MU) after closure. Repeat in 1 week with 5MU. Recurrence rate 18.7% in IFN group vs. 51.1% in excision alone. 2. IFNγ-1b (Actimmune®. 100mcg/0.5mL (1 million IU/50mcg); Intermune,. Brisbane, CA). 10–100mcg 3×/week for 3–10 weeks. Study with lower dose (10mcg) showed no benefit.[16] *Topical imiquimod 5% cream* 1. Imiquimod 5% cream (Aldara™; 3M Pharmaceuticals, Minneapolis, MN). Excision with same day imiquimod application q.h.s. ×8 weeks. No keloid recurrence after 6 months in 10 of 12 patients.	13–19
Steroids	**Benefits** Reduces scar elevation, thickness, pain, pruritus Prevents keloid scar recurrence when combined with excision **Side effects** Pain, cutaneous atrophy (may be permanent), telangiectasias, steroid precipitation (dermal yellowish deposits) *Primary therapy* 1. Intralesional steriods (ILS) [triamcinolone acetonide (TAC) 10–40mg/mL] at 4-week intervals. 2. Cordran tape to scar for at least 12-hour duration *Adjunctive therapy* 1. ILS intradermally at time of excision (TAC 10–20mg/mL) and postoperative ILS at 4-week intervals. 2. Combined with excision, silicone, pulse dye laser	20, 21, 22
5-fluorouracil (5FU)	**Benefits** Reduces scar elevation, thickness, pain, pruritus and redness. Increases scar pliability. **Side effects** Pain, ulceration, hyperpigmentation *Primary therapy* 1. 5FU (50mg/mL) combined with TAC (10mg/mL) in 9:1 ratio in same syringe. 2. 50–100mg 5FU per session. Start 3 sessions/week. Results usually seen by 5th injection. Taper frequency according to response. Hypertrophic scar respond better than keloid scar response.	23, 24, 25

TABLE 10-3. *Continued*

Options	Features	References
Cryotherapy	**Benefits** Reduces scar elevation, thickness **Side effects** Pain, ulceration, blistering, hypodepigmentation *Primary therapy* 1–2 freeze–thaw times of 15–20 seconds. Treat every 3rd week for 8–10 treatments *Adjunctive therapy* Causes temporary tissue edema, which facilitates ILS	26, 27
Radiation therapy	**Benefits** Reduces scar elevation, thickness, pain, redness, pruritus **Side effects** Acute and chronic radiation dermatitis Long-term potential of malignancy	28–30
Laser revision	**Nonablative lasers [pulse dye lasers (PDL)]** Decreases scar redness, thickness Increases scar pliability May be used *preemptively* to optimize scar cosmesis by starting PDL at time of suture removal, which remodels collagen during initial healing. May be used *therapeutically* with HS that are red and raised. **Side effects** Excessive fluences may cause blistering and worsen scar. Subpurpuric fluences are advisable.	31–34, 37

Interferon

Interferon (IFN) affects scar formation by inducing collagenase activity and inhibiting fibroblast production of collagen (type I and III) and glycosaminoglycan.[13] It may be directly injected or induced within a scar by topical imiquimod. When adjunctively combined with excision, IFN reduces the recurrence of keloids.[13–15] Primary therapy with IFN has not been studied. There are several effective regimens for IFN listed in Table 10-3. Systemic flulike symptoms may develop with injections, which may be largely abated by preinjection acetaminophen. For topical use, imiquimod application is initiated on the night of surgery and continued nightly for 8 weeks.[17] Local reactions of irritation, inflammation, burning and pain may occur and rest periods during the course may be necessary. Patients should also be monitored for bacterial impetiginization with symptoms of increasing pain, purulence, or malodor. In a small study of 12 patients with short-term follow-up (6 months), topical imiquimod prevented keloid recurrence in 10 patients who completed the trial.[18,19] Expense is the main limiting factor of IFN therapy.

Steroids

Intralesional steroids (ILS) have been the traditional mainstay of scar management in both primary and adjunctive roles (Table 10-3). As primary treatment, ILS alone may successfully reduce some elevated scars including HS, KS, and trapdoor elevations. Injections must be directed into the scar itself (elevated portion above skin) and not subcutaneously as tissue atrophy may develop.[20] Considerable resistance is common with initial injections and a larger gauge needle (25- to 27-gauge) is essential. A blanched appearance to the scar is the endpoint of each session (Fig. 10-1A,B), which is repeated at intervals until the scar flattens. For trapdoor elevations, triamcinolone 5 to 10 mg/mL is a safe starting point, whereas 20 to 40 mg/mL may be needed for HS or KS. Intervals between sessions will vary depending on the triamcinolone formulation. Longer acting triamcinolone acetonide (TAC) is injected every 4 weeks and shorter acting triamcinolone diacetate every 2 weeks. ILS into scars is typically painful and analgesics, local and topical anesthetics, or preinjection cryotherapy are helpful. Alternatively, Cordran tape (flurandrenolide impregnated tape, Oclassen Pharmaceuticals Cordan[R], San Rafel, CA) may be applied for at least 12 hours/day to soften the scars. Adverse effects of ILS include atrophy, dyschromias, yellowish precipitation, and telangiectasias. When used adjunctively, ILS is begun at the time of excision: either intradermally prior to closure or immediately after buried sutures and then continued at monthly intervals.[21] Encouragingly, incisional wound dehiscence has not been reported with intraoperative ILS.[22] The literature on ILS for scars is not uniformly supportive, with one study showing no statistical benefit in the ILS + excision group compared to excision

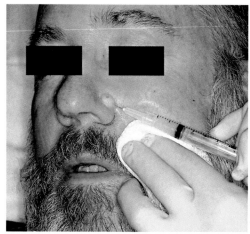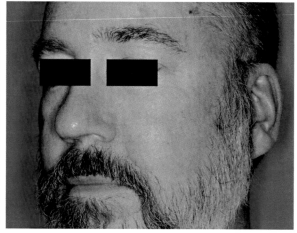

FIGURE 10-1. (A) Kenalog injection into a trapdoor scar (20 mg/cc). (B) Improvement after one injection session.

alone.[13] Most practitioners, however, advocate ILS as an important part of scar therapy.

5-Fluorouracil

5-Fluorouracil (5FU) works similarly to IFN in its effects on fibroblast activity and production of collagen and gly-cosaminoglycan. Fitzpatrick summarized his 9-year experience with 5FU and HS in over 1000 patients as follows: (1) 5FU is effective as primary therapy for HS and a subset of keloids (<2 cm diameter); (2) the effectiveness held true for a variety of scars (acne, laser, surgical); (3) younger and more symptomatic scars responded better than older, asymptomatic scars; (4) the response was faster with more frequent injections; (5) injections must be frequent (1–3/week) and up to 5 sessions may be needed to see benefits; (6) scar reduction is noted in the following order: pain and itching, scar softening, flattening, and redness; (7) safety profile was excellent and no hematologic suppression was observed at 5FU doses below 100 mg per injection; and (8) the pain of injection (main adversity) may be diminished by injecting with TAC–5FU combination.[23] Complications of 5FU include pain, ulceration, and hyperpigmentation, which have been transient.[24,25] The overall risk/benefit ratio with 5FU is favorable compared to ILS as tissue atrophy and telangiectasias do not occur. Results are enduring for HS but not for larger keloids.

Cryotherapy

With sufficient freezing, scar tissue becomes edematous, anoxic, and eventual cell death occurs. When repeated at regular intervals (every 3–4 weeks), cryotherapy may decrease scar elevation and thickness but will not change scar width. Blistering, ulceration, and permanent dyschromias are commonplace and patients should be fore-warned. Freezing a scar prior to ILS will cause scar tissue edema, which then facilitates needle penetration and steroid delivery.[26,27]

Radiation Therapy

When used alone, radiation therapy (RT) is no better than excision alone in treating KS. As an adjunct to excision, however, RT is an effective albeit rarely recommended treatment for KS.[28,29] The long-term potential for radiation-associated malignancies precludes the widespread usage of RT. As a result, RT is usually reserved for adult patients whose KS has failed previous therapies. RT may be delivered as external beam, interstitial implants, or high-dose brachytherapy.[30] In expert hands, RT will reduce scar elevation and thickness with minimal injury to surrounding and underlying healthy tissue.

Nonsurgical Laser

Laser revision for scars falls in both surgical and nonsurgical categories. The prototype nonsurgical (noninvasive) laser is the pulsed dye laser (PDL; 585 nm, 595 nm), which targets oxygenated hemoglobin. Most applications of the PDL are secondary interventions, in which an existing scar (HS or KS) is targeted to improve erythema, height, and pliability.[29,30] Preemptive uses of PDL to optimize scar appearance are promising.[31,32] By targeting the vascularity of an early scar, collagen remodeling occurs (especially at subpurpuric fluences) and the scar becomes less conspicuous. In a small study, Nouri and colleagues initiated PDL therapy on the day of suture removal and demonstrated improved cosmesis on the treated half. The PDL is also useful for treating postoperative telangiectasias that persist beyond 6 months. Timing for postoperative PDL therapy, therefore, may either be early (at 1 week) or late (>6 months). At excessive fluences, the PDL can precipitate blistering and HS. Energy densities, therefore, should be conservative and aim for minimal purpura or subpurpuric endpoints.

Surgical Options for Scar Revision

Surgical options for scar revision are outlined in Table 10-4.

Dermabrasion

The success of dermabrasion for scar revision is the gold standard by which other resurfacing techniques are compared. When performed 4 to 8 weeks postoperatively, surgical scars may be effaced.[33,34] Even older scars may be improved although enhancements are not as dramatic. Dermabrasion may be performed manually with various grades of sterilized sandpaper or machine diamond fraises of varying coarseness. Freezing the skin prior to machine dermabrasion (but not necessary for manual) is essential to produce a firm surface for sanding. Soft, thin skin (periorbital) and free margins cannot be dermabraded easily and other resurfacing techniques (laser, discussed below) are available. Hypopigmentation should be expected and may be problematic in darker skin types (Fig. 10-2A,B). Dyschromias are partially minimized by manual compared to machine dermabrasion (the latter requires a cryogen which further injures melanocytes). Patients should be advised that visible skin pores within the resurfaced region will not be smaller. In fact, these dilated pores may be more accentuated by dermabrasion (Fig. 10-2B). Dermabrasion is ideal for mild contour and suture line irregularities (Fig. 10-3A–C). Tapering shallow elevations or depressions to the surrounding skin, for example, is an ideal use of dermabrasion. Whenever possible, entire subunits should be resurfaced. For these surgical scars, dermabrading to achieve fine pinpoint bleeding is the endpoint. This correlates histologically to the junction of the papillary and upper reticular dermis. In no instance should dermabrasion extend beyond the level of the sebaceous glands. Dermabrasion is generally not effective and may even worsen HS or widely spaced scars.

Surgical Lasers

Surgical lasers such as the CO_2 and erbium:YAG target water and ablate the epidermis and dermis to varying depths. This resurfacing is similar to manual dermabrasion and may blend textural scar and surface irregularities at 4 to 8 weeks postoperatively. Both techniques achieve similar degrees of scar improvement and have similar side effects. Compared to dermabrasion, however, CO_2 laser resurfacing is unique in that a residual zone of thermal damage (RTD) extends beyond the ablated layer.

TABLE 10-4. Surgical options for scar revision.

Options	Features	References
Dermabrasion	Improves scar contour, textural irregularities, and overall blending to adjacent skin	35–39
	Will not address scar width or trapdooring	
	Ideal period for dermabrasion is 6–8 weeks postoperatively	
	Residual hypopigmentation may be seen	
Ablative lasers (CO_2, erbium:YAG)	Similar to dermabrasion in benefits	
	CO_2 laser has added feature of heat induced collagen remodeling	
	Resurfacing lasers lack tactile control available with dermabrasion	
	May be used *preemptively* after buried sutures to deepithelialize wound edges. Subsequent reepitheliallization of incision then seals scar line.	
	May be used *therapeutically* to address mild textural irregularities.	
	Side effects	
	Hypo- and depigmentation (which may be delayed) may develop. Excessive thermal damage may worsen scar.	
Broken line techniques		
Geometric broken line (GBL)	Similar to W-plasty in scarline disruption.	40, 41
W-plasty	Lengthens and disrupts scar continuity into multiple angulated segments	42, 43
	Overall scar orientation not affected	
Z-plasty	Achieves scar lengthening and reorientation	44–48
	May correct contractile scars	
Miscellaneous		
Surgical debulking	Corrects trapdoor scars, thick flaps, and grafts.	
Reexcision (including staged excision)	May be staged and combined with broken line techniques	
Scalpel sculpting	Addresses focal contour elevations	
Subcision	Releases vertical tethers to overlying skin and creates a broad plane of new scar formation	49
	Improves focally depressed adherent scars	

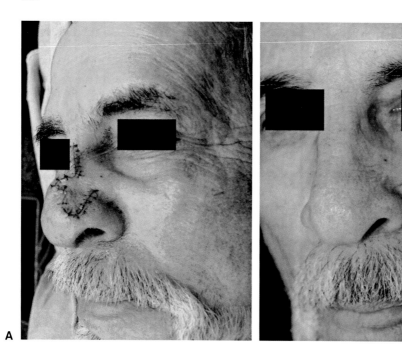

FIGURE 10-2. (A) Bilobed transposition flap on the nasal tip. (B)
Hypopigmentation and accentuated
pores following dermabrasion.

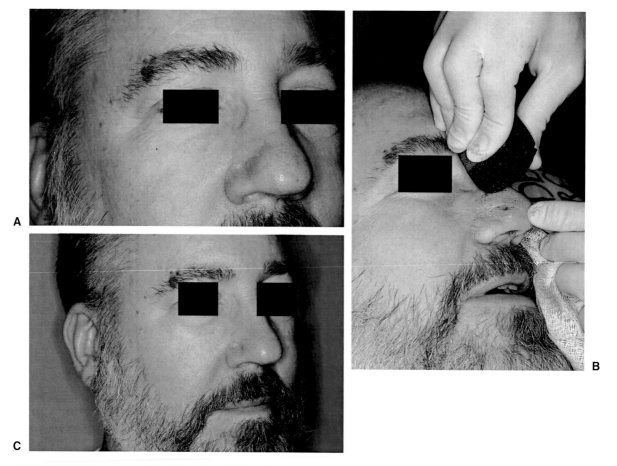

FIGURE 10-3. (A) Mild contour and incision line visibility. (B) Manual dermabrasion at 8 weeks after surgery. (C) Scar and improvement 2 months after dermabrasion.

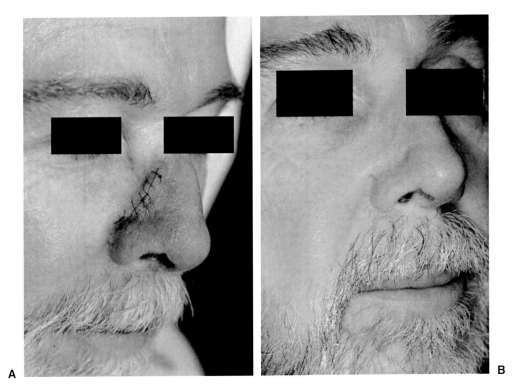

FIGURE 10-4. (A) CO_2 laser resurfacing of incision line following dermal sutures and before epidermal sutures. (B) Scar is practically invisible.

This RTD contracts underlying collagen and may be manipulated to even further improve cosmesis. Other advantages of laser scar revision include (1) freezing the skin, which is vital in dermabrasion, is not necessary with laser; (2) laser may address scars where dermabrasion is not possible or difficult (periorbital, small crevices); (3) skin resurfacing is more precise (lasers may achieve either partial- or full-thickness epidermal ablation); and (4) intraoperative hemostasis is better with laser (less exposure to blood spraying with laser). Resurfacing lasers may also be used intraoperatively to achieve an almost invisible scar. Following buried sutures, this author uses the CO_2 laser to resurface the incisional skin (suture line plus 5 mm of peripheral skin) (Fig. 10-4A,B). CO_2 laser settings are in the ultrapulse mode, 300 mJ, 5 to 7 W, using a 3-mm handpiece. A computer pattern generator may also be used. With reepithelialization, the suture lines are sealed and even at 1 week, the scar is barely visible. Linear closures, skin grafts, and flap incisions have all been treated accordingly with exceptional long-term outcomes (Fig. 10-5A–C).

Broken Line Techniques

Methods under this category include geometric broken lines (GBL), W-plasty, and Z-plasty. As a rule, these techniques require an incision or excision of the original scar. The scar is surgically transformed into multiple smaller linear or curvilinear segments. They are effective in improving both function and cosmesis and sometimes are the only options for revising a distorted anatomy. Table 10-5 compares the features and applications of these techniques.

Geometric Broken Lines (GBL) and W-Plasty

Given their similarities, GBL and W-plasty technique will be discussed together. Their common benefits for scar revision include: (1) the central scar is excised in the revision; (2) the scar is divided into multiple smaller segments; (3) angulated lines and shapes are used to disrupt the scar's visual continuity; (4) the scar is lengthened to some degree; and (5) the scar's original direction is preserved.[40–43] These techniques are ideal for scars that already parallel relaxed skin tension lines (RSTL) and do not require a change in direction. They are not used to revise free margin distortion. The GBL and W-plasty are designed by first dividing the scar with multiple cross-marks. These cross-marks are lines that are drawn across and perpendicular to the scar (Fig. 10-6A–D). The lines are outlined 5 mm apart and in a tapering fashion (shorter lines at either ends of the scar and longer lines towards the center). No cross-mark should extend more than 1 cm

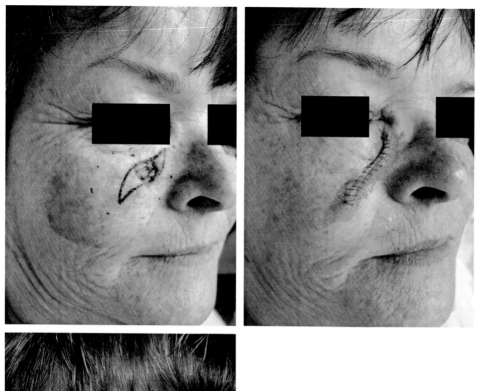

FIGURE 10-5. (A) Curvilinear closure design. (B) CO_2 laser resurfacing of incision line intraoperatively. (C) Exceptional long-term results.

TABLE 10-5. Broken line techniques compared.

Technique	Lengthens scar	Tissue sparing	Changes scar direction	Tension and distortion	Application
Z-plasty	+++	+++	+++	+++	Transposition of flaps Contracted/webbed scar Scar opposing relaxed skin tension lines Free margin distortion Combination with W-plasty
W-plasty	+	+	Not applicable	+	Does not involve transposition of flaps Milder contracted scar Camouflage long scars along RSTL Revise suture railroad tracks
Geometric broken line(GBL)	+	+	Not applicable	+	Similar to W-plasty More camouflage effect than W-plasty

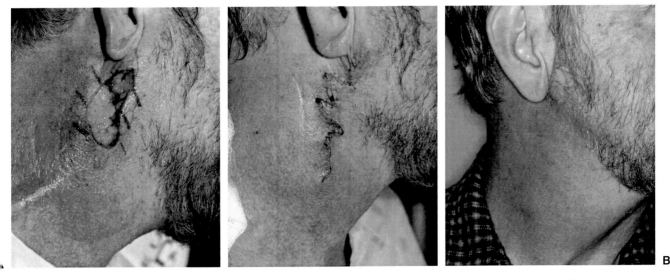

FIGURE 10-16. (A) Skin cancer defect at the mandibular angle with multiple Z-plasties designed in the closure. (B) Closure completed. (C) Long-term results.

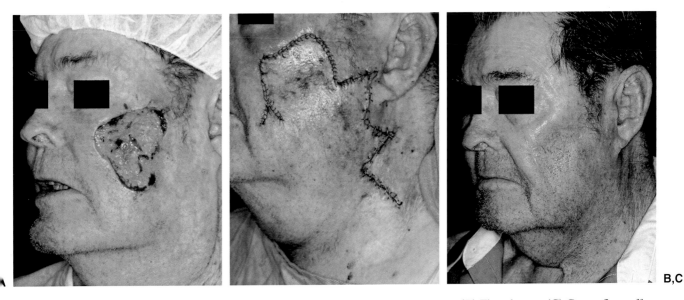

FIGURE 10-17. (A) Cheek defect to be repaired with a rhombic flap and double Z-plasty. (B) Flap closure. (C) Camouflage effects of Z-plasty application during closure (2 months postoperatively).

Surgical Debulking

Surgical debulking is most appropriate for contour prominences that resist nonsurgical interventions. Intralesional steroids, massage, and time, for example, will improve most scars and should always precede surgery, especially because they give patients options for scar revision. Scar revision instruments are useful adjuncts to the surgical tray (Fig. 10-18). The bulkiness of a paramedian forehead flap commonly requires some surgical debulking (Fig. 10-19A). The flap should be elevated to leave the bulk of the scar at the wound base and not at the flap's underside. This precaution permits maximal visualization and prevents flap perforation. Trimming should also be performed in calculated strips or layers to avoid excessive thinning (Fig. 10-19B,C). Bolster dressings are helpful in securing the new contour changes.

Scar Excision

On occasion, a suboptimal scar cannot be salvaged, and its excision becomes necessary. The most critical decision in removing the old scar is whether to reapproximate the wound as before or to revise with adjunctive techniques. A direct excision and reclosure is appropriate if the scar already lies within RSTL and if tension is minimal (Fig. 10-20A–C). At other times, a skin graft or flap may be needed for optimal scar revision (Fig. 10-21A–D).

Scalpel Sculpting

This technique is the application of a shave excision. Using a Schick blade or similar malleable edge, a contour elevation may be sculpted flush with the surrounding skin. Scalpel sculpting may be combined with dermabrasion where the former may address the elevated scar and the latter may blend in the surrounding skin. Simple and effective, this technique is best for focal contour elevations (Fig. 10-22A–C).

Subcision®

One etiology for depressed scars is the tethering of overlying skin by vertical fibrous bands. Subcision® is an effective technique for elevating such scars by surgically releasing these vertical tethers.[49] A 1-inch Nokor™ needle (16- to 19-gauge; Becton-Dickinson, Franklin Lakes, NJ) is inserted peripheral to the scar and advanced underneath it. The needle is then swept widely underneath the scar in a fanlike horizontal motion, disrupting the vertical fibrous adhesions (Fig. 10-23). The level of release is usually mid- to deep dermal, or rarely in the subdermal–fat interface. Subcision® is more or less a method of focused undermining that is less traumatic than open techniques. The procedure usually requires multiple sessions. With each treatment, the depressed scar is progressively elevated as new collagen forms in a platelike plane underneath the scar.

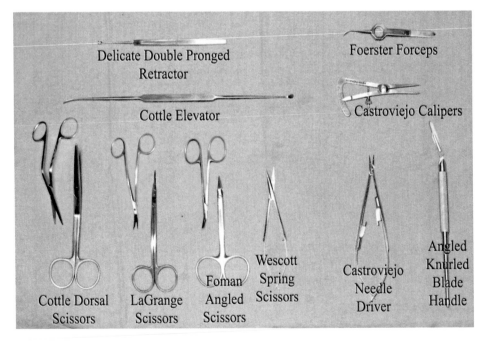

FIGURE 10-18. Instruments commonly used by author for scar revision.

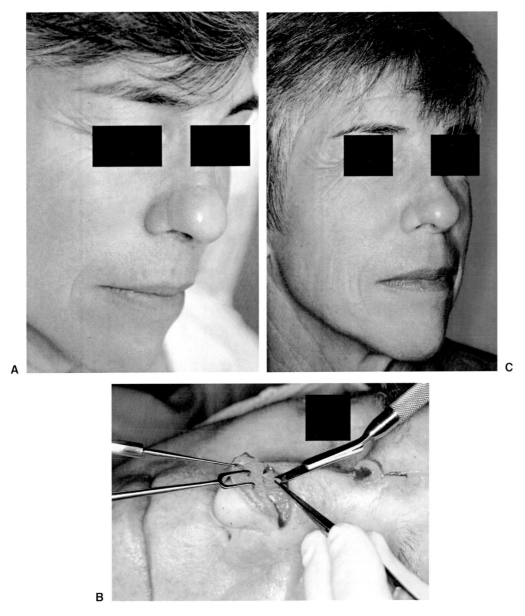

FIGURE 10-19. (A) Bulkiness of nasal tip from paramedian forehead flap. (B) Flap elevation and debulking of scar at the base. (C) Improved contour following surgical debulking.

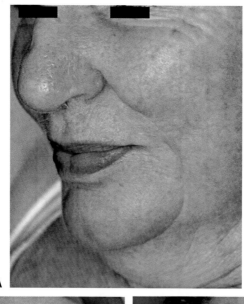

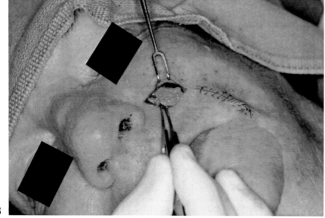

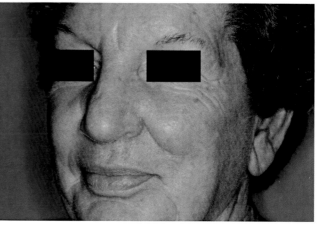

FIGURE 10-20. (A) Hypertrophic scar (HS) at lower melolabial fold and cheek fullness following cheek-to-nose pedicled flap. (B) Excision of HS and reclosure, fat debulking of upper cheek fullness. (C) Results after revision.

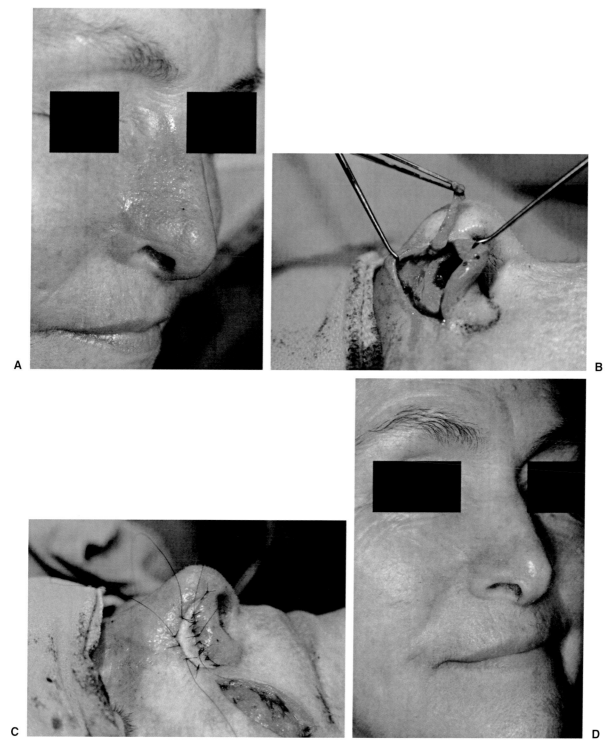

FIGURE 10-21. (A) Alar notching and blunting of alar sulcus from a melolabial transposition flap. (B) Scar debulking at alar sulcus to re-create groove. (C) Full-thickness skin graft to displace ala inferiorly in correct notching. (D) Results at 6 months.

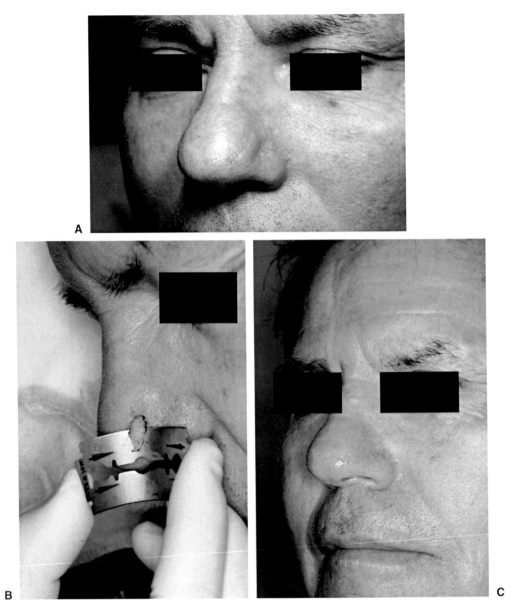

FIGURE 10-22. (A) Focal contour elevation from paramedian forehead flap. (B) Scalpel sculpting or shave excision. (C) Improved contour.

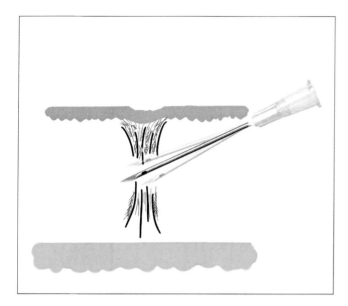

FIGURE 10-23. Subcision® technique for revising depressed scars. A Nokor™ needle is inserted peripheral to the depressed scar and undermining is performed beneath the scar in a sweeping motion.

Conclusion

There are a myriad of scar revision techniques. Note two scars are alike and each option is effective for a given scar and indication. Methodically analyzing the scar is the most critical part of successful scar revision. Equally essential is open patient communication and an informed consent. Patience and time will yield fruitful dividends. Surgical techniques are wonderful adjuncts when properly applied.

References

1. Teot L. Clinical evaluation of scars. Wound Repair Regen 2002;10:93–97.
2. Rogues C. Massage applied to scars. Wound Repair Regen 2002;10:126–128.
3. Field T, Peck M, Hernandez-Reif M, Krugman S, Burman I, Ozmen L. Postburn itching, pain, and psychological symptoms are reduced with massage therapy. J Burn Care Rehabil 1999;20:268–271.
4. Rogues C. Pressure therapy to treat burn scars. Wound Repair Regen 2002;10:122–125.
5. Kerckhove EV, Stappaerts K, Fieuws S, et al. The assessment of erythema and thickness on burn related scars during pressure garment therapy as a preventive measure for hypertrophic scarring. Burns 2005;31(6):696–702.
6. Chang CH, Song JY, Park JH, Seo SW. The efficacy of magnetic disks for the treatment of earlobe hypertrophic scar. Ann Plast Surg 2005;54:566–569.
7. Russell R, Horlock N, Gault D. Zimmer splintage: as simple effective treatment for keloids following ear piercing. Br J Plast Surg 2001;54:509–510.
8. Kerckhove EV, Stappaerts K, Boeckx W, et al. Silicones in the rehabilitation of burns: a review and overview. Burns 2001;27:205–214.
9. Hamanova H, Broz L. Topigel in the treatment of hypertrophic scars after burn injuries. Acta Chir Plast 2002;44:18–22.
10. Gold MH. A controlled clinical trial of topical silicone gel sheeting in the treatment of hypertrophic scars and keloids. J Am Acad Dermatol 1994;30:506–507.
11. Borgognoni L. Biological effects of silicone gel sheeting. Wound Repair Regen 2002;10:118–121.
12. Hirshowitz B, Lindenbaum E, Har-Shai Y, Feitelberg L, Tendler M, Katz D. Static-electric field induction by a silicone cushion for the treatment of hypertrophic and keloid scars. Plast Reconstr Surg 1998;101:1173–1183.
13. Berman B, Flores F. Recurrence rates of excised keloids treated with postoperative triamcinolone acetonide injections or interferon alfa-2b injections. J Am Acad Dermatol 1997;37:755–757.
14. Granstein RD, Rook A, Flotte TJ, et al. A controlled trial of intralesional recombinant interferon-gamma in the treatment of keloidal scarring. Clinical and histologic findings. Arch Dermatol 1990;126:1295–1302.
15. Larrabee WF, East CA, Jaffe HS, Stephenson C, Peterson KE. Intralesional interferon gamma treatment for keloids and hypertrophic scars. Arch Otolaryngol Head Neck Surg 1990;116:1159–1162.
16. Broker BJ, Rosen D, Amsberry J, et al. Keloid excision and recurrence prophylaxis via intradermal interferon-gamma injections: a pilot study. Laryngoscope 1996;106:1497–1501.
17. Kaufman J, Berman B. Topical application of imiquimod 5% cream to excision sites is safe and effective in reducing keloid recurrences. J Am Acad Dermatol 2002;47:S209–S211.
18. Berman B, Villa A. Imiquimod 5% cream for keloid management. Dermatol Surg 2003;29:1050–1051.
19. Jacob SE, Berman B, Nassiri M. Topical application of imiquimod 5% cream to keloids alters expression genes associated with apoptosis. Br J Dermatol 2003;149(Suppl 66):62–65.
20. Ketchum LD, Smith J, Robinson DW, Masters FW. The treatment of hypertrophic scar, keloid scar and scar contracture by triamcinolone acetonide. Plast Reconstr Surg 1996;38:209–218.
21. Kelly PA. Medical and surgical therapies for keloids. Dermatol Ther 2004;17:212–218.
22. Giovannini UM. Treatment of scars by steroid injections. Wound Repair Regen 2002;10:116–117.
23. Fitzpatrick RE. Treatment of hypertrophic scars using intralesional 5FU. Dermatol Surg 1999;25:224–232.
24. Apikian M, Goodman G. Intralesional 5-fluorouracil in the treatment of keloid scars. Australas J Dermatol 2004;45:140–143.
25. Nanda S, Reddy BSN. Intralesional 5-fluorouracil as a treatment modality for keloids. Dermatol Surg 2004;30:54–57.

26. Rusciani L, Rosse G, Bono R. Use of cryotherapy in the treatment of keloids. J Dermatol Surg Oncol 1993;19: 529–534.
27. Ceilley RI, Barin RW. The combined use of cryosurgery and intralesional injections of suspension of fluorinated adrenocorticosteroids for reducing keloids and hypertrophic scars. J Dermatol Surg Oncol 1979;5:54.
28. Garg MK, Weiss P, Sharma AK, et al. Adjuvant high dose rate brachytherapy (Ir-192) in the management of keloids which have recurred after surgical excision and external beam radiation. Radiother Oncol 2004;73:233–236.
29. Guix B, Henriquez I, Andres A, et al. Treatment of keloids by high-dose brachytherapy: a seven year study. Int J Radiat Oncol Biol Phys 2001;50:167–172.
30. Clavere P, Bedane C, Bonnetblanc JM, Bonnafoux-Clavere A, Rousseau J. Postoperative interstitial radiotherapy of keloids by iridium 192: a retrospective study of 46 treated scars. Dermatology 1997;195:349–352.
31. Alster TS. Improvement of erythematous and hypertrophic scars with 585 nm flashlamp pulsed dye laser. Ann Plast Surg 1994;32:186–190.
32. Alster TS, Williams CM. Improvement of keloid sternotomy scars by the 585 nm pulsed dye laser: a controlled study. Lancet 1995;345:1138–1200.
33. McCraw JB, McCraw JA, McMellin A, Bettencourt N. Prevention of unfavorable scars using early pulse dye laser treatments: a preliminary report. Ann Plast Surg 1999;42: 7–14.
34. Nouri K, Jimenez GP, Harrison-Balestra C, Elgart GW. 585 nm pulsed dye laser in treatment of surgical scars starting on the suture removal day. Dermatol Surg 2003;29: 65–73.
35. Katz BE, Oca AG. A controlled study of the effectiveness of spot dermabrasion ("scarabrasion") on the appearance of surgical scars. J Am Acad Dermatol 1991;24:462–466.
36. Yarborough JM Jr. Ablation of facial scars by programmed dermabrasion. J Dermatol Surg Oncol 1988;14:292–294.
37. Nehal KS, Levine VJ, Ross B, Ashinoff R. Comparison of high-energy pulsed carbon dioxide laser resurfacing and dermabrasion in the revision of surgical scars. Dermatol Surg 1998;24:647–650.
38. Tanzi EL, Alster TS. Treament of atrophic facial acne scars with dual-mode Er:YAG laser. Dermatol Surg 2002;287:551–555.
39. Ammirati CT, Cottingham TJ, Hruza GJ. Immediate postoperative laser resurfacing improves second intention healing on the nose: 5 year experience. Dermatol Surg 2001;27:147–152.
40. Davidson TM, Horlbeck DM. The geometric broken line technique. In: Harahap M, ed. Surgical techniques for cutaneous scar revision. New York: Marcel Dekker; 2000:407–423.
41. Lee KK, Mehrany K, Swanson NA. Surgical revision. Dermatol Clin 2005;23:141–150.
42. Onizuka T, Ohkubo F. The W-plasty technique. In: Harahap M, eds. Surgical techniques for cutaneous scar revision. New York: Marcel Dekker; 2000:397–405.
43. Rodgers BJ, Williams EF, Hove CR. W-plasty and geometric broken line closure. Facial Plast Surg 2001;17:239–244.
44. Frodel JL, Wang TD. Z-plasty In: Swanson NA, Baker SR, eds. Local flaps in facial reconstruction. St. Louis: Mosby; 1995:131–149.
45. Rohrich RJ, Zbar Ross IS. A simplified algorithm for the use of Z-plasty. Plast Reconstr Surg 1999;203:1513–1518.
46. Furnas DW, Fischer GW. The Z-plasty: biomechanics and mathematics. Br J Plast Surg 1971;24:144–160.
47. Seno H, Yanai A, Hirabayashi S. The Z-plasty technique. In: Harahap M, eds. Surgical techniques for cutaneous scar revision. New York: Marcel Dekker; 2000:381–395.
48. Johnson SC, Bennett RG. Double Z-plasty to enhance rhombic flap mobility. J Dermatol Surg Oncol 1994;20:128–132.
49. Orentreich DS, Orentreich N. Subcutaneous incisionless (Subcision®) surgery for the correction of depressed scars and wrinkles. In: Harahap M eds. Surgical techniques for cutaneous scar revision. New York: Marcel Dekker; 2000:245–257.

11
Miscellaneous Complications

Mary E. Maloney and Nathaniel J. Jellinek

This chapter will cover a wide variety of complications without a common uniting theme. Some topics are well established in the literature, whereas others are well recognized, common problems that have not been researched extensively. References may be sparse or nonexistent in some areas. These miscellaneous complications are still important and the cutaneous surgeon should be capable of avoiding them before they occur and treating them once they arise.

Contact Dermatitis

Contact dermatitis is one of the most frequent complications in dermatologic surgery.[1] In one series of surgical patients, 2% of evaluated patients had contact dermatitis and 12% had an irritant dermatitis to preoperative agents or postoperative dressing regimens.[2] These reactions interfere with wound healing and require early recognition and prompt therapy to prevent impaired healing and scarring. Contact reactions may be divided into three subsets: irritant contact dermatitis, allergic contact dermatitis (type IV), and immediate (type I) reactions, which include both contact urticaria and anaphylaxis.

Irritant reactions are nonimmunologic and can be expected after a single exposure. They result from contact between the skin and an exogenous toxic agent. Anyone with enough exposure will react. One common example is adhesive tape, which may cause an irritant reaction in a significant portion of the population, although the length of exposure necessary for dermatitis varies widely. Most irritant reactions are mild to moderate in intensity, but can be severe enough to cause full-thickness injury (Fig. 11-1A–C).

Allergic contact dermatitis is a type IV delayed hypersensitivity reaction requiring prior or prolonged exposure for the first reaction (sensitization.) Subsequent reactions will occur with shortened intervals after repeated exposures. Type IV reactions are T-lymphocyte–mediated inflammatory processes and require a functioning immune system.

Type I reactions result from antigens causing IgE-mediated mast cell degranulation, with release of active mediators such as histamine. This cascade can lead to contact urticaria or full-blown anaphylaxis.

Surgical Preparations

The common preparatory agents used in the surgical setting include chlorhexidine, povidone–iodine, and alcohol. Hexachlorophene has been seldom used because of its neurotoxicity in the infant population. Benzalkonium chloride is rarely used, in part because of its potential for causing allergic contact dermatitis.

Chlorhexidine

Chlorhexidine has become a popular skin-prepping agent because it has broad spectrum antibacterial activity, rapid onset, and is not inactivated by body fluids. The risk of sensitization is significantly increased in patients with leg ulcers or eczematous dermatitis where exposure is repeated or prolonged.[3] Some have estimated the rate of sensitivity at 2.5% to 5.4%.[4,5] Reports of contact reactions, which can be severe, are still relatively rare but well documented.[6,7]

There are a number of reports of type I reactions to chlorhexidine.[8–10] In many instances, there has been prior mucosal contact to the agent, but any route of exposure can cause type I sensitization.[10] Because chlorhexidine is available over the counter in many compounds, it is difficult to identify all previous exposures. However, anaphylaxis has been documented after contact with unbroken skin.[11] Interestingly, there are reports of patients with both type I and type IV sensitivity.[12,13] If the surgeon is unaware of the possibility of chlorhexidine anaphylaxis, correct identification of the offending agent can be significantly delayed.

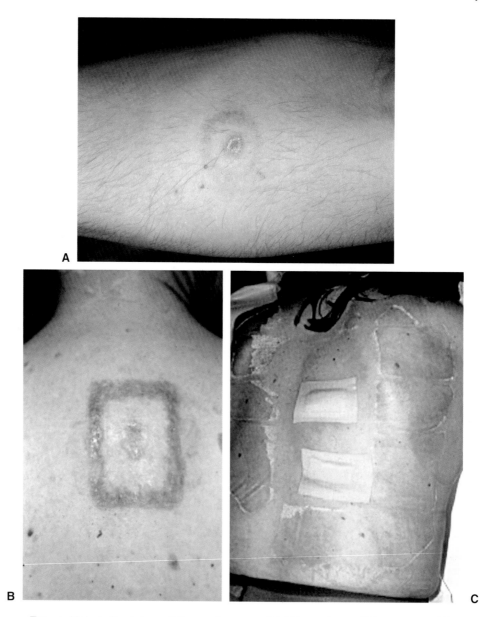

FIGURE 11-1. Irritant dermatitis may be very mild (A), moderate (B), or severe (C).

Chlorhexidine is an ocular irritant, and the toxicity can be quite severe. In addition, exposure to the eye may cause corneal damage ranging from transient epithelial defects to ulceration, and on occasion, opacification.[14] Other agents are more appropriate for the periorbital location.

Chlorhexidine's ototoxicity to the inner ear is well documented in several studies.[15,16] Any small perforation of the tympanic membrane could allow access to the inner ear. Therefore, it is not an appropriate preparatory agent for ear surgery.

Iodophors

Povidone–iodine is an iodophor, a complex of iodine and a carrier molecule, which releases iodine slowly. Povidone itself is a polymer that resembles a plasma protein. The iodophor has the germicicdal activity of iodine, but greatly reduces the toxicity of iodine by its slow release from the complex.[17] Reports of contact dermatitis, while rare, do occur.[6,17] Severe irritant dermatitis has been reported after a patient had prolonged contact with drapes saturated with povidone–iodine. The reaction was so extensive that it resembled a burn.[18]

Several systemic reactions have been documented. Burn patients have been reported to have a severe metabolic acidosis as a result of extensive topical povidone–iodine exposure.[19] Another patient developed iododerma as a result of wound irrigation with povidone–iodine.[20] Iodophors are also felt to be toxic to human cells, and use on open wounds may not be appropriate.[21] Because free iodine is released from povidone–iodine, it should not be used as a preoperative preparatory agent in patients with a known allergy to iodine.[17]

Alcohol

Alcohol is a very rapidly acting and efficient antimicrobial agent. It is both volatile and flammable. Therefore, to prevent burns during electrosurgery or laser surgery, the surgical site must fully dry before surgery is begun. Alcohol will not possess bacteriocidal activity until it has dried.

Fisher's text reports a low rate of allergic reactions to alcohol,[22] but more frequent prolonged use will promote irritation through induction of xerosis. Alcohol is both drying and defatting and can cause varying amounts of irritant dermatitis. Moisturization after repeated use may prevent dryness and the resultant dermatitis.

Less well recognized is alcohol's role as a contact allergen. There are reports of contact sensitivity: both contact dermatitis and contact urticaria to alcohol itself or its denaturing additives.[22–25] When allergy develops, there is usually cross-reactivity to amyl, butyl, methyl, and isopropyl types. In these individuals, ingestion of alcohol may cause stomatitis, urticaria, generalized morbilliform eruption, or a flare of eczematous dermatitis. However, not all contact reactions are associated with a reaction to ingested alcohol.[26]

Topical Antibiotics

Contact allergy to topical antibiotics is a well-recognized problem. The 2000 report of the North American Contact Dermatitis Group lists the top 50 allergens. Two topical antibiotics place in the top 10: Neomycin is the second most common allergen and bacitracin is number 10.[27] These medications can be a significant problem.

Neomycin

Long-term use of neomycin in the setting of chronic ulcers or chronic eczematous dermatitis has lead to sensitization. Fraki showed that 34% of leg ulcer patients become allergic over time.[28] However, leg ulcers alone could not lead to neomycin's place as the second most common allergen. Neomycin is present in a multitude of over-the-counter products, making routine exposure extremely common.[1] Prystowsky found that use of neomycin for more that 1 week for an eczematous dermatitis increased the risk of developing allergic contact dermatitis to neomycin.[29] Neomycin was also found to be the most common sensitizer (16%) when used in the treatment of chronic external otitis.[30] Intermittent use on wounds, however, is not associated with an increased risk of sensitization.[31]

Cross-reactivity of neomycin with aminoglycosides such as gentamycin (40%–66% cross-reactivity), tobramycin (25%–65%), kanamycin (43%–60%), and amikacin (33%) can be significant.[1,32]

Neomycin, which has been used as an oral prep agent for bowel surgery, is not significantly absorbed from the bowel. In spite of this, there have been reports of generalized eczematous dermatitis in patients with known contact sensitivity to neomycin in patients taking oral neomycin.[32]

Bacitracin

Bacitracin, originally thought to have a very low risk of sensitization, has risen to number 10 on the sensitization list.[27] It is well documented that allergic contact dermatitis can result from topical exposure to bacitracin. As in the case of neomycin, exposure to chronic wounds or dermatitis provides the greatest risk for the development of sensitivity.[33]

It has been demonstrated that many patients will have sensitivity to both neomycin and bacitracin.[34] The two compounds do not have structural similarity to account for cross-reactivity. Animal studies had supported that the sensitivity is a cosensitization (patients develop sensitivity to both chemicals independently, but usually at the same exposure) as opposed to a cross-sensitivity. This concomitant sensitization was demonstrated in a large Finish study.[35] Bacitracin has been shown to cause anaphylaxis.[36–38]

Other Topical Antibiotics

Mupirocin, erythromycin sulfate and sterate, and polymixin B are all rare sensitizers, though allergic contact dermatitis has been reported to each of them.[32,39,40] In the sensitized patient, these products can cause the same set of problems as those of the more common allergens.

Diagnosis and Wound Care Implications

Contact dermatitis in the sensitized patient will occur 24 to 96 hours after exposure with redness, vesiculation, and, usually, pruritus. Early in the course, when redness alone is present, it may be difficult to distinguish contact allergy from early infection. Pruritus may help differentiate the two. One of the keys to the diagnosis is that contact dermatitis involves the wound margin, whereas reactions to tape usually spare the wound margin (Fig. 11-2A,B). When there is extensive vesiculation and drainage, secondary infection is frequently present. Treatment of the secondary infection will help the reaction to respond to discontinuation of neomycin and the addition of topical steroids.

The surgeon must decide if the presence of contact dermatitis should change the schedule of suture removal.

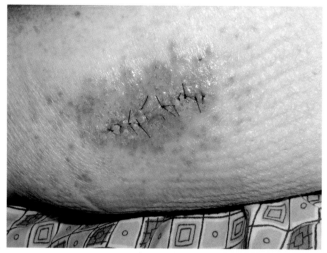

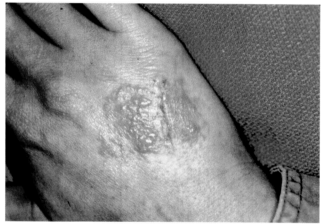

FIGURE 11-2. Contact dermatitis to neomycin which fully involves the suture line (A). Tape reaction sparing the suture line (B).

Because early wound strength depends on epidermal cell cohesion, vesiculation and disruption of the epidermis may significantly interfere with wound integrity. If there is good wound support with buried sutures, percutaneous sutures can be removed on schedule. If there is not sufficient dermal support, percutaneous sutures should not be removed. A compromise is to remove some of the sutures on schedule, leaving others (particularly the sutures carrying the greatest tension) in place for another week.

Whether topical antibiotics should be a part of routine wound care continues to be debated. Gette showed that 5.3% of a series of surgical patients had an allergic contact dermatitis to neomycin. Only 2% of this series were sensitive to bacitracin, and all of those patients used a combination (neomycin/bacitracin) antibiotic ointment.[41] The conclusion of that study was that bacitracin without neomycin should be safe for postoperative wound care.

A study comparing petrolatum with bacitracin showed 2% postoperative infections in the petrolatum group (8 of 9 by *Staphylococcus aureus*) compared to 0.9% in the bacitracin group (0 of 4 with *Staphylococcus aureus*). Another four patients in the bacitracin group had contact dermatitis.[42] Results suggest that petrolatum can be used instead of antibiotic ointment in routine wounds, though topical antibiotics may decrease the risk of staphylococcal infections when the risk of infection is high.

Complications of Suture Material and Technique

Extrusion of Buried Sutures

Buried sutures are an important part of wound closure. The final surgical result depends in large part on relieving wound tension, and buried sutures are important in "carrying" this tension. "Breaking strength" of a wound at 7 days without buried sutures is less than 10% of final wound strength and wound cohesiveness depends largely on epidermal cellular adhesion.[43] Therefore buried sutures are necessary to prevent dehiscence and carry wound tension.

One of complication of buried sutures is suture extrusion, known commonly as spitting sutures. Buried sutures may move to the surface, either as tufts of suture (Fig. 11-3) or small sterile abscesses that appear in the suture line. There may be only small fragments of suture, but most commonly the sutures and knots are extruded fully intact.

There are a number of potential risk factors for the extrusion of sutures. Buried sutures are present long after they have lost their tensile strength. The longer they are present, the greater the risk of extrusion, so that the longer-acting sutures have a greater chance of spitting.

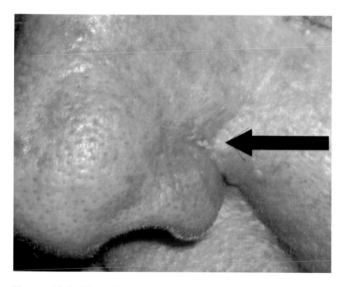

FIGURE 11-3. Extrusion of a buried suture without an inflammatory reaction.

Similarly, the larger the diameter of the suture used, and thereby the greater the time to full hydrolysis for synthetic sutures (or enzymatic degradation for gut), the greater the chance of extrusion. Knot tying, too, may affect suture extrusion. One intriguing study showed that the number of throws on the knot correlated directly with extrusion, with five throws leading to 30% extrusion rate while three throws lead to only 10% extrusion rate.[44] In addition, sutures placed close to the surface, or knotted at the surface rather than at the depth of the wound will lead to a higher rate of extrusion. New sutures have been recently developed may extrude less. Poliglecaprone 25 is a monofilament absorbable suture that seems to extrude less than the braided sutures in its class, such as polyglactin 910.

To minimize extrusion, the surgeon should bury the knot and choose the smallest appropriate diameter suture with the shortest appropriate time to absorption. Nevertheless, some patients will consistently extrude some or all of the buried sutures.[45]

Suture extrusion routinely occurs anywhere from 2 to 6 weeks postoperatively. On rare occasions, it can occur as late as 6 months after surgery. When the sutures extrude they frequently form a small papule that will erode and drain. Occasionally wisps of suture are seen by the patient (Fig. 11-3). At other times the surgeon will identify the suture with gentle probing with forceps. The suture may be snipped or cut with a #11 blade and removed. The area will heal rapidly once the offending suture has been extracted.

Stitch Abscess

Stitch abscesses may be the result of an inflammatory reaction to either the buried or cutaneous suture, the epithialization of a suture track, or true infection. The most common cause is a sterile inflammatory reaction to a suture (Fig. 11-4), which may be accompanied by the

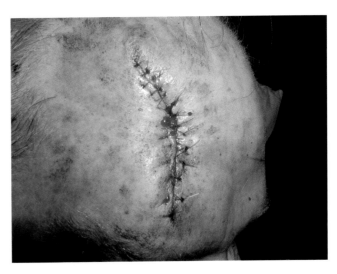

FIGURE 11-5. The degree of tension on this wound is a risk factor for cross-hatching.

extrusion of the buried suture. Simple removal of the stitch will allow resolution.

The epithialization of a suture track may cause the formation of a milium or keratinatous material that causes inflammation. In either case, opening the lesion with a #11 blade with expression of the material should allow rapid healing.

The last type of stitch abscess is a true infection, which will have a more significant surrounding inflammatory reaction. While rare, true abscesses occur most commonly with braided suture that allows wicking of bacteria into the depth of the suture track. For this reason, it may be prudent to use a monofilament suture in patients with a preexisting cutaneous infection, or in those suspected of being colonized (patients with active folliculitis or atopic dermatitis) with bacteria. A true abscess should be opened and drained. Because of the increase in community-acquired infections such as methicillin-resistant *Staphylococcus aureus* (MRSA), cultures should be sent before the initiation of antibiotic therapy.

Railroad Tracking

Railroad tracking or cross-hatching is almost always the result of excess wound tension. For this reason, it is not uncommon to see both cross-hatching and scar spread in the same final scar.

Tension on a wound requires the surgeon to use a large diameter suture and to leave the suture in place for a longer period of time to allow the wound to gain its own tensile strength. Suture material under tension may "bite" into the tissue, and this may be accentuated with wound swelling (Fig. 11-5). These depressed marks form cross-hatched tracks and may leave permanent scars. Needle puncture sites may also leave scars when sutures are left

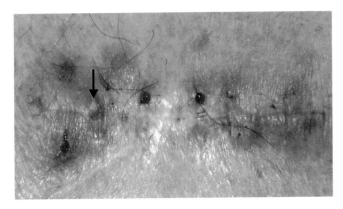

FIGURE 11-4. Suture irritation with a single intact sterile suture abscess.

intact for long periods. While no wound is immune from this complication, the most common sites include the back, chest, and extremities, where wound tension is notably increased with movement, lifting, or exercise. Railroad tracking tends to fade slowly with time but may be permanent.

The most important factor in preventing railroad tracking is the removal of tension on the wound. Orientation of closure to minimize tension, such as vertical orientation of a wound over the spine, is an obvious initial step. Defatting the wound, extension of the wound deep into the subcutaneous tissue, undermining extensively and at the appropriate depth, and the removal of large standing cones when present will also reduce tension on a wound.

The placement of adequate buried sutures relieves and shares tension along the wound and can carry tension so that smaller diameter cutaneous sutures can be simply coapt the wound margin rather than carry tension. Occasionally, closing a wound under tension is preferable to second intent healing, flap, or graft closure. Lower legs of elderly patients can be an especially complex area for healing with any closure technique. In these patients, keeping the closure as simple as possible is prudent. The scalp similarly may do best with a wound under tension to minimize alopecia associated with a graft of second intent healing, or the redirection of hair orientation with a flap. Patients on multiple anticoagulants may be at high risk for hematoma if extensive undermining or flap movement is performed. Wounds under tension may actually tamponade small vessels and prevent postoperative bleeds. In each of these instances, it is appropriate to discuss the reasons for wound closure selection with the patient before the procedure.

Allergy to Suture Material

Irritation from suture material is common as all sutures are foreign bodies. Many materials have been designed to be less reactive (polypropelene, polyester, and even nylon) and will cause less reaction than a foreign protein like silk.

True allergic reactions to suture materials are rare. Two examples include stainless steel (found in suture and staples) and chromic sutures. Stainless steel contains varying amounts of nickel, and in the nickel-sensitive patient, an allergic dermatitis can occur. Chromic suture is composed of gut treated with a chromate-containing compound designed to delay enzymatic degradation and prolong the tensile strength of the suture. Patients with a chromate allergy may react to these sutures.[1] There is no evidence presently that either of these sutures act as the sensitizing agent. These reactions may look like a wound infection or irritant reaction. The surgeon must be aware of patient sensitivity to these materials and avoid these sutures (or staples) in this population.

Excessive Granulation Tissue

Excessive granulation tissue occurs most commonly at the site of wounds healing by second intention (including failed grafts that require second intention healing), wounds closed with guiding sutures alone (another form of second intention healing), and, rarely, at the site of wounds closed with primary layered closure, simple closure, or flaps. Excessive granulation tissue, known to lay people as "proud flesh," is composed of connective tissue and vascular tissue with varying amounts of inflammation (Fig. 11-6). It is raised above the level of the surrounding tissue, often covered with a pseudomembrane composed of dried serum and exudates, and is frequently colonized with bacteria, but not truly infected. The exophytic nature and pseudomembranous surface prevent reepithelialization. Migrating epithelial cells during wound healing can easily grow and migrate along a flat surface or down a depression but have significant difficulty migrating up a raised edge, resulting in a nonhealing wound that bleeds with trauma.

There are two approaches to the treatment of excess granulation tissue. First, the gellataneous material can be curetted to a firm healthy base. While this can occasionally be performed without local anesthesia (as the granulation tissue itself contains little or no nerve endings), this technique will frequently cause bleeding which will necessitate obtaining hemostasis with electrosurgery and thereby require local anesthesia. However, the curettage method affords complete removal of this material with the reinstitution of more normal healing.

The second approach is treatment with silver nitrate. Complete treatment of the entire area of excessive granulation is required, resulting in the formation of a grayish membrane overlying the granulation tissue which will

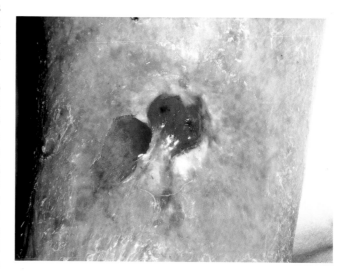

FIGURE 11-6. Excessive granulation tissue interferes with the re-epithialization of this leg wound.

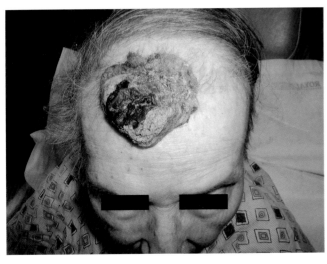
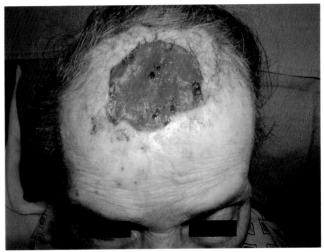

FIGURE 11-7. Erosive pustular dermatosis has a thick crust (A) overlying the granulation tissue base (B).

slough off during routine wound care. However, the patient needs to be informed of the nature of this grayish material or they can be quite startled at the next dressing change. Use of silver nitrate avoids local anesthesia and any further cautery but may require a second or even third treatment to get full healing of the wound. The other possible side effect of silver nitrate is silver tattooing of the wound, which does not occur routinely (because the silver nitrate membrane is removed with cleansing) but can complicate the occasional healing wound. In the nail unit, it may lead to longitudinal melanonychia.[46]

Erosive pustular dermatosis of the scalp is disorder of excess granulation tissue.[47] This disorder occurs in the elderly and presents as a bed of granulation tissue with overlying thick crust and prurulent material (Fig. 11-7A,B). It occurs in thin, atrophic, sun-damaged skin or at the site of previous surgery (including skin grafting, cryosurgery, and resurfacing) or radiation. Unlike hypergranulation tissue, it responds poorly to silver nitrate or destructive modalities. However, topical steroids or tacrolimus may be beneficial. Its presentation is frequently confused with a cutaneous malignancy, especially because of the possibility of pseudoepitheliomatous hyperplasia at the epidermal margin.

Milia

Milia are 1- to 2-mm white cysts arising from the infundibulum of vellus hairs that are lined by thin stratified squamous lining with a granular layer. They may form primarily in disorders characterized by recurrent epidermal regeneration, such as epidermolysis bullosa or porphyria. Postoperatively, milia may arise as a complication of ablative and resurfacing procedures, as well as incisional surgery. The pathogenesis varies, however.

Incisional surgery may be complicated by milia as the suture tract reepithelializes. Resurfaced wounds feature hypersebaceous and hyperproliferative epidermal regrowth, often coupled with occlusive dressings. This combination may result in disorders of the follicle, including acne and milia in up to 11% of cases.[48,49] Dermabrasion may implant epidermal debris, leading to postoperative milia as well.

Over time, many milia resolve spontaneously. For persistent cysts, treatment is straightforward. Incising the cyst roof with a #11 blade and expressing the contents with a comedo extractor or two tongue depressor blades is effective. Gentle electrocautery to the cyst roof may also be used. Alternatively, superficial peels with glycolic acid or light abrasion with a buff puff may unroof the cyst surface. For extensive and persistent milia, therapy with topical retinoids may gradually normalize the skin.

Complications of Extracellular Fluid

Edema

Edema, a potential complication of any surgical procedure, is caused by capillary leakage of fluids with concominant soft tissue swelling. Almost all surgical procedures are accompanied by a small amount of postoperative swelling. It is the degree of swelling that may cause complications.

Thin tissues, such as the eyelid or genital area, show edema much more easily than thicker areas, such as the back or chest (Fig. 11-8). Clinically evident swelling can lead to further complications, such as increased wound tension, dehiscence, and pain.

Chronic eyelid lymphedema secondary to periocular surgery occurs presumably as a result of blockage of the

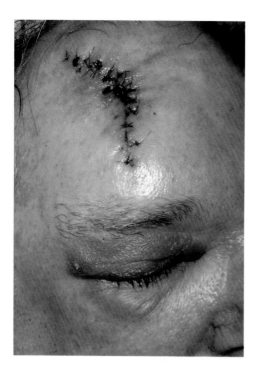

FIGURE 11-8. Moderate periorbital edema following surgery on the forehead.

lymphatic channels by postsurgical fibrosis. This potentially distressing condition, seen predominantly in elderly patients with loose skin, may be effectively managed by frequent, gentle massage and reassurance. Surgical intervention to reduce periocular lymphedema should be avoided because it may increase the amount of fibrosis, resulting in further lymphedema and swelling.

Prevention of edema is much more effective than treatment. Exercise causes vascular dilatation and increases the heart rate. These factors can exacerbate capillary leakage and, therefore, strenuous activity or exercise should be avoided in the 24- to 48-hour postoperative period. The application of ice or cooling agents postoperatively, especially in areas prone to swelling, will also help diminish edema. Ice is particularly important in the periorbital area after surgery on the eye, on the forehead, or underlying cheek. The usual recommendation is now for "soft ice" — a commercially available soft ice pack that will conform to the body area. These bags should never be placed directly on the skin to prevent over cooling of the skin and cold injury. An alternative to a commercially available ice pack is a package of frozen vegetables, usually peas or corn. The small kernels will again conform to the wound site and be soft and supple. They can be refrozen and used repeatedly. However, it is important to remind the patient to discard these vegetables after use as an ice pack as the freezing and thawing will leave them inedible.

The final measure to prevent edema is elevation of the affected area. For leg wounds, the patient should be instructed to either walk or sit with their foot elevated, but not to stand for long periods of time or sit with their foot dangling. Surgery on the forearm or hand requires elevation and surgical sites of the hand, in particular, may require a sling to facilitate that elevation. Elevation of any extremity wound should also be maintained at bedtime by placing the affected limb on a pillow. Facial surgery around the eye may cause periorbital edema. This may be delayed 24 to 36 hours postoperatively and is almost always exacerbated by lying flat while sleeping. Patients should be instructed to sleep on several pillows rather than in a more supine position to avoid this complication.

Once swelling has developed, all the preventive measures should be used to assist in reducing and resolving the swelling: avoidance of exercise, ice, and elevation. Pain associated with swelling should be reevaluated by the surgeon as it may indicate infection or hematoma.

Seroma

A seroma is the accumulation of serous fluid within or underlying a wound. Although this is a relatively rare event, there is a dearth of original literature on the development of seromas in dermatologic surgery.

The most common circumstance for seroma development is the presence or development of a dead space in a wound, underlying a skin graft, or following liposuction. A dead space may occur when a mass-occupying lesion such as a cyst is removed. Closure of the dead space with buried sutures should prevent the accumulation of serous fluid. If the dead space is not closed or the buried sutures do not fully close this space, serous fluid can accumulate and cause a seroma. If all bleeding has not been stopped, a hematoma could also form.

Seromas may develop under a skin graft if the graft bed leaks serous fluid, which may float the graft off the vascular bed and contribute to graft failure. To prevent this complication, it is common to place some type of pressure dressing over a graft. The most common is the tie-over dressing, in which a xeroform or cotton dressing is sutured in place. Occasionally a bulky dressing alone secured with pressure can be used instead of a tie-over dressing, especially in areas where it is difficult or impossible to tie a dressing securely (e.g., nasal ala and canthus of the eye). Basting sutures may also hold a graft firmly to the wound bed. "Pie crusting," while designed to prevent hematoma, will also prevent seroma.

A seroma may be difficult to distinguish from a hematoma, especially in a deep wound. Seromas tend to be softer and more "blotable" than hematomas, which tend to become firmer as the blood clots and organizes. An easy diagnostic test is to insert a large-bore needle to along the suture line. Serous fluid can be easily extracted with this technique, while aspiration is difficult to impossible in an organized hematoma. The removal of the fluid may not fully resolve the problem in a deep wound. Unless the dead space is obliterated in some way, the seroma will simply reform. Occasionally, evacuation followed by a pressure dressing will close the dead space. However, for a large or recurrent seroma, a small opening of the incision line can be made, and the cavity packed to both allow serous fluid to wick out and cause granulation to occur, thereby closing the dead space. The entire wound does not need to be reopened, only a small enough opening to allow the placement of packing. This technique should maximize the cosmetic result. When necessary the scar can be revised at a later date, but this is seldom required.

Grafts overlying seromas should be nicked with a #11 blade to drain the fluid. The graft will then again sit on the vascular base, and have the potential for a "take." A pressure dressing should be reapplied for 24 hours to facilitate this process, but the initial incision used to promote drainage will also prevent the reaccumulation of fluid.

Neurosensory Complications

Pain

Pain as such is not a complication of surgery. It is an anticipated result of incisional, ablative, and resurfacing types of surgical procedures. It is important to predict the amount of pain that a procedure will produce and treat appropriately. A simple excision with a wound closed in a layered side-to-side fashion with little or no tension should produce minimal pain that can be adequately treated with acetaminophen as needed. As the size of the wound enlarges and the tension of closure increases, the possibility of pain will also rise. It is not uncommon for a grafted site to be relatively painless for the patient while the graft donor site, a wound closed under some tension, or a split-thickness skin graft donor site may cause the patient a moderate discomfort requiring an analgesic. It is also important to remember that pain tolerance of patients varies quite widely. Where one patient will complain of virtually no pain following a procedure, another patient may have exquisite pain to the exact same procedure. For any surgery done under local anesthesia, the patient's tolerance to local anesthesia injection will be an excellent guide to their overall pain threshold.

Injection of a long-acting anesthetic after closure is completed can provide more than 6 hours of pain relief, and is especially appropriate in wounds under tension. Occlusive dressings have also been shown to reduce postoperative pain, especially in wounds left to heal by second intention.[50]

Before discharging the patient, the surgeon should evaluate the need for pain medication. That evaluation should include the patient's pain threshold, the location and size of the wound, the type of surgery performed, and the tension on the wound. Postoperative instructions should outline what to take for pain and what to do if pain exceeds expectation, including phone numbers to call for assistance.

Late Pain

Once a pain level or plateau has been reached postoperatively, the expectation is that pain will diminish on a daily basis. When pain status suddenly changes, it is an indication that there has been a change in the wound status. A rapidly expanding hematoma either early or late in the postoperative period will cause exquisite pain as well as swelling. A wound infection will cause increasing pain and a deep wound infection may cause pain long before erythema or purulent drainage appears. Escalation of pain is an indication for the surgeon to reevaluate the wound for other complications.

Late postoperative pain in scar tissue is uncommon. When it occurs, it is generally attributed to a neuroma or nerve entrapment in dense scar tissue. Treatment of such a scar with intralesional corticosteroids will frequently soften the scar and resolve the pain. A more serious cause of late postoperative pain in the setting of tumor treatment is the recurrence of tumor, particularly in a perineural location. Perineural basal carcinoma or squamous cell carcinoma may cause sharp pain that may be fleeting or long lasting. It may radiate along a nerve or cause pain, paresthesias, or itching at the nerve-ending site rather than at the site of actual tumor involvement. In this setting, a deep biopsy, usually an incisional biopsy that obtains a good sample of the deep portion of the scar, is necessary to fully rule out the possibility of perineural recurrent tumor.

Reflex Sympathetic Dystropy

Reflex sympathetic dystrophy (RSD) is a debilitating condition of pain following injury. It has been called several names, including causalgia, erythromelalgia, and complex regional pain syndrome. Recently, it has been subdivided into types I and II. RSD type I is that syndrome associated with minor inciting injuries including dermatologic surgery.

Reflex sympathetic dystrophy is characterized by intense pain out of proportion to, and often extending over a greater distribution than the original injury. The pain may be sharp, burning, throbbing, or aching. Classically, it has been divided into three stages. The first, or acute, stage (1–3 months) is characterized by hyperalgesia and allodynia out of proportion to clinical signs of inflammation. The second, or dystrophic, stage (3–6 months) is associated with signs attributable to local sympathetic hyperactivity; the skin may be cool, edematous, and hyperhidrotic, showing pallor, cyanosis, and even livedolike changes. The hair growth may slow, and nail plates may demonstrate a variety of changes including thickening, brittleness, or rigidity. Unlike the first stage, the hallmark of which is pain, the second stage may exhibit variable discomfort. The third, or atrophic, stage (8–18 months) is characterized by progressive, often irreversible tissue damage. Changes include muscle, subcutaneous, and pilar atrophy with fixed mottling of the skin, fibrous joint ankylosis, and Sudeck's atrophy: diffuse osteoporosis with skeletal cystic and subchondral erosions.[51]

The exact pathogenesis is unknown. Theories abound, most under the uniting theme of autonomic nerve dysfunction.[4] Others, however, blame immunologic, inflammatory, or central nervous system involvement for this syndrome. Diagnosis depends on the presence of clinical features appropriate to the syndrome stage, including an initial traumatic event, and is a diagnosis of exclusion. X-rays, bone scans, and magnetic resonance imaging may be helpful in showing musculoskeletal changes.[52]

Treatment is difficult, and often best accomplished by a pain specialist. Over 60 treatment strategies have been described in the literature! Therapeutic options include physical therapy, counseling, analgesics, sympathetic blockade (either medical or surgical), calcitonin, anti-inflammatory agents, and α- and β-blockers.

Pruritus

It is surprising that the healing wound does not induce more pruritus. The healing wound is awash with neutrophils, macrophages, epidermal, fibroblast, transforming, platelet-derived, and vascular endothelial growth factors, as well as proteases, tumor necrosis factor, histamine, kinins, and prostaglandins. Many of these substances, in particular histamine, kinins, and prostaglandins, induce pruritus.[43,53,54] Many or most of these factors are also involved with inflammatory or eczematous dermatoses that have significant associated pruritus. Nevertheless, the mild pruritus associated with normal wound healing seldom requires significant attention and quickly will resolve spontaneously. When significant pruritus occurs, one must suspect another cause such as a contact or irritant dermatitis.

Late pruritus of scars is most commonly seen in keloid or hypertrophic scars, and less commonly in more normal scars. There is a well-documented increase in mast cells and histamine content in keloids that parallel the rate of collagen synthesis. This may well account for much of the pruritus seen in keloids.[55,56]

Treatment of the pruritus involved with hypertrophic or keloidal scarring involves treatment of the abnormal scar itself with one of a long list of treatment options, including intralesional steroids, cryotherapy, interferon, imiquimod, laser, radiation, intralesional 5-fluorouracil (5FU), topical tacrolimus, pressure dressings, silicone dressings, or reexcision.[57] Pruritus and pain resolve as the scars soften, even if there is not full resolution of the scar thickness, presumably because histamine is reduced in parallel with the end of collagen synthesis.

Nerve regrowth into or through the scar may also be associated with abnormal sensations including pruritus. Immature scars may have an increased number of thinly myelinated or unmyelinated C fibers and this may cause pruritus in many patients. As scars mature and innervation is completed, this sensation should resolve.[55]

Telangiectasias

Telangiectasias are another complication of cutaneous surgery, and may be seen after both ablative and incisional procedures. They are more common in photodamaged skin and may be a sequela of chronic ultraviolet exposure independent of cutaneous surgery. Telangiectasias develop more frequently in wounds under tension. While the specific etiology and pathogenesis are unknown, older data suggests that the persistent vascular dilation results from lack of nerve regeneration into the new blood vessels.[58] More recent data from rosacea research has implicated vascular endothelial growth factor (VEGF) in the production of telangiectasias.[59] Alternatively, nitric oxide and nitric oxide synthases may be involved, and have been studied in rosacea, although definitive data is currently lacking for their role in postoperative telangiectasias. Certain patients appear to be predisposed to developing telangiectasias, demonstrating telangiectasias elsewhere on the body. Some, indeed, have erythematotelangiectatic rosacea. This population is at higher risk for developing this complication.

Postoperative telangiectasias will often resolve spontaneously over 6 to 12 months and can be followed conservatively and treated with only makeup. There are multiple approaches for treatment for persistent telangiectasias. The 585 to 595 nm pulsed dye lasers may be used with small spot size to precisely target individual vessels. Alternatively, a larger spot size can field treat an area with telangiectasias as well as underlying persistent erythema. Similarly, the 532 nm KTP laser may accurately treat the telangiectasias. Deeper vessels may be targeted with the longer wavelength, long-pulsed 1064 nm Nd:YAG laser. All of these lasers demonstrate more selective photothermolysis for blood than the earlier argon or CO_2 lasers, which were associated with unwanted thermal tissue injury and subsequent scarring. In addition, electrodessication and sclerotherapy may used to ablate individual vessels.

Nasal Valve Compromise

The nasal valve is the soft tissue underlying the lateral alar cartilage. It is responsible for controlling air movement on inspiration and flaring the nostril for full inspira-

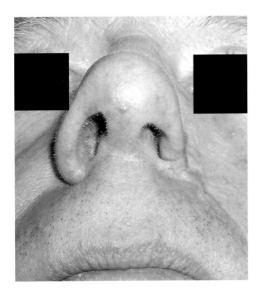

FIGURE 11-9. The nasal valve has collapsed, causing difficulty with inspiration, and requiring repair.

tion. When this structure no longer lies in its anatomic location, but buckles or is distorted into the vestibule, it disrupts air flow and causes nasal stuffiness that is accentuated when the patient is recumbent.[60,61] Nasal valve compromise can be caused by a wide variety of nasal surgeries, including grafts, flaps, and second intention healing of deep alar defects[62] (Fig. 11-9).

For the majority of patients, this defect causes nasal fullness and the sense that one side of the nose is blocked. Patients with any compromise of the other nostril will become obligate mouth breathers, losing the benefits of air filtration, humidification, and warming provided by the nose.

As Robinson points out, the best treatment is prevention.[62] Cartilage struts or battens should be used whenever the alar wall is thinned to prevent collapse or potential collapse. Second intention healing should be avoided when it would allow buckling of the valve at the time of final scar maturation. Care should be taken that any sliding flap does not put buckling tension on the alar cartilage. When such tension does occur, further undermining or flap redesign should be undertaken. The use of a nasal trumpet has been reported to maintain pressure on the nasal valve during healing (preventing buckling), while allowing a patent airway.[63]

There are multiple procedures and variations on procedures described for correction of the deformity or obstruction once it has occurred, including auricular composite grafting,[64] suspension of the alar cartilage from the orbit,[65] or suspension of the cartilage from the periosteal SMAS layer of the upper lateral nose.[66] It is the goal of each of these repairs to reestablish normal air flow through the nose.

Postoperative Pigmentary Changes

There is no dermatologic surgical procedure that completely avoids potential pigmentary change as a complication. These procedures include cryosurgery, sclerotherapy, electrodessication and curettage, excisional surgery with repair, resurfacing, and laser therapy. By understanding the risks for any particular patient, steps can be taken to minimize the result and fully prepare the patient for potential postoperative pigment problems. Different techniques have different risks for both hypopigmentation and hyperpigmentation.

Incision/Electrodessication and Curettage

Incisional, excisional, and flap surgery only rarely produce pigmentary changes. When changes occur, they tend to be mild and resolve spontaneously. Scars that result from electrodesiccation and curettage are notorious for being starkly hypopigmented and permanent (Fig. 11-10).

Cryosurgery

Cryosurgery has been most frequently associated with hypopigmentation. Melanocytes are more sensitive to cold than keratinocytes. Hence, melanocytes become innocent bystanders of tumors treated with cryosurgery. Zacarian reported permanent loss of pigment to be unavoidable after treating 4228 tumors with cryosurgery,

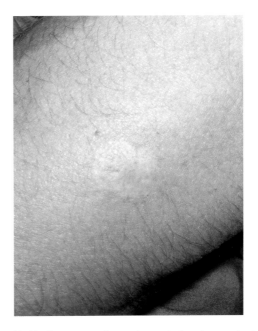

FIGURE 11-10. Permanent hypopigmentation in an electrodessication and curettage scar.

although some patients had full repigmentation over time. His expectation was of permanent hypopigmentation, most notable in patients with dark skin. Hyperpigmentation was an infrequent occurrence, which resolved spontaneously in several months.[67]

Grafting

Grafts may heal with either hypo- or hyperpigmentation. The hypopigmentation is usually permanent, while hyperpigmentation is not permanent and will fade over several months. Resolution may be more rapid with the use of retinoic acid and hydroquinone. Graft dyschromia will also be improved with spot dermabrasion in spite of the fact that resurfacing itself can cause pigmentary changes. Grafts may have a poor color match, regardless of the donor site or care during surgery. These color mismatches are not truly hypo- or hyperpigmentation, but rather relative color changes. While the color match may improve with time, it seldom will fully match surrounding tissue.[68]

Resurfacing

Resurfacing-associated postinflammatory hyperpigmentation occurs frequently, developing during the first 6 to 8 weeks after the procedure. Stratigos states the rate to be 36% of all patients,[69] while Nanni has shown that the incidence approaches 100% in Fitzpatrick types IV to VI.[49] Patients with a history of melasma are at an even increased risk.

Some authors recommend pretreatment of patients with retinoic acid and/or hydroquinone,[68,70,71] while others feel pretreatment with bleaching agents is ineffective.[48,72] Early treatment with a combination of retinoic acid and hydroquinone with vigorous sun protection will speed resolution of this complication. Some authors start treatment for potential hyperpigmentation in high-risk patients as early as 2 weeks following therapy, and continue for 6 weeks as a prophylactic measure.[48]

There are two types of hypopigmentation that develop after resurfacing procedures. The first is a relative hypopigmentation when compared to pretreatment mottled photodamaged skin. The second type is a more significant, delayed hypopigmentation that develops 3 to 12 months after surgery and after an initial return to normal skin color. This complication spans all skin types, and is not limited to darker pigmented patients.[73] Goldberg has noted that the greater the depth of resurfacing, the denser the resulting fibrosis and the greater the possibility of hypopigmentation. He also points out that the neck seems to have the greatest risk of hypopigmentation. Treatment is ineffective and the hypopigmentation is usually permanent.[72]

Other Laser Therapies

There are a growing number of lasers used for hair removal, tattoo removal, and vascular anomalies. All may cause temporary hypo- or hyperpigmentaton that will resolve spontaneously. The one exception is hypopigmentation that may result from the Q-Switched ruby laser, which may persist indefinetly.[72]

Sclerotherapy

The incidence of postinflammatory hyperpigmentation ranges from 11% to 35%, with some authors reporting up to 80% with the use of sodium tetradecyl sulfate.[5] Many factors play a role in the development of hyperpigmentation, including technique, the sclerosing agent and concentration of the agent used, factors that elevated intravascular pressure, use of postprocedure compression to decrease intravascular pressure, vessel diameter, and the patient's medications.[74] In spite of the high incidence of this complication, only 1% to 2% have hyperpigmentation after 1 year.[75]

Histology of hyperpigmented areas shows hemosiderin deposition and not increased melanin. However, some experts still feel there is a component of melanocytic hyperactivity contributing to the hyperpigmentation.[76]

Prevention may be achieved with the use of compression stockings postoperatively.[77] Effective treatment is limited because the pigment is dermal hemosiderin and not melanin. Some success in the treatment of hyperpigmentation has been reported with 20% trichloroacetic acid, chelation,[78] and laser therapy (including intense pulsed light) that targets hemoglobin rather than melanin.[74,79] Laser therapy has been useful in spite of the fact that laser itself can cause hyperpigmentation. However, because most hyperpigmentation resolves with time and without treatment, watchful, supportive waiting is a reasonable approach.

References

1. Lawlor K, Taylor JS. Contact allergy. In: Wheeland RG, ed. Cutaneous surgery. Philadelphia: Saunders; 1994:76–90.
2. Marks JG, Rainey MA. Cutaneous reactions to surgical preparations and dressings. Contact Dermatitis 1984;10:1–5.
3. Reynolds NJ, Harman RRM. Allergic contact dermatitis from chlorhexidine diacetate in a skin swab. Contact Dermatitis 1990;22:103–128.
4. Lasthein AB, Brandrup F. Contact dermatitis from chlorhexidine. Contact Dermatitis 1985;13:307–309.
5. Osmundsen PE. Contact dermatitis to chlorhexidine. Contact Dermatitis 1982;8:81–83.
6. Rietschel RL, Fowler JF. Antiseptics and disinfectants. In: Rietschel RL, Fowler JF, eds. Fisher's contact dermatitis. 5th ed. Philadelphia: Lippincott Williams & Wilkins; 2001:162–163.

7. Goon AT, White IR, Rycroft RJ, et al. Allergic contact dermatitis from chlorhexidine. Dermatitis 2004;15:45–47.

8. Kautheim AB, Jermann THM, Bircher AJ. Chlorhexidine anaphylaxis: case report and review of the literature. Contact Dermatitis 2004;50:113–116.

9. Beaudouin E, Kanny G, Morisset M, et al. Immediate hypersensitivity to chlorhexidone: literature review. Allerg Immunol (Paris) 2004;36:123–126.

10. Snellman E, Rantanen T. Severe anaphylaxis after a chlorhexidine bath. J Am Acad Dermatol 1999;40:771–772.

11. Autegarden JE, Pecquet E, Huet S, et al. Anaphylactic shock after application of chlorhexidine to unbroken skin. Contact Dermatitis 1999;40:215.

12. Bergqvist-Karlsson A. Delayed and immediate-type hupersensitivity to chlorhexidone. Contact Dermatitis 1988;18:84–88.

13. Lauerma AI. Simultaneous immediate and delayed hypersensitivity to chlorhexidine digluconate. Contact Dermatitis 2001;44:59.

14. Nasser RE. The ocular danger of Hibiclens (chlorhexidine). Plast Reconstr Surg 1992;89:164–165.

15. Igarashi Y, Suzuki J. Toxicity of chlorhexidine gluconate in cats. Arch Otorhinolaryngol 1985;242:167–176.

16. Igarash Y, Oka Y. Vestibular ototoxicity following intratympanic applications of chlorhexidine gluconate in the cat. Arch Otorhinolaryngol 1988;245:210–217.

17. Marks JG. Allergic contact dermatitis to poidone-iodine. J Am Acad Dermatol 1982;6:473–475.

18. Corazza M, Bulciolu G, Spisanil L, et al. Chemical burns following irritant contact with providone-iodine. Contact Dermatitis 1997;36:115–116.

19. Pietsch J, Meakins JL. Complications of povidone-iodine absorption in topically treated burn patients. Lancet 1976;1:280–282.

20. Bishop ME, Garcia RL. Iododerma from wound irrigation with povidone-iodine. JAMA 1978;240:249–250.

21. Lineaweaver W, Howard R, Soucy D, et al. Topical antimicrobial toxicity. Arch Surg 1985;120:267–270.

22. Rietschel RL, Fowler JF. Contact dermatitis in health personnel. In: Rietschel RL, Fowler JF, eds. Fisher's contact dermatitis. 5th ed. Philadelphia: Lippincott Williams & Wilkins; 2001:451–465.

23. Ludwig E, Hansen BM. Sensitivity to isopropyl alcohol. Contact Dermatitis 1977;3:240–244.

24. Melli MC, Giorgini S, Sertoli A. Sensitization from contact with ethyl alcohol. Contact Dermatitis 1986;14:315.

25. Kanzaki T, Hori H. Late phase allergic reaction of the skin to ethyl alcohol. Contact Dermatitis 1991;25:252–253.

26. VanKetel WG, Tan-Lim KN. Contact dermatitis from ethanol. Contact Dermatitis 1975;1:7.

27. Marks JG, Belsito DV, Fowler JF, et al. North American Contact Dermatitis Group patch test results, 1996–1998. Arch Dermtol 2000;136:272–273.

28. Fraki J, Petonen L, Hopsu-Havu K. Allergy to various components of topical preparations in stasis dermatitis and leg ulcer. Contact Dermatitis 1979;5:97–100.

29. Prystowsky S, Nonomura J, Smith R, et al. Allergic hypersensitivity to neomycin. Arch Dermatol 1979;115:713–715.

30. Prystowsky S, Nonamura J, Smith R, et al. Contact allergy to various components of topical preparations for treatment of external obitis. Acta Otolaryngol 1985;100:414–418.

31. Leyden JJ, Kligman AM. Contact dermatitis to neomycin sulfate. JAMA 1979;242:1276–1278.

32. Rietschel RL, Fowler JF. Reactions to topical antimicobials. In: Rietschel RL, Fowler JF, eds. Fisher's contact dermatitis. 5th ed. Philadelphia: Lippincott Williams & Wilkins; 2001:167–184.

33. Katz B, Fisher A. Bacitracin: a unique topical antibiotic sensitizer. J Am Acad Dermatol 1987;17:1016–1024.

34. Epstein S, Wenzel FJ. Cross-sensitivity to various "mycins." Arch Dermatol 1962;86:183–194.

35. Pirla V, Forstrom L, Rouhunkoski S. Twelve years of sensitization to neomycin in Finland. Acta Derm Venercol 1967;47:419–425.

36. Roup G, Stennegard O. Anaphylactic shock elicited by topical administration of bacitracin. Arch Dermatol 1969;100:450–452.

37. Elsner P, Penny I, Burg G. Anaphylaxis induced by topically applied bacitracini. Am J Contact Derm 1990;1:162–164.

38. Schecter J, Wilkinson R, Carpio J. Anaphylaxis following the use of bacitracin ointment. Arch Dermatol 1984;120:909–911.

39. Zappi E, Brancaccio RR. Allergic contact dermatitis from Mupirocin ointment. J Am Acad Dermatol 1997;36:266–267.

40. VanKetel WG. Polymixine 8-sulfate and bacitracin. Contact Dermatitis News 1974;15:445.

41. Gette MT, Marks JG, Maloney ME. Frequency of post operative allergic contact dermatitits to topical antibiotics. Arch Dermtol 1992;128:365–367.

42. Smack DP, Harrington AC, Dunn C, et al. Infection and allergy incidence in ambulatory surgery patients using white petrolatum vs. bacitracin ointment. JAMA 1996;276:972–977.

43. Clark RAF. Cutaneous tissue repair; basic biologic considerations I. J Am Acad Dermatol 1985;13:701–725.

44. Drake DB, Rodeheaver PF, Edlich RF, et al. Experimental studies in swine for measurement of suture extrusion. J Long Term Eff Med Implants 2004;14:251–259.

45. Dufresne RG. Surgical complication: prevention, recognition, and treatment. In: Ratz JL, ed. Textbook of dermatologic surgery. Philadelphia: Lippincott-Raven; 1998:59–73.

46. Haneke E, Baran R. Longitudinal melanonychia. Dermatol Surg 2001;27:580–584.

47. Laffitte E, Gurkan K, Piguet V, et al. Erosive pusturlar dematosis of the scalp: treatment with topical tacrolimus. Arch Dermatol 2003;139:712–714.

48. Weinstein C, Ramirez OM, Pozner JN. Postoperative care following CO2 laser resurfacing: avoiding pitfalls. Plast Reconstr Surg 1997;100:1855–1866.

49. Nanni CA, Alster TS. Complications of cargon dioxide laser resurfacing: an evaluation of 500 patients. Dermatol Surg 1998;24:315–320.

50. Hebda PA, Lee CI. Occlusine dressings for surgical and other acute wounds. Wounds 1992;4:84–87.

51. Phelps RG, Wilentz S. Reflex sympathetic dystrophy. Int J Dermatol 2000;39:481–486.

52. Turner-Stokes L. Reflex sympathetic dystrophy – a complex regional pain syndrome. Disabil Rehabil 2002;24:939–947.

53. Singer AJ, Clark RAF. Cutaneous wound healing. N Engl J Med 1999;371:738–746.

54. Clark RAF. Basics of cutaneous wound repair. J Dermatol Surg Oncol 1993;19:693–706.

55. Herman E. Itching in scars. In: Berhhard JB, ed. Itch: mechanisms and management of pruritus. New York: McGraw-Hill; 1994:153–160.

56. Cohen IK, Beaver MA, Horakova Z, et al. Histamine and collagen synthesis in keloid and hypertrophic scar. Surg Forum 1972;23:509–510.

57. Burton CS. Dermal hypertrophies. In: Bolognia JL, Jorizzo JL, Rapini RP, ed. Dermatology. New York: Mosby; 2003: 1531–1537.

58. Remensnyder JP, Majno G. Oxygen gradients in healing wounds. Am J Pathol 1968;52:301–323.

59. Kosmadaki MG, Yaar M, Arble BL, Gilchrest BA. UV induces VEGF through a TNF-alpha independent pathway. Fed Am Soc Exp Biol J 2003;17:446–448.

60. DeLara Galindo S, Cuspinera E, Ramirez LC. Anatomical and functional account of the lateral nasal cartilages. Acta Anat 1977;97:393–399.

61. Howard B, Rohrich R. Understanding the nasal airway: principles and practice. Plast Reconstr Surg 2002;109:1128–1146.

62. Robinson JK, Burget GC. Nasal valve malfunction resulting from resection of cancer. Arch Otolaryngol Head Neck Surg 1990;116:1419–1424.

63. Jones E, Youker S, Fosko S. A nasal trumpet orthosis to maintain nares opening during a melolabial interpolation flap. Dermatol Surg 2006;32(1):96–99.

64. Karen M, Chang E, Keen MS. Auricular composite grafting to repair nasal vesibular stenosis. Otolaryngol Head Nec Surg 2000;122:529–532.

65. Friedman M, Ibrahim H, Syed Z. Nasal valve suspension: an improved, simplified technique for nasal valve collapse. Laryngoscope 2003;113:381–385.

66. Rizvi SS, Gauthier MG. How I do it: lateralizing the collapsed nasal valve. Laryngoscope 2003;113:2052–2054.

67. Zacarian SA. Cryosurgery of cutaneous carcinoma. J Am Acad Dermatol 1983;9:947–956.

68. Skouge JW. Skin grafting. New York: Churchill Livingstone; 1991:44–45, 61–63.

69. Stratigos AJ, Dover JS, Arndt KA. Laser therapy. In: Bolognia JL, Jorizzo JL, Rapini RP, eds. Dermatology. New York: Mosby; 2003:2153–2175.

70. Waldorf HA, Kauvar ANB, Geronemus RG. Skin resurfacing of fine to deep rhytides using a char-free carbon dioxide laser in 47 patients. Dermatol Surg 1995;21:940–946.

71. Ho C, Nguyen Q, Lowe NJ, et al. Laser resurfacing in pigmented skin. Dermatol Surg 1995;21:1035–1037.

72. Goldberg DJ. Complications in cutaneous laser surgery. New York: Taylor & Francis; 2004.

73. Bernstein LJ, Kauvar AB, Grossman MC, Geronemus RG. The short and long term side effects of carbon dioxide laser resurfacing. Dermatol Surg 1997;23:519–525.

74. Goldman MP, Bergow JJ. Complications and adverse sequelae of sclerotherapy. In: Sclerotherapy: treatment of varicose and telangiectatic leg veins. 3rd ed. St Louis: Mosby; 2001:191–197.

75. Georgiev M. Post sclerotherpy hyperpigmentation: a one-year follow up. J Dermatol Surg Oncol 1990;16:608.

76. Ramelet AA. Complications of ambulatory phlebectomy. Dermatol Surg 1997;23:947–954.

77. Weiss RA, Sadick NS, Goldman MP, et al. Post-sclerotherapy compression: controlled comparative study of duration of compression and its effects on clinical outcome. Dermatol Surg 1999;25:105.

78. Myers HL. Topical chelation therapy for varicose pigmentation. Angiology 1966;17:66.

79. Goldman MP. Post sclerotherapy hyperpigmentation treatment with a flash-lamp excited pulsed dye laser. J Dermatol Surg Oncol 1992;18:417.

Section III
Complications of Cosmetic Procedures

Evaluating the psychosocial status of a patient is a crucial component of every medical specialty. However, dermatologists and cosmetic surgeons undoubtedly encounter patients with certain psychological disorders at a much higher frequency than many of their colleagues. At its most superficial level, the underlying goal of any cosmetic surgery procedure is to provide some sort of psychological benefit to the patient from the completion of the procedure.[1] More specifically, the surgeon should be able to lead the patient to greater emotional health.[1] Because of this inextricably intertwined relationship of cosmetic surgery and psychology, the psychosocial health of every cosmetic surgery patient must be thoroughly evaluated in order to ensure that no serious underlying psychological disorders exist that would preclude a specific patient from an aesthetic procedure. As such, any doctor performing cosmetic procedures should have a working knowledge of the presentation, etiology, and treatment options for many of the common diseases that may be encountered. With this knowledge the cosmetic surgeon will also be able to aid in the identification of patients in need of counseling or psychiatric treatment and avoid performing surgeries that would otherwise be contraindicated due to the presence of these various mental conditions. Consequently, the team will be able to develop the most appropriate plan of action for the treatment of the patient, ultimately helping him or her attain a more physically and emotionally appealing state.

Many individuals whom we consider to be typical cosmetic surgery patients most likely suffer from at least one diagnosable psychological disorder including, but not limited to, social inhibition, moderate self-consciousness, anxiety, and depression.[2] Older, interview-based studies that investigated the mental status of patients seeking cosmetic surgery showed that 70% of these patients had an Axis II personality disorder, and 19.5% had and Axis I disorder, as defined by the *Diagnostic and Statistical Manual of Mental Disorders, Third Edition* (DSM-III-R).[3] It is important to note that more recent studies that utilized the psychometric assessment Minnesota Multiphasic Personality Inventory (MMPI) have shown that only 25% of patients seeking cosmetic surgery had a psychological abnormality.[3] In fact, aesthetic surgery can be contraindicated in any patient whose psychological health could not be improved in one way or another through the desired operation. These patients may be much more psychologically disturbed, suffering from severe depression, personality disorders, neurosis, and other psychoses. In most cases, however, upon completion of an appropriately indicated treatment and possibly some minor psychological counseling, the patient should have a positive outlook on the procedure and he or she should be able to function as a normal member of society. In all of these cases, it is important that the surgeon be able to immediately recognize the presence of these more severe conditions so that appropriate treatment can be obtained.

This chapter will commence with a case scenario to better illustrate some of the more common psychological conditions frequently seen in patients seeking cosmetic surgery. For each condition, the most common features of the initial presentation usually detectable in the preoperative consultation will be examined. Focusing on some of the more common psychological comorbidities (i.e., body dysmorphic disorder) of cosmetic surgery patients, there will be a description of what tools (i.e., questionnaires) may be helpful in the identification of different personalities as one considers a patient's candidacy for surgery. A discussion will follow of the current therapies and treatment options available to these patients, and whether or not cosmetic surgery is indicated. Finally, a review will be conducted of the psychological complications of cosmetic surgery that can be encountered and pitfalls that every physician should try to avoid.

Case Scenario 1

A 46-year-old male is seen in consultation for his complaint of "horrible scarring on his face." The patient has a past medical history significant for hypertension. The patient writes on his intake form that his past surgical history includes liposuction, rhinoplasty, and, most recently, a full-face laser resurfacing. The patient writes next to the resurfacing that the procedure was performed by "Dr. Quack." Upon entering the examination room you find a moderately cachectic, middle-aged man in no apparent distress.

During your review of the patient's intake form and further questioning of his chief complaint, the patient states he is unhappy with the scarring on his cheeks due to "acne as a kid." As you examine the patient's skin he repeatedly points to multiple areas on his face. Your examination reveals no abnormal scarring. He actually looks younger than his age would dictate.

When offered a mirror to point out his scarring, the patient grabs the mirror from your hand and aggressively points to multiple random areas on his face stating "look doc, can't you see them?" To be continued . . .

Preoperative Cosmetic Consultation

Within the first few moments of meeting a patient seeking a cosmetic consultation, the physician should begin to focus on some basic determinants of the patient's candidacy for cosmetic surgery. These determinants include the patient's request, the physical examination, the medical examination, and, most importantly, the psychological assessment.[4]

The patient's request should be completely guided by the patient. The physician should allow the patient to speak freely about the complaint and any pertinent history without interruption. It may be useful to offer a mirror and pointer to aide the patient in physically pointing out his or her complaint. At that point, a patient can be physically examined and the complaint can be addressed. Other additional problems can be pointed out to the patient by the surgeon. A medical history and psychiatric exam are performed to assess if any procedures are medically feasible. With this information, the surgeon relates what can be done for the patient's complaint, including nothing at all, and what results can be expected from a procedure. It is important during the consultation to fully detail the wound healing process and possible need for additional procedures.[4]

The Psychiatric Exam

The importance of obtaining the mental status of a patient is unique in its ubiquity. It is a mainstay of every examination regardless of where the patient encounter takes place: the examination table in the emergency room or on the psychiatrist's couch. Even though the psychiatrist and the emergency room physician will undoubtedly have very different goals for their evaluations, the general structure of the examination and the information obtained are generally the same. The basic steps to the psychological evaluation of a patient and the information that is necessary for the cosmetic surgeon to obtain before proceeding with any cosmetic procedure will be described subsequently.

The psychological exam is also unique in that it begins the moment the patient walks into the office. Astute nurses and office staff should watch for the patient that may be acting strange or unusually. The physician should begin evaluating the mental status of the patient from the moment they meet, throughout the visit, and to the moment the patient walks out of the door. For most cosmetic surgeons and physicians in general, this is a simple task, as a highly developed power of observation is warranted by their chosen occupation.

The first thing any physician should notice is the appearance of the patient. Taken alone, appearance means next to nothing in our society as fashion and grooming style are no longer accurate indicators of occupation, intelligence, or mental status. However, the appearance of a patient may give the physician clues as to the line of questions that will be most appropriate in obtaining information about this particular patient. More often than not, the most informative indicator of appearance is that of clothing, for example, dirty, disheveled, tight, flashy, grotesque, gothic, seductive, etc. For instance, a patient who comes in very neat and well dressed with a blouse that exactly matches the earrings, nail polish, and shoes might be one you would consider screening for obsessive–compulsive disorder. It is important to remember that these are not concrete associations that can be stereotyped, but rather observations that may lead a physician to specific lines of questioning.

The next attribute the physician should typically notice is the patient's orientation to time and place. Normally, orientation is not an issue that needs direct questioning unless the patient appears to be noticeably confused or vague about his or her surroundings. Even in cases where this does appear to be a problem, a few simple questions can often confirm whether or not this lack of orientation will significantly impact the outcome of the procedure to be performed. In situations where questioning is warranted, directly asking the patient if he or she knows the year or who the current president of the United States is

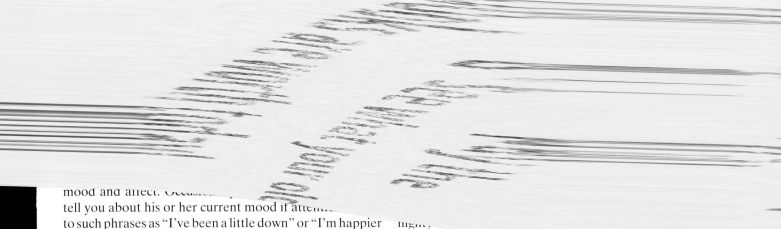

mood and affect. Occasionally a patient will tell you about his or her current mood if attentive to such phrases as "I've been a little down" or "I'm happier than I've been." When not told directly, the physician must rely on observation. In some cases, such as mania or severe depression, the behavioral signs are straightforward. With depression, there may be signs of sadness, indifference to the questioning, reluctance to answer questions at length, or use of a monotonous voice. At the other extreme, manics often express inappropriate happiness and extreme eagerness to answer questions, sometimes preventing the doctor from getting a word in edgewise. At this point, it may be appropriate to question the patient about his or her use of psychiatric or other mental health services. Even though this may seem like a very direct, personal question, those who are not being treated will simply say no, while those who are will usually not be any more embarrassed than a person seeking treatment for a disease such as diabetes or hepatitis. The information gained by asking this question is far more valuable than any temporary embarrassment or discomfort one would cause to the patient. It may be useful to have questions on a medical intake form that assesses current and past psychiatric conditions. Naturally, this would not replace the techniques described above but would give the physician an indication that something may be awry.

As mentioned above, depression and mania are usually very readily recognized by physicians. Other conditions, such as schizophrenia, require a heightened level of observational psychiatric skill. In identification of schizophrenics, the doctor should look for what are called colorless affects. These affects include monotonous speech and other nonreactive, nonresponsive behaviors. It is very important to distinguish patients truly suffering from schizophrenia from those who may simply be too scared or too nervous to ask many questions or to respond appropriately. The physician should be cognizant not guide the patient in his or her answers too much, and that close attention is paid not just to the content of the speech, but *how* the patient is speaking as well.

Questioning of lifestyle can be useful in understanding the patient's mood, motives, and goals. Occupation and job changes, separations or divorces, illness or death of loved ones, and passing of milestones, such as birthdays, empty nesting, and the marriage of offspring are exam-

ability to stay focused on one topic. On the other hand, severely depressed individuals typically find it harder to answer questions and will have slower response times. Other psychological comorbidities may be noted if the patient is excessively concerned with details or is not interested in anything past an overly generalized description of the procedure. Understanding the patient's background may also be helpful in investigating these attributes. The purpose of evaluating the patient's thought processes, judgment, and insight is to determine if the patient is able to independently arrive at a rational decision. In all these areas, it is important for the physician to focus on asking specific but open-ended questions so that more of the patient's personality and character will come through in the answers.

Another aspect of the psychological exam is the evaluation of the patient's intelligence and level of comprehension. If a patient is to undergo an extensive procedure that may lead to dramatic alterations of appearance or may have severe untoward effects, the physician must be confident that the patient possesses the intellect to process and understand the details of the procedure, and the intricacies of the wound healing process. Most of the time, the screening described above will give the physician a reasonable assessment of the patient's cognitive ability. If there is doubt, however, several mental status exams have been developed that can be used by non-psychiatrists to screen patients with limited cognitive function. One of the more widely used is that developed by M.F. Folstein called the Mini-Mental Status Exam.[6] Tools such as these provide a simple and efficient way for physicians to ensure that the mental competence of the patient fits the complexity of the procedure.

By the end of the first appointment, using the above listed techniques and the appropriate questions pertinent to the requested procedure, the doctor should be able to ascertain the following:

1. How long has the patient been dissatisfied with the relevant body part?
2. Why is the surgery is requested at this particular time?

3. What are the motivations for surgery?
4. Is the patient requesting the procedure due to someone else's wish?
5. What are the expectations? What will the surgery do for the patient and how will it influence his or her life?
6. What surgeries/procedures has the patient undergone in the past? How was the patient's experience? Were there real or perceived problems with the procedures or physician?
7. Has the patient sought consultation and/or treatment for this specific complaint from another physician? Is this a second opinion or did they not want to proceed with the other surgeon for a specific reason?
8. Is the patient in some form of life crisis?
9. Does the patient suffer from any known psychiatric condition that would preclude him or her from undergoing the procedure?
10. Is the physician or office staff suspicious of an unreported or unrecognized psychiatric condition that would likewise reduce surgical candidacy?
11. Do family and friends support the surgery and how will they react?

By taking the time to go through these aspects of the initial interview and finding the answers to these questions, the surgical team will be able to significantly reduce the amount of complications due to the psychiatric comorbidities of the patient. The very best time to screen patients for the presence of these conditions is during the preoperative consultation sessions. There will be a discussion later in the chapter regarding psychiatric problems that may arise during the intraoperative and postoperative periods and recommendations on dealing with these issues.

Case Scenario 2

A 52-year-old woman seeks improvement of aging skin. You see many lentigos and irregular pigmentation that you feel are amenable to a chemical peel. The patient seems to be a good candidate and has no medical contraindications.

During the consultation you ask a very broad question: "Tell me about what is happening in your life right now?" The patient reveals she is going through a divorce, and that her husband left her for a "younger woman." The patient begins to cry and with gentle probing it becomes evident that at present the patient is very unhappy with every aspect of her life. Signs of depression are noted.

At this point it is determined that a chemical peel is a good procedure for the patient, but not at this time. Her

generalized unhappiness could easily be transferred to her procedure, her subsequent outcome, and the physician. She reluctantly agrees to wait until she is more emotionally stable. Eight months later after a second consultation, the peel is successfully performed on a better-adjusted woman.

Psychiatric Comorbidity and Personality Identification in Cosmetic Surgery Settings

Over the years, there has been a growing interest in determining the actual rates of psychiatric conditions present in a typical cosmetic surgery practice. One such study by Ishigooka and colleagues indicates that just under half (47.7%) of a sample of 415 patients seeking cosmetic surgery suffer from at least one serious mental disorder.[7] Among the major diagnoses were schizophrenia, persistent delusional disorders, major depressive episodes, neurotic disorders, hypochondriacal disorder, paranoid personality disorder, and histrionic personality disorder. In addition, over half of the patients surveyed suffered from poor social adjustment (56%), indicating that many patients are turning to surgery as a way of obtaining social acceptance. Furthermore, the researchers also found that men tend to suffer from a greater number of mental conditions, including dysmorphophobia, a disease that will be discussed in great length later in this chapter.

Below are some generalizations of true psychiatric illnesses that patients may carry, for which psychiatric consultation is warranted and necessary. A patient with a diagnosis of a psychiatric illness is not a contraindication to cosmetic surgery. On the contrary, a surgeon can perform the procedure with consultation of mental health professionals during a period of psychotic remission, or if the patient is under tight therapeutic control.[8]

Schizophrenia

- Delusions and hallucinations about their appearance.
- Nonspecific and vague requests regarding the desired result.
- Cause of disfigurement placed on nonrealistic forces and/or people, or a conspiracy to prevent the correction of the disfigurement.

Anxiety Disorders

- Difficulty resolving feelings if there is an imperfect surgical result.
- Preoperative consultation and day of surgery can actually trigger anxiety disorder relapse.
- Request cosmetic surgery to "feel better" rather than to correct a physical imperfection.

ough psychiatric screening in a cosmetic surgery setting. Under most conditions, the personality type of the patient will have little or no effect on the major outcome of the indicated procedure. However, by identifying certain personality characteristics in patients, the physician will be able to estimate what level of care the patient will require throughout the course of treatment, how to best handle any questions or problems that may arise, and how to ensure that both doctor and patient view the procedure as a success. Below we will describe some common personality characteristics and some generalizations about the type of care each type of personality prefers.

Passive–Aggressive Patient

- Increased need for postoperative nurturing.
- Whining and childish behavior may frustrate nursing and supporting staff.
- Important to remember that a higher level of nurturing and comfort should be provided within reason.
- Physician may need to direct staff to withdraw somewhat from patient as to not indulge the behavior.

Hostile and Angry Patient

- Paranoid patient will project feelings onto doctor and staff.
- In reality, the vast majority of these patients are simply frightened.
- Strong and confident reassurance is needed in the postoperative period.
- Honest and thorough answers should be given to all the patient's questions.
- Do not simply tell patient "everything will be alright." Patients will do much better if all information is given forthrightly.

Sociopath

- The doctor must maintain an authoritative presence.
- The doctor is in charge in regards to the surgical treatment and postoperative management.

Obsessive–Compulsive Patient

- Patients will need a concrete plan.
- Details are extremely important to the patient (How long? How severe? How much?).

including dysmorphic syndrome, dermatologic hypochondriasis, dermatologic nondisease, monosymptomatic hypochondriasis nondisease, and monosymptomatic hypochondriasis. According to the *Diagnostic and Statistical Manual of Mental Disorders, Fourth Edition* (DSM-IV), the American Psychiatrics Association's diagnostic manual, a diagnosis of body dysmorphic disorder is based upon three major criteria.[11] Although the DSM-IV criteria maintain that the patient may be preoccupied with any part of the body, the most common areas of complaint tend to be the skin, face, and nose.[12] First, the patient must show a preoccupation and excessive concern with an imagined defect, or a defect that is slight and unnoticeable at normal conversational distance. Second, this preoccupation must cause some hindrance to the patient in terms of normal social or occupational functioning. Examples of this include poor performance at school or work and difficulty in dating or maintaining other relationships. Finally, this preoccupation must not be explainable by another comorbid condition such as anorexia nervosa or transsexualism. Body dysmorphic disorder is listed under the rubric of hypochondriasis, although the difference lies in that there is no other underlying mental disorder resulting in this disease. As with most other psychological disorders, the exact physiologic cause of body dysmorphic disorder has yet to be determined. Unfortunately, even though this disorder is one of the most commonly seen, it can also be one of the most difficult to treat.

Epidemiology

Although several studies have been conducted to establish the prevalence of body dysmorphic disorder, a tremendous amount of disagreement exists. The best estimate for the prevalence of this disorder in the general population is around 2% in the United States,[13] with reported rates ranging from 0.7% to 2.3%.[14] As would be expected, the overall rates of body dysmorphic disorder appear to be much higher in dermatological and cosmetic surgery settings. In cosmetic surgery, rates have been reported ranging from 7% to 15%,[15] while in dermatology, one of the largest studies, which involved screening 268 patients for body dysmorphic disorder, revealed a rate of 11.9% (95% confidence interval, 8.0%–15.8%).[16] It is believed

BDDQ

This questionnaire asks about concerns with physical appearance. Please read each question carefully and circle the answer that is true for you. Also, write in answers where indicated.

NAME: _____ TODAY'S DATE: _____

1. Are you very worried about how you look? Yes No

> **If yes:** Do you think about your appearance problems a lot and wish you could think
>   about them less? Yes No

> **If yes:** Please list the body areas you do not like:

> _____

> _____

Examples of your disliked body area include: your skin (forexample: acne, scars, wrinkles, paleness, redness); hair; the shape or size of your nose, mouth, jaw, lips, stomach, hips, etc.; or defects of your hands, genitals, breasts, or anyother body part.

If the answer to either of the above questions was **No**, you are finished with this questionnaire. Otherwise, please continue.

2. Is your *main* concern with how you look that you are not thin enough or that you might get too fat? Yes   No

3. How has this problem with how you look affected your life?

> Has it often upset you *a lot*? Yes No

> Has it gotten in the way of doing things with friends or dating? Yes   No

> **If yes**, please describe how: _____

> _____

> Has it ever caused problems with school? Yes   No

> **If yes**, what are they? _____

> _____

> Are there things you avoid because of how you look? Yes No

> **If yes**, what are they? _____

> _____

4. How much time a day do you usually spend thinking about how you look? Please circle one.

> a) Less than 1 hour a day

> b) 1 - 3 hours a day

> c) More than 3 hours a day

You're likely to have BDD if you give the following answers on the BDDQ:

> Question 1: Yes to both parts

> Question 3: Yes to any of the questions

> Question 4: Answer b or c

FIGURE 12-1. A body dysmorphic disorder questionnaire (BDDQ).

that body dysmorphic disorder effects men at an equal, or slightly higher, rate than women, although presentations of the disease in each gender can vary slightly.[17] With a rough average of 1 in every 10 patients, it is apparent that cosmetic surgeons see a great number of patients suffering from this disorder, many of whom continue to be undiagnosed.

Evaluation

The first step in diagnosing the disease lies in listening to the patient. Most physicians have already discovered that listening to the patient can often be both the best and worst thing you can do while in practice. One of the most common "red flags" is that the patient has been to countless doctors for the same problem. If, after listening to the patient's chief complaint, you can find no sign of the defect to which he or she is referring; the best plan of action is to probe the patient through further questioning to elicit what about the defect bothers them. Another choice is to have the patient complete a standard body dysmorphic disorder questionnaire (BDDQ). Many forms of questionnaires have been published, but most are aimed at establishing the presence of the criteria set forth by the DSM-IV. An example of a typical BDDQ is shown in Figure 12-1.

The results of this questionnaire in no way serve as a way to definitively diagnose body dysmorphic disorder. The survey simply attempts to determine if a severe physical preoccupation exists, the severity of the preoccupation, and if the preoccuption can be attributed to another condition such as anorexia nervosa. Upon completion, the physician should have a fairly good understanding as to whether or not the patient meets the DSM-IV criteria for body dysmorphic disorder and if treatment should be pursued. The physician should be aware that patients suspected of body dysmorphic disorder are most likely not going to be very amenable to any discussion that makes them seem mentally ill. Therefore, great care must be taken to ensure that enough evidence is present to confront any patient with the possibility of this diagnosis.

We will now focus our attention on the complexities of dealing with the psychological comorbidities of cosmetic patients, including body dysmorphic disorder, as it relates to postoperative complications.

Psychological Complications of Cosmetic Surgery

Postoperative complications are an inherent risk of any procedure. The nonpsychological complications of surgery will be covered in other chapters of this book. Psychological complications of surgery can be as devastating to the patient as, for example, a wound dehiscence. A strong

patient–physician relationship that was establishe[d during the] preoperative consultation and extends through[out the course] of surgery into the postoperative period will de[crease the] likelihood of postoperative psychological com[plications.] Psychological support is an important fact[or in postop]erative care.

In the postoperative period, the three [most common] reasons of patient dissatisfaction are [a failure of rapport] between the physician and [the patient, (2) unrealistic] psychological expectations on the part of the pa[tient,] and (3) a physical complication or disappointment with the anatomic change.[4] Patients who have psychological comorbidities need to be screened prior to the surgery. With the help of mental health professional consultation and treatment these patients can be prepared for the postoperative phase of their surgery and the psychological complications that can arise. Unfortunately, no surgeon can be prepared for hidden psychological disease that can be uncovered following a cosmetic surgery. Postoperative psychological complications that can arise, or be exacerbated, in patients with or without psychiatric disease include body dysmorphic disorder, anxiety disorders, posttraumatic stress disorder, depression, and suicide.

Body Dysmorphic Disorder

A very common preoperative comorbidity of patients seeking cosmetic surgery can also be one of the more common postoperative psychological complications. Although body dysmorphic disorder may sound fairly trivial, the comorbid conditions associated with this disease are not only damaging to the patient's quality of life, but also carry the risk of physical harm to the patient and others. One such example occurred when a 48-year-old woman who suffered from body dysmorphic disorder almost inflicted a mortal wound through skin picking, as reported by O'Sullivan and colleagues.[18] Skin picking, also called neurotic excoriations, is a fairly common finding with body dysmorphic disorder, but can also be present with various other conditions such as trichotillomania and obsessive compulsive disorder.[18] At the time of the incident, the patient had had a 4-year history of skin picking and had been seen by several dermatologists and family practitioners for the treatment of severe skin wounds and infections. The patient claimed to be trying to eradicate pimples and bumps from her face, arms, and legs, which she would think about for 2 to 4 hours daily. On several occasions, it was necessary to hospitalize the patient for treatment of wounds that would not resolve on their own. Even though the patient received psychiatric therapy for her condition, the symptoms of body dysmorphic disorder did not seem to improve and the picking continued. After the removal of a small occlusion cyst of the neck (unrelated to body dysmorphic disorder), the patient continued to pick at the surgical defect because she thought it "just didn't feel right." Described by her as a pimple, she proceeded to pick at the wound with her fingernails and eventually a pair of tweezers. She continued to dissect through her dermis, subcutaneous tissue, and musculature until she had exposed her carotid artery. When the patient's husband discovered her, he noted what he described as a "bullet hole" in her neck and immediately rushed her to the hospital where the wound was properly treated. In this dangerous incident, the patient suffered from no other psychiatric conditions other than body dysmorphic disorder.

Despite the danger body dysmorphic disorder patients pose to themselves through skin picking and other compulsive disorders, there is significant overlap with other psychiatric diseases that can place the patient in mortal danger through suicide, and the physician in danger through feelings of frustration and retribution. Being strongly related with severe depression, patients with body dysmorphic disorder have rates of suicidal tendencies that far exceed the general population. In one study, 22% of patients who had presented to a dermatology clinic with body dysmorphic disorder had attempted suicide.[16] Furthermore, when patients with body dysmorphic disorder are assessed for mental health status, they frequently score lower than patients suffering from a variety of severe chronic illnesses such as diabetes, depression, and myocardial infarction.[19] Along with suicide and depression, body dysmorphic disorder has also been shown to be positively correlated with other psychiatric and medical illnesses such as anxiety disorder, heart disease, diabetes, panic disorder, obsessive–compulsive disorder, substance abuse, and other manic–depressive conditions.[19] In most cases, the social phobias develop prior to body dysmorphic disorder, while depression and substance abuse begin after the onset of the disease.[20] Some studies have also reported gender differences regarding specific comorbid conditions. More specifically, women with body dysmorphic disorder are often reported to suffer from panic attacks, bulimia, and generalized anxiety disorder, while men are more likely to suffer from bipolar disorder.[21]

Along with risk to the patient, there may also be significant danger to the patient's family as well as the physician. As might be expected, the continuous doctor shopping and seeking out of treatments can often lead to a heightened level of frustration on the part of the patient. As treatments continue to fail, patients often tend to lash out at their loved ones, especially the spouse, for being unable to help them find the treatment they feel they need. In addition, surgeons who have performed cosmetic surgery on patients with body dysmorphic disorder, especially male patients, have reported cases of extreme violence after being disappointed with the outcome of the surgery. In some of these more tragic cases, the aggression toward the surgeon has even lead to murder.[15]

Anxiety Disorders

Anxiety is a normal response to surgery and is seen in varying degrees in all surgery patients. In cosmetic surgery patients, anxiety can be particularly apparent because patients worry that the operation may not satisfy personal expectations for improved self-image.[22] In a recent report that looked at anxiety disorders in plastic surgery patients, the authors describe a 43-year-old woman who underwent blepharoplasty. One week postoperatively the patient began complaining of nausea, dizziness, insomnia, and the fear of having a "stroke." With the help of psychological consultation and treatment, none of these complaints were linked to a preexisting psychological illness, and the patient was diagnosed as having a panic attack. The patient recovered within three months of the onset of symptoms.[23] According to the DSM-IV, a panic attack is a condition that involves the abrupt development of symptoms, such as palpitations, shortness of breath, trembling, nausea, and chest pain, within 10 minutes.[11]

Posttraumatic Stress Disorder

Another psychological complication likely to be encountered after cosmetic surgery is posttraumatic stress disorder. Posttraumatic stress disorder is a condition that can develop in patients who have experienced an event that is life threatening, associated with serious injury, or that caused intense fear, horror, or helplessness in the patient.[13] These patients are usually survivors of motor vehicle accidents, natural disasters, sexual assault, or military combat. Symptoms include persistent symptoms of increased arousal, outbursts of anger, or an exaggerated startle response. Cosmetic surgeons are faced with the complications of this disorder when performing surgery on patients that have been sexually abused, assaulted, or have sustained a traumatic injury. Proper screening for these patients during the preoperative consultation will aid in referring these patients to mental health professionals. In the above-mentioned study that looked at anxiety disorders in plastic surgery patients, the authors give an example of a 22-year-old woman who at 2 weeks after a rhinoplasty began complaining of nightmares, anxiety, and feelings of suffocation. After referral to a psychologist the patient was found to have a posttraumatic stress disorder to an incident of sexual abuse that occurred 10 years prior.[23] This patient also recovered without complications with the aide of psychological intervention.

Depression

Depression is another psychological disorder that can be related to a patient's preoperative psychological comorbidities, or can occur after a cosmetic surgery de novo without a prior psychological basis. Studies evaluating plastic surgery patients have shown that varying degrees of depression after surgery can occur at a rate as high as 57%. Nineteen percent of these patients required hospitalization for their depression.[4] Cosmetic surgeons should be aware of the signs of depression as denoted earlier in this chapter. In our experience, procedures that incur longer postoperative healing and slower overall results, like laser resurfacing, deep chemical peels, and dermabrasion, lead to more feelings of disappointment, even if the patient is aware of this truth preoperatively. The patients who take part in procedures that are more involved or have delayed healing seem to be more likely to experience feelings of depression postoperatively.

Suicide

The most devastating of any postoperative psychological complication to cosmetic surgery is suicide. Unfortunately, in the rare patient where psychological comorbidities are known and are felt to be in control preoperatively, postoperatively these patients have been found to be more susceptible to postoperative anxiety, depression, or psychological decompensation. This can be manifested as violent behavior toward the surgeon, health care staff, or the patient themselves.[22] These patients tend to be male and react to surgery with pursuit of additional surgery, delusional fixation on an imperfection, paranoid attitudes toward future physicians, and suicide attempts.[4] The value of preoperative screening for psychological comorbidities should not be understated, for the referral for proper treatment could inevitably save a life.

Treatment Options

Most cosmetic surgeons are not trained in current pharmacological, psychological, and behavioral therapy for the psychological comorbidities or complications that have been addressed in this chapter. Therefore, consulting a mental health professional to evaluate a patient preoperatively or postoperatively will be the best approach to these patients. Working as a team of mental health professional, cosmetic surgeon, and patient will only maximize the patient's outcome, no matter their psychological comorbidities. To elucidate on current treatment options for patients with psychological comorbidities or complications, current protocols for the treatment of body dysmorphic disorder will be utilized due to its high prevalence in cosmetic surgery patients. Some of these techniques are useful in the treatment of other psychological disorders due to their overlap. What follows are some general guidelines adapted from Katharine Phillps' guide for dermatologists and plastic surgeons as to how one should proceed with a patient suspected of having body dysmorphic disorder[24]:

- Provide education
- Inform the patient of your suspicion of body dysmorphic disorder, explaining in simple terms what that means.
- Recommend reading material (fliers, the Internet, etc.) where the patient may obtain more information. A list of appropriate websites is given below.
- Do not downplay any of the patient's appearance concerns as this may have a significant negative impact on his or her recovery.
- If appropriate, educate any family members who may be involved or are able to help.
- Behavior modifications
- Do not try to talk the patient out of picking their skin or being worried about their appearance.
- Attempting to end the patient's compulsive behaviors often leads to further depression, frustration, and lack of recovery.
- Do not encourage the patient to use make up or any other concealing methods to hide their deformity as this has also been shown to interfere with recovery.
- Appropriate referrals
- Explain to the patient that the disorder cannot be effectively treated by dermatologists or with cosmetic procedures.
- Attempt to refer the patient to a psychiatrist, emphasizing the amount of time they spend worrying about their appearance and how it affects their mentality.
- If the patient is worried about taking antipsychotic medications, explain that therapies that do not include the use of medications may be available.
- If the patient is suicidal or severely depressed, attempt no other referral than to a psychiatrist as treatment with antipsychotic medications is the best approach.

Once referred to a psychiatrist or other mental health professional, the patient can expect to encounter two forms of treatment: pharmacotherapy and cognitive–behavioral therapy (CBT), a form of psychotherapy. For over 10 years, the mainstay of treatment for body dysmorphic disorder has been pharmacological with selective serotonin reuptake inhibitors.[25] Two studies that investigated the use of fluvoxamine in body dysmorphic disorder showed a reduction in the severity of symptoms in approximately two thirds of patients.[26] In most situations, cosmetic surgeons are not qualified to monitor the patient's progress under the influence of these medications. If the physician feels that treatment for a psychological comorbidity or complication is warranted, a referral to a qualified psychiatrist is most likely the best course of action.

Although most research indicates that surgery should be contraindicated in patients with severe psychological conditions such as body dysmorphic disorder, there are some physicians who feel that surgeons are "passing up"

15. Phillips KA, Grant J, Siniscalchi J, Albertini RS. Surgical and nonpsychiatric medical treatment of patients with body dysmorphic disorder. Psychosomatics 2001;42:504–510.
16. Phillips KA, Dufresne RG Jr., Wilkel CS, Vittorio CC. Rate of body dysmorphic disorder in dermatology patients. J Am Acad Dermatol 2000;42:436–441.
17. Phillips KA, Diaz SF. Gender differences in body dysmorphic disorder. J Nerv Ment Dis 1997;185:570–577.
18. O'Sullivan RL, Phillips KA, Keuthen NJ, Wilhelm S. Near-fatal skin picking from delusional body dysmorphic disorder responsive to fluvoxamine. Psychosomatics 1999; 40:79–81.
19. Phillips KA. Quality of life for patients with body dysmorphic disorder. J Nerv Ment Dis 2000;188:170–175.
20. Gunstad J, Phillips KA. Axis I comorbidity in body dysmorphic disorder. Compr Psychiatry 2003;44:270–276.
21. Perugi G, Akiskal HS, Giannotti D, Frare F, Di Vaio S, Cassano GB. Gender-related differences in body dysmorphic disorder (dysmorphophobia). J Nerv Ment Dis 1997;185:578–582.
22. Hasan JS. Psychological issues in cosmetic surgery: a functional overview. Ann Plast Surg 2000;44:89–96.
23. Rankin M, Borah G. Anxiety disorders in plastic surgery. Plast Reconstr Surg 1997;100:535–542.
24. Phillips KA, Dufresne RG. Body dysmorphic disorder. A guide for dermatologists and cosmetic surgeons. Am J Clin Dermatol 2000;1:235–243.
25. Phillips KA, Najjar F. An open-label study of citalopram in body dysmorphic disorder. J Clin Psychiatry 2003;64: 715–720.
26. Wilson JB, Arpey CJ. Body dysmorphic disorder: suggestions for detection and treatment in a surgical dermatology practice. Dermatol Surg 2004;30:1391–1399.
28. Phillips K. The broken mirror: understanding and treating body dysmorphic disorder. New York: Oxford University Press; 1996.
29. Pope HG, Phillips K, Olivardia R. The Adonis complex: the secret crisis of male body obsession. New York: The Free Press; 2000.

13
Complications of Ablative and Nonablative Lasers and Light Sources

Elizabeth L. Tanzi and Tina S. Alster

Complications of cutaneous laser surgery can be understood by reviewing the evolution of laser technology over the past several decades. Lasers initially were designed to operate in a continuous-wave (CW) mode, which produced a continuous beam of radiation that subsequently was absorbed by a tissue chromophore. Although particular skin structures could be destroyed using these early lasers, their use was limited because the energy emitted not only altered the target, but also conducted heat into adjacent nonirradiated tissue. The nonselective thermal injury produced in adjacent tissue resulted in significant side effects and complications; specifically, dyspigmentation, and scarring.[1-3]

The safety and efficacy expected from modern laser systems can be attributed to the revolutionary work of Anderson and Parrish in the 1980s.[4] Their theory of selective photothermolysis outlined the mechanism for specific tissue destruction through manipulation of the type of laser energy produced and the manner in which it was delivered. Through application of their theory, a specific chromophore or target can be selectively destroyed with minimal thermal tissue damage when the laser wavelength matches that absorbed by the chromophore and when the target is exposed to the laser energy for an interval shorter than its thermal relaxation time, defined as the time required for the target to cool to half its peak temperature after laser irradiation.

Lasers designed based on the theory of selective photothermolysis are more specific and have a lower risk profile in terms of scarring; however, they have their own unique side-effect profiles. Depending upon the wavelength and pulse durations delivered, skin dyspigmentation, epidermal cell injury, textural changes, as well as crusting and tissue splatter potentially can occur. It is imperative to recognize that even the safest lasers can cause injury if used improperly. Application of inappropriately stacked pulses or scans, use of excessive energy or power settings, and improper patient selection potentially can result in a high rate of morbidity with any laser system.

Ablative Laser Resurfacing: Pretreatment Considerations

Because of the varied side effects and complications possible after cutaneous laser surgery, it is essential that each patient receive consultation and counseling before treatment to assess his or her specific risk of adverse sequelae. Dermasurgeons must spend time educating patients on the realities of laser treatment and the potential side effects that may occur. During the consultation, clinical photographs and written material can enhance the patient's understanding of the procedure, expected clinical outcome, and potential complications. It is also important that patients understand the importance of good wound care after a laser procedure. Preoperative laser evaluation should include a basic medical history, including documentation of medications and allergies. A history of smoking, abnormal scarring, excessive sun exposure, allergic or inflammatory conditions, herpes simplex virus outbreaks, immune disorders, or previous cosmetic procedures within the involved area should also be ascertained. Proper pretreatment education and close physician follow-up helps to reduce morbidity and allows for early recognition and management of potential problems.[5-7]

Ablative Laser Skin Resurfacing

Since the introduction of the high-energy, pulsed carbon dioxide (CO_2) and erbium:yttrium-aluminum-garnet (Er:YAG) lasers in the mid-1990s, cutaneous laser resurfacing has become an accepted method for effective facial skin rejuvenation.[8-16] These ablative lasers enable the treatment of photodamaged facial skin, specifically photoinduced facial rhytides, lentigines, and dermal elastosis. Although reported rates of serious complications associated with the use of these systems are low, adverse reactions can occur even in the hands of the most experienced laser surgeons. Fortunately, most adverse reactions are transient and, if detected early, are amenable to treatment without permanent sequelae. All laser surgeons should be familiar with the signs of an impending problem and cognizant of appropriate remedies when such a reaction does occur.

The frequency and severity of adverse reactions associated with cutaneous resurfacing lasers depends on multiple factors, including the type of laser system being used. Early laser technology consisted solely of CW lasers systems for resurfacing, which were associated with unacceptably high rates of scarring and permanent pigmentary alterations due to prolonged tissue exposure to laser energy.[1,2,8] The pulsed and scanned CO_2 and Er:YAG systems were developed taking into account the principles of selective photothermolysis, so that high laser energies and short pulse durations best effected tissue ablation with minimal thermal injury of residual skin.[17–33]

Other factors affecting the risk of adverse reactions with laser resurfacing include the number of laser passes performed, the energy densities used, the degree of pulse or scan overlap, the skin type and pretreatment condition of the individual patient, the anatomic location to be resurfaced, and the individual expertise of the laser surgeon. True adverse reactions, however, are rare and must be differentiated from the normal posttreatment morbidity that all patients experience after ablative laser skin resurfacing, including erythema, edema, crusting, and serous discharge.[6,34]

Normal Healing Process

After cutaneous ablative laser resurfacing, all patients experience some degree of immediate posttreatment morbidity. Because laser ablation involves complete epidermal vaporization and upper papillary dermal destruction and remodeling, the most common immediate posttreatment reactions include intense erythema, edema, and copious serous discharge that persist until reepithelialization is complete (Fig. 13-1). If a pulsed CO_2 laser is used to deliver multiple passes to the skin, reepithelialization is complete in an average of 7 to 9 days, compared with 4 to 5 days after short-pulsed, Er:YAG laser treatment.[10,26,35] The degree of erythema correlates directly with the number of laser passes delivered due to the increasing depth of penetration and degree of residual thermal injury. The pulsed CO_2 laser ablates tissue to a depth of 20 to 60μm with each consecutive pass and produces zones of thermal damage ranging 20 to 150μm after a typical skin resurfacing procedure, compared with 20 to 50μm of residual thermal damage with the

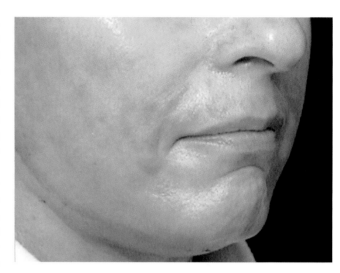

FIGURE 13-1. Erythema is an expected consequence of ablative CO_2 or Er:YAG laser skin resurfacing, but has a tendency to be more prolonged in patients after multiple-pass CO_2 laser procedures. No specific treatment is generally indicated.

short-pulsed, Er:YAG laser.[8,10,18–20,24–28] Therefore, patients treated with a traditional multiple-pass CO_2 laser technique experience more persistent and intense erythema, especially in the immediate postoperative period. Maximum erythema intensity occurs 8 to 10 days after CO_2 laser skin resurfacing and lasts an average of 3 to 6 months, compared with 2 to 4 weeks for short-pulsed, Er:YAG laser–treated patients.[3,6,11,26,29,34] Edema is another normal consequence of cutaneous laser treatment and is most pronounced on the second and third postoperative days with either laser. Application of cool compresses and ice alleviates the edema, which resolves after several days.

Trends in ablative facial resurfacing have emerged that offer more modest clinical improvement in rhytides and atrophic facial scars with reduced postoperative morbidity and shorter recovery times than traditional, multipass CO_2 laser skin resurfacing. Less aggressive techniques include single-pass CO_2 laser ablation and use of modulated (variable-pulsed Er:YAG or combined Er:YAG/ CO_2) laser systems.[36–42] The single-pass CO_2 laser technique involves application of a single set of nonoverlapping scans to the skin. The partially desiccated tissue is left intact to serve as a biologic wound dressing. At standard treatment parameters, the aforementioned method ablates the entire epidermis. The modulated Er:YAG laser systems emit light with extended pulse durations up to 500μs, producing larger zones of thermal damage compared with traditional short-pulsed Er:YAG laser systems.[31,33,42] In addition, increased thermal coagulation of dermal vessels is effected, permitting deeper tissue penetration and improved intraoperative field visualization. These larger zones of collateral tissue damage result in beneficial tissue effects that approximate those of the CO_2 laser.[40,42] The use of these advanced techniques are associated with shorter and less severe erythema, edema, and postinflammatory hyperpigmentation compared with traditional, multiple-pass CO_2 laser skin resurfacing.[35,43]

A meticulous postoperative wound care regimen is the best measure to ensure proper healing and rapid resolution of symptoms during the recovery process. Two different recovery regimens are available to patients after resurfacing: the open and closed wound dressing techniques. The open technique involves the liberal application of a healing ointment or plain petrolatum with cool water compresses every 2 to 3 hours for the first several days after the procedure. The open technique is labor intensive and may be associated with increased patient discomfort, but allows excellent visibility of the resurfaced skin and permits early detection of untoward side effects.[44,45] The closed technique involves the placement of a semiocclusive biosynthetic dressing over the irradiated skin in an attempt to decrease patient discomfort and speed reepithelialization by limiting crust development. The closed system is relatively easy for patients to use and thus has greater compliance.[46] However, if wound dressings are left in place for extended periods of time, potentially higher rates of infection may occur.[6,47,48] In addition, the use of semiocclusive dressings may contribute to wound maceration and, if opaque, render direct visualization of the resurfaced skin difficult. Some laser surgeons advocate using a combined open and closed wound care approach to maximize postoperative healing. The closed technique is used for the first 2 days postprocedure when the edema, serous drainage, and discomfort are greatest, followed by an open technique for the remainder of the recovery period until reepithelialization is completed. Proper pretreatment education and close physician follow-up, in addition to a carefully executed home recovery regimen, ensures minimal posttreatment morbidity and allows for complications to be detected and addressed expeditiously.

Complications of Ablative Laser Skin Resurfacing

Complications of ablative laser skin resurfacing can be categorized according to severity (Table 13-1). Mild side effects or complications include prolonged erythema and edema, acne or milia formation, irritant or allergic contact dermatitis, and persistent pruritus. Moderate complications include reactivation of herpes simplex virus (HSV), superficial bacterial or fungal infection, transient postinflammatory hyperpigmentation, and permanent, delayed-onset hypopigmentation. The most serious complications of laser skin resurfacing are rare and include hypertrophic scarring, ectropion formation, and disseminated infections. The risk of these untoward side effects are

TABLE 13-1. Complications of ablative laser skin resurfacing.

Mild
Prolonged erythema
Acne and milia formation
Allergic/irritant contact dermatitis
Petechiae
Pruritus

Moderate
Herpes simplex virus reactivation
Superficial cutaneous infection
Postinflammatory hyperpigmentation
Delayed-onset hypopigmentation

Severe
Hypertrophic scarring
Ectropion formation
Disseminated infection

significantly reduced when appropriate pretreatment patient selection is made, proper surgical technique is used, and when the posttreatment recovery period occurs under optimal healing conditions.

Prolonged Erythema

Posttreatment erythema is an expected consequence of laser skin resurfacing and occurs in every patient after treatment. Erythema is most intense after CO_2 laser resurfacing and may persist for 6 months or longer.[6,16,34] Short-pulsed, Er:YAG laser-induced erythema is usually less severe and of shorter duration, lasting several weeks on average.[6,25,29] The risk of prolonged erythema is increased when multiple laser passes or inadvertent stacking or overlapping of laser pulses are performed, producing greater depths of tissue injury.[22,23] It has also been proposed that aggressive debridement of the skin to remove partially desiccated tissue during surgery may also contribute to excessive erythema.[36] Postoperative wound infection and dermatitis irritate the skin and may also result in persistent erythema.[34,49] Patients who have active rosacea or who regularly use topical tretinoin prior to ablative resurfacing may be predisposed to intensified erythema.

Topical ascorbic acid has been shown to decrease the severity and duration of postoperative erythema.[50,51] It is best applied when reepithelialization has been completed in order to avoid irritation of the denuded surface, which could further aggravate skin erythema. Application of topical corticosteroids will not reduce normal postoperative erythema and could potentially retard wound healing and therefore should not be prescribed with the intention of speeding resolution of erythema. However, focal areas of erythema with induration and tenderness may herald incipient scar formation and should be promptly and aggressively treated with potent (class I) topical corticosteroid preparations and/or pulsed dye laser irradiation.[7,52]

Acne and Milia

Acne flares and milia formation are relatively common side effects of cutaneous laser resurfacing due to the use of occlusive healing ointments and biosynthetic dressings during the acute recovery process.[7,22,34] Aberrant follicular epithelialization during healing may also contribute to acne exacerbation within 1 to 2 weeks postoperatively. Patients with a prior history of acne are at particular risk of its development after resurfacing.

Acne has been reported to occur in as many as 80% of patients and milia in upwards of 14% of patients who undergo ablative laser skin resurfacing. Treatment is usually not necessary for mild flares because spontaneous resolution is commonly observed once use of the occlusive ointments and dressings are discontinued. Short courses of oral antibiotics such as doxycycline or minocycline may be necessary for moderate-to-severe acne flares, especially in patients with a strong acne predisposition.[15,34,47] Once the skin has reepithelialized, topical antibiotics (e.g., erythromycin, clindamycin) can be used without fear of allergic or irritant contact dermatitis. Milia typically resolve spontaneously during continuation of the reepithelialization process, but can also be remedied with topical application of retinoic acid or manual extraction. Intralesional corticosteroids may be necessary for the rare inflamed cyst.[6,7]

Contact Dermatitis

Contact dermatitis after cutaneous laser resurfacing can occur in over 50% of patients and is usually irritant in nature. Because of the deepithelialized state of newly resurfaced skin, the normal protective epidermal barrier is impaired, rendering the skin more susceptible to irritation.[34] An allergic or irritant reaction to fragrances or allergens contained within a wide variety of topical ointments, soaps, moisturizers, or cosmetics may develop.[49] Topical antibiotics (e.g., neosporin, polysporin, or bacitracin) are the most common offending agents, so their use should be avoided during the reepithelialization process. It is also imperative that patients refrain from application of self-prescribed remedies during recovery because many herbal or other "natural" compounds may exacerbate irritation and contribute to postoperative morbidity.

Signs and symptoms suggestive of an irritant or allergic contact dermatitis include diffuse and intense facial erythema and/or pruritus (Fig. 13-2). The eczematous eruptions observed are not usually the result of a true type IV allergic reaction, as patch tests fail to reveal allergy in the majority of cases.[53] Because most reactions are of the irritant variety, only the sole use of bland, non-fragrance-containing emollients is necessary during recovery. When an allergic or irritant contact dermatitis is suspected, all potential inciting agents must be immediately discontin-

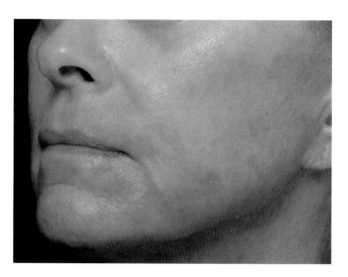

FIGURE 13-2. Contact dermatitis is a relatively common side effect of laser skin resurfacing because of the impairment of the protective epidermal barrier that occurs with skin ablation. Topical antibiotics and other irritants should be avoided in the immediate postoperative period until reepithelialization is completed.

ued. Although most reactions will clear once the offending agents are removed, the use of strong corticosteroids and oral antihistamines may speed the resolution of the dermatitis and reduce the risk of scarring. In severe cases, oral corticosteroids can be prescribed to decrease the inflammatory response. Frequent application of cool compresses can also alleviate pruritus.[34,53]

Infection

Viral, bacterial, and fungal infections may complicate any ablative laser resurfacing procedure with development of signs and symptoms during the first postoperative week before reepithelialization is complete.[48,54] These infections must be promptly identified and treated so as to avoid scarring, delayed wound healing, infection with other opportunistic pathogens, or dissemination. Reactivation of HSV is the most frequently occurring infectious sequela of cutaneous ablative laser resurfacing.[22,34] Because of the high rate of asymptomatic carriers of HSV infection, all patients must be assumed to be carriers of the virus. Therefore, any patient, regardless of prior HSV history, planning to undergo full-face or perioral resurfacing should receive prophylactic oral antiviral therapy. Despite adequate antiviral prophylaxis, 2% to 7% of laser-treated patients experience HSV reactivation.[3]

Detection of a postoperative herpetic infection may be difficult because of the lack of intact epithelium. Whereas a herpetic infection on normal skin typically presents as intact vesicopustules on an erythematous base, an outbreak on laser-treated skin may only appear as superficial erosions. There may also be associated symptoms of pruritus or dysesthesia with delayed reepithelialization. Because dissemination of the herpes virus may result in atrophic scarring, suspected HSV infection should be treated aggressively with an appropriate antiviral agent.[6,7,53]

Oral antiviral agents (e.g., acyclovir, famciclovir, valacyclovir) should be initiated at the time of the resurfacing procedure and continued for another 7 to 10 days until reepithelialization is complete. If a herpetic outbreak occurs despite adequate prophylaxis, drug dosages should be increased to maximum zoster levels or a change to a different antiviral should be made, as viral resistance to the initially prescribed drug may have occurred. For the rare case of herpetic dissemination, intravenous administration of acyclovir with hospitalization becomes necessary.[53]

Superficial cutaneous bacterial and fungal infections may also complicate recovery from cutaneous laser resurfacing. Bacterial infections are often due to excessive wound occlusion during the initial postoperative recovery period and therefore are more commonly seen when a closed wound technique is used. The moist environment of newly resurfaced skin provides an ideal medium for overgrowth of opportunistic pathogens. *Staphyloccocus aureus* and *Pseudomonas aeruginosa* are the most commonly isolated bacteria, whereas *Candida albicans* is the most commonly isolated fungus, although many wounds have multiple contaminating organisms on culture.[44,48] Patients with nasal colonization of staphylococci may be more susceptible to infection; however, it has not been proven that prophylactic topical antibiotic ointment decreases this risk.[54]

Signs and symptoms of an acute bacterial process include focal areas of increased erythema, purulent discharge, pain, delayed healing, and erosions with crusting (Fig. 13-3). A meticulous postoperative wound care regimen is essential to decrease the risk of bacterial infection. Patients should be advised to wash their hands with antibacterial soap before dressing or ointment application. Washcloths and other linens should not be reused during the recovery process. Frequent dressing changes and dilute acetic acid compresses are additional measures that keep the wound clean and free of infection. If an infection is suspected, patients should be given broad-spectrum antibiotics (e.g., semisynthetic penicillins or first-generation cephalosporins) until results of bacterial cultures with antibiotic sensitivities are obtained. Although antibiotic prophylaxis remains standard practice for those patients at increased risk of infection (e.g., immunosuppression, mitral valve prolapse with regurgitation, valvular heart disease), its routine use is controversial. Large-scale prospective and controlled studies are indicated to determine if antimicrobial coverage is warranted in all patients.[54]

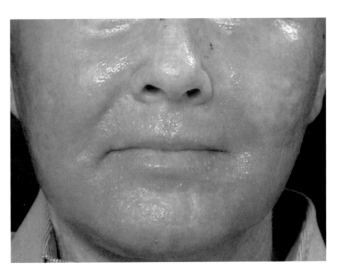

FIGURE 13-3. Excessive crusting, discharge, and slow wound healing are signs of infection. Appropriate bacterial, viral, and fungal cultures should be obtained prior to placement on oral antibiotics.

Pigmentary Alteration

Transient postinflammatory hyperpigmentation is one of the most common side effects of cutaneous laser resurfacing, occurring in one third of all treated patients regardless of skin tone[7,34] (Fig. 13-4). Individuals with darker skin phototypes (Fitzpatrick IV–VI) almost universally hyperpigment after ablative skin resurfacing and should be warned of this potential reaction prior to the procedure. Hyperpigmentation usually develops 3 to 4 weeks postoperatively and can persist for several months without intervention.[6,7,34] Although postinflammatory hyperpigmentation following variable-pulsed Er:YAG laser skin resurfacing can last longer than that seen after treatment with a short-pulsed Er:YAG laser, it is not as persistent as that observed after multiple-pass CO_2 laser skin resurfacing (average: variable-pulsed Er:YAG laser, 10.4 weeks; CO_2 laser, 16 weeks).[6,29,35,39] Because the cutaneous dyspigmentation is so conspicuous, most patients seek treatment to hasten its resolution. Treatment options for hyperpigmentation include topical bleaching agents (hydroquinone, kojic acid), retinoic, azelaic, ascorbic and glycolic acid compounds, as well as broad-spectrum sunscreens to prevent further ultraviolet light–induced melanin synthesis. Mild glycolic acid peels (30%–40%) may also hasten pigment resolution and can be repeated at 2- to 4-week intervals for more efficient results.[44,53] Because any of these topical remedies has the potential to irritate the skin and thus further contribute to the abnormal pigmentation, their use should be avoided during the first postoperative month.[34,53]

Careful preoperative screening is necessary to determine which patients are at greatest risk of developing hyperpigmentation after laser skin resurfacing. Patients

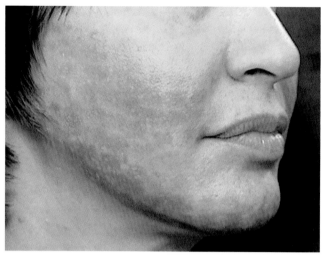
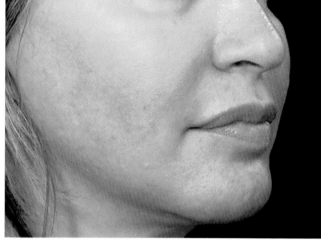

A

B

FIGURE 13-4. Daily use of topical bleaching agents and in-office glycolic acid (30%–40%) peels at 2- to 4-week intervals hasten resolution of postinflammatory hyperpigmentation. Hyperpigmentation observed 1 month after laser skin resurfacing (A) was effectively cleared after a series of glycolic acid peels (B).

should regularly use sunscreens with a sun protection factor of 30 or higher for a minimum of 4 weeks preoperatively in preparation for the procedure. Patients with a suntan should not be resurfaced because they have a much higher risk of postoperative hyperpigmentation due to stimulation of their melanocytes. It is also important for patients to get into the practice of regular sunscreen use prior to laser resurfacing because it will be necessary to limit their ultraviolet exposure postoperatively. Daily sunblock use also becomes important so that the benefits obtained with the laser procedure can be maintained.

Although many laser surgeons recommend pretreating patients with topical bleaching agents and retinoic or glycolic acid compounds prior to cutaneous laser resurfacing, no studies to date have demonstrated any reduction in the rate of postinflammatory hyperpigmentation with this practice. In fact, a prospective study that examined the effects of application of either glycolic acid or hydroquinone with tretinoin versus no treatment at all in 100 patients prior to CO_2 laser resurfacing showed equivocal incidence of postinflammatory hyperpigmentation between the three groups, giving further evidence that pretreatment is unnecessary.[55] Topical agents primarily exert their effects on the superficial epithelium and do not reach the deeply situated melanocytes located within hair follicles or adnexal structures which potentiate the hyperpigmentation.

Hypopigmentation is an uncommon complication of cutaneous laser resurfacing and does not usually manifest until 6 to 12 months after the procedure[1,7,34] (Fig. 13-5). Once residual erythema and hyperpigmentation have faded, conspicuous skin lightening becomes more appar-

ent. The risk of hypopigmentation postresurfacing appears to be directly related to the depth of penetration and degree of thermal injury imparted on the tissue. True hypopigmentation is rare; most cases of skin lightening represent "relative hypopigmentation" due to the removal of photodamaged skin (appearing paler than that of adjacent nontreated dyspigmented skin). In order to reduce the appearance of relative hypopigmentation, it is important to treat within appropriate cosmetic units. When

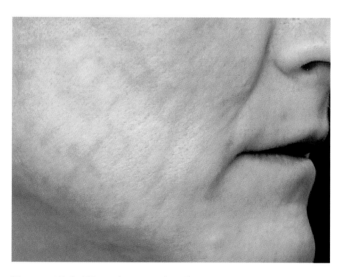

FIGURE 13-5. Hypopigmentation becomes more apparent as postoperative erythema fades, often taking several months to observe. It is related to increased thermal injury to skin during laser treatment, destructive prior procedures (such as phenol peels or dermabrasion), or incomplete treatment within a cosmetic unit (relative hypopigmentation).

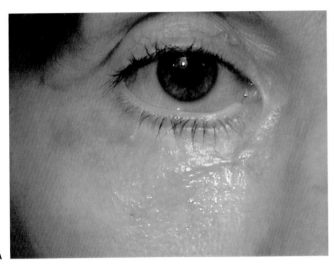 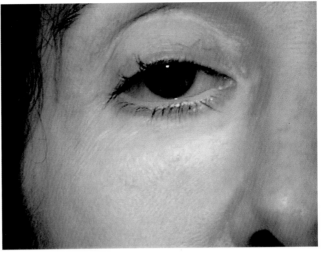

A   B

FIGURE 13-6. Periocular, mandible, and neck regions are more prone to scarring and should, thus, be carefully treated. Pulsed dye laser (585 nm) irradiation can be applied at 6- to 8-week intervals to improve scar color, pliabilility, texture, and bulk.

Hypertrophic scarring and ectropion, while rare after laser skin resurfacing, is seen as early as 1 month postoperatively (A). Significant improvement after two sessions using a 585 nm pulsed dye laser system is typical (B).

more than one facial area requires treatment, it may be best to resurface the entire face in order to minimize obvious lines of demarcation. True hypopigmentation is more common in patients who have had previous dermabrasion or phenol peeling, as fibrosis from the prior procedures may become unmasked.[22,34] Treatment for relative or true hypopigmentation involves the use of chemical peels (glycolic acid or trichloroacetic acid) to help blend lines of demarcation. Irradiation with an excimer (308 nm) laser or application of topical oxsoralen and limited exposure of the skin to ultraviolet light have also been used to induce melanogenesis in these areas.[56,57]

Hypertrophic Scarring

Hypertrophic scarring and textural changes are rare but serious complications of cutaneous ablative laser resurfacing. The use of excessively high energy densities, stacking or overlapping of pulses or scans, or failure to completely remove desiccated tissue between laser passes are known causes of excessive residual thermal necrosis in treated tissue that may eventuate in scar formation.[3,6,22,23,34] Patients who experience postoperative wound infection or contact dermatitis or those with a history of radiation therapy, isotretinoin use within the previous 6 months, or keloid tendency are also at increased risk of scarring. Additionally, certain anatomic locations are more prone to scar formation, including the mandible, neck, and periorbital areas, and should, therefore, be treated with conservative parameters and fewer laser passes.

Focal areas of increased erythema or induration are the first signs of impending scar formation. The skin may be tender in these locations and the prompt initiation of treatment is warranted. Application of potent topical corticosteroids or silicone gel products, as well as intralesional corticosteroid injections, can halt or slow scar progression.[34,44] A vascular-specific 585 nm pulsed dye laser (PDL) can also be used to treat erythematous and hypertrophic scars (Fig. 13-6). Numerous reports in the literature have demonstrated its ability to improve scar color, pliability, texture, and bulk.[52,58–61] Pulsed dye laser irradiation of scars also alleviates associated symptoms of pruritus or dysesthesia. Treatment sessions are repeated at 6- to 8-week intervals with laser parameters similar to those used for benign vascular lesions.

Ectropion Formation

Ectropion of the eyelids is another potentially serious complication following cutaneous laser resurfacing, often requiring surgical correction.[7] Patients who have undergone previous lower blepharoplasty or other surgical manipulation of the eyelids are at increased risk.[44,53] A preoperative evaluation of each patient with a manual "snap" test of the lower eyelid should be performed in order to determine the risk of lid eversion. While application of lower energy densities and fewer laser passes are advocated for infraorbital treatment in order to reduce the risk of scar formation and/or potential compromise of the eyelid margin, it is important to also observe laser–tissue interaction intraoperatively in order to detect excessive collagen contraction that could potentiate lid eversion.

Nonablative Laser Skin Remodeling

In an attempt to limit the prolonged postoperative recovery period associated with ablative laser skin resurfacing and in response to growing public interest in minimally invasive treatment modalities, nonablative laser and light source technology was developed. Rapid advances in this technology have produced several lasers and light-based sources capable of improving fine facial rhytides, dyspigmentation, and telangiectasia associated with cutaneous photodamage. Many of the nonablative laser systems currently in use emit light within the infrared portion of the electromagnetic spectrum (1000–1500 nm).[60,61] At these wavelengths, absorption by superficial water-containing tissue is relatively weak, thereby effecting deeper tissue penetration. Because nonablative remodeling involves creation of a dermal wound without epidermal injury, all of these laser systems employ unique methods to ensure epidermal preservation during treatment. These methods typically include contact cooling handpieces or dynamic cryogen devices capable of delivering variable duration spray spurts either before, during, and/or after laser irradiation. Because laser beam penetration and dermal wounding must be targeted to the relatively superficial portion of the dermis, contact cooling devices that theoretically lead to excessive dermal cooling may affect the level or degree of energy deposition in the skin. As such, there remains no general consensus concerning which method of cooling is most efficacious during treatment.

Nonablative Laser Remodeling: Pretreatment Considerations

Proper patient selection is critical to the success of nonablative laser skin remodeling. Patients with mild-to-moderate facial photodamage with realistic expectations of treatment are the best candidates for nonablative procedures. Patients seeking immediate improvement in photodamaged skin or those who desire a dramatic result may be less than satisfied with the overall clinical outcome.

For patients with a strong history of herpes labialis, prophylactic oral antiviral medications should be considered when treating the perioral skin. Reactivation of prior herpes simplex infection can occur after nonablative laser skin remodeling due to the intense heat produced by the laser or light source.[44]

Prior to nonablative laser procedures, sun exposure should be avoided, particularly when using shorter-wavelength systems such as the pulsed dye laser or an intense pulsed light source. Unwanted absorption of laser energy by activated epidermal melanocytes can increase the risk of side effects, including crusting, blistering, and dyspigmentation.

In general, treatment of facial photodamage with nonablative technology does not produce results comparable to those of ablative CO_2 and Er:YAG lasers; however, many patients are willing to accept modest clinical improvement in exchange for fewer associated risks and shorter recovery times.

Pulsed Dye Laser

Clinical studies have demonstrated the ability of 585 nm and 595 nm pulsed dye laser (PDL) to reduce mild facial rhytides with few side effects.[62] The most common side effects of PDL treatment include mild edema, purpura, and transient postinflammatory hyperpigmentation. Although increased extracellular matrix proteins and types I and III collagen and procollagen have been detected following PDL treatment, the exact mechanism whereby wrinkle improvement is effected remains unknown.[63] One theory states that vascular endothelial cells damaged by the yellow laser light release mediators that stimulate fibroblasts to produce new collagen fibers.[64]

Intense Pulsed Light Source

Several investigators have shown successful rejuvenation of photodamaged skin after intense pulsed light (IPL) treatment.[65,66] The IPL source emits a broad, continuous spectrum of light in the range of 515 to 1200 nm. Cutoff filters are used to eliminate shorter wavelengths depending on the clinical application, with shorter filters favoring heating of melanin and hemoglobin. Several investigators report signs of photoaging, including telangiectasias and mottled pigmentation of the face, neck, and chest, improved by a series of IPL treatments, with minimal side effects and complications.[65–67] Postoperative erythema and mild edema typically last less than 6 hours with desquamation and dyspigmentation as uncommon side effects. However, patients with darker skin phototypes must be treated with caution due to the increased risk of epidermal injury with subsequent hyperpigmentation, and, in rare cases, permanent hypopigmentation and scarring after IPL treatment.[68]

Mid-Infrared Lasers

The 1064 nm Q-switched (QS) neodymium:yttrium-aluminum-garnet (Nd:YAG) laser was the first mid-infrared laser system used for nonablative remodeling. Although absorption of energy by tissue water is relatively weak at the 1064 nm wavelength, it was possible to achieve dermal penetrative depths that could potentially induce neocollagenesis. The nanosecond range pulse duration of the QS Nd:YAG laser was also determined to limit significant thermal diffusion to surrounding structures, thereby making it suitable for nonablative rejuvenation.

In 1997, Goldberg and Whitworth[69] published their experience using a 1064 nm Nd:YAG laser for facial rhytide reduction. Eleven patients (skin phototypes I, II) with mild-to-moderate periorbital or perioral rhytides underwent treatment on one side of the face with a QS Nd:YAG laser at a fluence of 5.5 J/cm², 3 mm spot size, and CO_2 laser ablation on the contralateral side as a split-face comparison. Pinpoint bleeding was used as the clinical endpoint of treatment on the QS Nd:YAG laser-treated facial half. On the QS Nd:YAG laser-treated side, only three patients demonstrated improvement. These three patients had also developed prolonged posttreatment erythema (lasting up to 1 month), suggesting that the amount of dermal wounding (with subsequent collagen remodeling) was directly related to the degree of cutaneous injury. Another study using the QS Nd:YAG laser for rhytide reduction in 61 patients (242 sites) was conducted using a topical carbon solution for improved optical penetration of the 1064 nm light.[70] At least slight improvement was seen in 97% of class I rhytides and 86% of the class II rhytides. Side effects of treatment were mild and limited, including transient erythema, purpura, and postinflammatory hyperpigmentation.

A long-pulsed Nd:YAG laser has also been used for photorejuvenation. Investigators[71] used a combination technique using a long-pulsed 1064 Nd:YAG laser and long-pulsed 532 nm potassium-titanyl-phosphate (KTP) laser, both separately and combined, for noninvasive photorejuvenation in 150 patients, skin phototypes I through V. Patients treated with the combined laser approach showed at least 70% improvement in erythema and pigmentation and 30% to 40% improvement in fine rhytides.

A 1320 nm Nd:YAG laser was the first commercially available system marketed solely for the purpose of nonablative laser skin remodeling.[72–74] The 1320 nm wavelength is associated with a high scattering coefficient that allows for dispersion of laser irradiation throughout the dermis. The 1320 nm Nd:YAG laser handpiece contains three portals: the laser beam itself, a thermal feedback sensor that registers skin surface temperature, and a dynamic cryogen spray apparatus used for epidermal cooling. When skin surface temperatures are maintained at 40°C to 45°C, dermal temperatures reach 60°C to 65°C during laser irradiation, thereby effecting collagen contraction and neocollagenesis. In order to prevent unwanted sequelae (e.g., blistering) from excessive heat production, it is imperative that epidermal temperatures be kept lower than 50°C. A series of three or more treatment sessions are scheduled at regular time intervals (typically once a month) for maximum mitigation of fine rhytides.[60,75]

The 1320 nm Nd:YAG laser produces mild subclinical epidermal injury that leads to enhanced skin texture and new papillary collagen synthesis by stimulation of cyto-kines and other inflammatory mediators. Thus, the long-term histologic improvement seen in photodamaged skin may not be based solely on direct laser heating of collagen, but by further stimulation of cytokine release by heating the superficial vasculature. In addition, the histologic findings suggested that multiple passes with fluence and cooling adjusted to a T_{max} of 45°C to 48°C can yield improved clinical results, as compared to those specimens in which epidermal temperatures above 45°C were not achieved.[76]

The 1450 nm mid-infrared wavelength diode laser targets dermal water and penetrates the skin to an approximate depth of 500 μm. This low-power laser system achieves peak powers in the 10 W to 15 W range with relatively long pulse durations of 150 ms to 250 ms. Because of these long exposure times, epidermal cooling must be delivered in sequence during the application of laser energy in order to avoid excessive thermal buildup within the superficial layers of the skin. Multiple studies have demonstrated its efficacy in treating mild-to-moderate rhytides, atrophic facial scarring, and active acne vulgaris.[77–80]

Goldberg and colleagues[77] reported on the effects of 1450 nm diode laser irradiation in 20 patients with class I to II rhytides. Two to four treatment sessions were delivered with 6 months follow-up evaluation. Patients were treated with laser and cryogen spray cooling on one facial half and cryogen spray cooling alone on the contralateral side. On the laser-treated facial halves, 7 did not demonstrate any improvement, 10 showed mild improvement, and 3 had moderate improvement. None of the sites treated with cryogen alone showed any improvement after 6 months. Side effects of treatment were mild and included transient erythema, edematous papules, and one case of postinflammatory hyperpigmentation persisting for 6 months. The authors concluded that the 1450 nm diode laser was effective for treatment of mild to moderately severe facial rhytides with minimal morbidity. Additionally, their study demonstrated that nonablative laser treatment alone was responsible for the clinical improvements and that the nonspecific injury induced by cryogen spray cooling could not effect the changes seen. In a controlled clinical and histologic study, other investigators[79] demonstrated improvement in mild-to-moderate perioral or periorbital rhytides in 25 patients treated with four consecutive 1450 nm diode laser treatments. Peak clinical improvement was seen 6 months after the series of laser treatments. Side effects were limited to transient erythema, edema, and postinflammatory hyperpigmentation.

Because of the minimal postoperative recovery and few associated side effects, nonablative skin remodeling with a mid-infrared laser is an attractive procedure to patients and physicians alike. The most common side effects of treatment include postoperative erythema

E.L. Tanzi and T.S. Alster

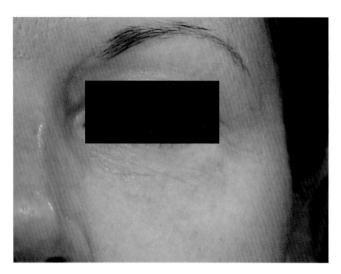

FIGURE 13-7. Mild transient erythema and edema is typical after nonablative laser skin treatment.

and mild edema, typically lasting less than 24 hours (Fig. 13-7). Transient postinflammatory hyperpigmentation is observed far less commonly than after ablative laser skin procedures and may be attributed to excessive cryogen cooling of the epidermis during treatment. Topical bleaching agents and light glycolic acid peels can hasten the resolution of postinflammatory hyperpigmentation (Fig. 13-8). Development of atrophic, pitted scars after nonablative laser skin resurfacing is rare and the risk minimized by proper functioning of the equipment (particularly the epidermal cooling device) and by careful placement of non-overlapping laser pulses.

Although nonablative lasers are not yet capable of results comparable with those of ablative laser systems,

they have been shown to improve mild-to-moderate atrophic scars, rhytides, and acne vulgaris with virtually no external wound. Therefore, nonablative laser resurfacing is ideal for patients with either mild cutaneous pathology or in those who are unwilling or unable to undergo a labor-intensive procedure associated with considerable postoperative morbidity such as ablative laser skin resurfacing. In the weeks following a series of nonablative laser procedures, follow-up visits can help identify patient concerns and increase the overall satisfaction with treatment. Because clinical improvement after a series of nonablative laser procedures often take several weeks to realize, reassurance by the laser surgeon regarding the patient's progress can be particularly important.

Short-Contact Photodynamic Therapy

Photodynamic therapy (PDT) with topical 5-aminolevulinic acid (5-ALA) is an evolving, noninvasive treatment for a variety of dermatologic conditions. Several reports have documented the successful use of PDT in the treatment of acne vulgaris, nonmelanoma skin cancers, psoriasis, verrucae, sebaceous hyperplasia, and cutaneous T-cell lymphoma.[81–92] Photodynamic therapy involves the application of a photosensitizing chemical to a specific cutaneous lesion which, when exposed to visible light, results in excitation of the photosensitizer and consequent production of a reactive oxygen species that leads to cytotoxicity. Topical application of 20% aminolevulinic acid (ALA) initiates time-dependent accumulation of the endogenous photosensitizer, protoporphyrin IX (PpIX) in dysplastic and neoplastic dermatologic lesions and epidermal appendages such as sebaceous glands and hair

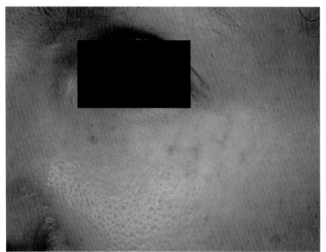

A

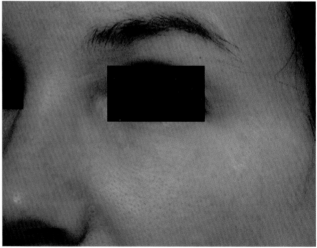

B

FIGURE 13-8. Postinflammatory hyperpigmentation is observed far less commonly than after ablative laser skin procedures and may be attributed to excessive cryogen cooling of the epidermis

during treatment, resulting in an arclike pattern (A). Complete resolution after a series of 30% glycolic acid peels (B).

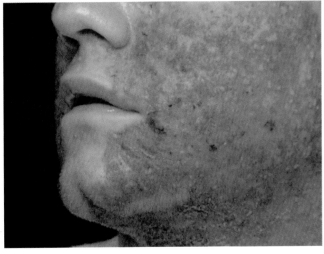
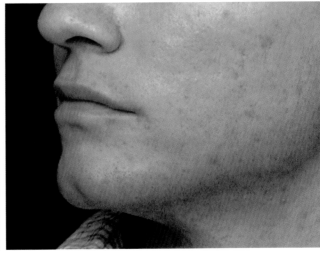

FIGURE 13-9. Severe phototoxic reactions after short-contact photodynamic therapy are rare and are often due to noncompliance with posttreatment avoidance of ultraviolet light exposure for 36 hours (A). Crusting and erythema typically resolve within a week with the use of cool compresses and bland healing ointment (B).

follicles. Because hyperproliferative cells are metabolically more active than normal cells, they convert more ALA to PpIX. Protoporphyrin IX has a large absorption peak in the Soret band (400–430 nm) and smaller absorption peaks at longer wavelengths (509, 544, 584, 630, 690 nm), therefore many different light sources can be utilized for 5-ALA photodynamic therapy. Shorter blue light wavelengths are most effectively absorbed by 5-ALA, but have limited skin penetration. On the other hand, the longer yellow and red wavelengths can activate 5-ALA deeper in the skin, potentially reducing the number of treatments needed to exert a positive clinical effect.

Short contact (typically 1- to 4-hour incubation), photodynamic therapy has been used most recently for enhanced photorejuvenation and acne vulgaris.[93–96] In a split-face comparison study, investigators[97] reported that short-incubation, topical 20% 5-ALA PDT with intense pulsed light (IPL) was an effective, well-tolerated method of photorejuvenation that resulted in greater clinical improvement than IPL treatment alone. More substantive improvement of skin color, tone, and texture was evident within two treatment sessions using the combination therapy. Other split-face studies have demonstrated similar findings for the treatment of photodamage and rhytides.[98] Furthermore, short-contact PDT can be used to effectively improve acne vulgaris following a series of treatments with few side effects.[99,100]

After treatment, patients are instructed to use a mild hypoallergenic cleanser and moisturizer, followed by a broad-spectrum sunscreen and strict avoidance of UVA and UVB light for 36 hours in order to avoid a severe phototoxic reaction. Although short-contact PDT with 5-ALA and IPL is well tolerated, it can be associated with more side effects than treatment with traditional IPL treatment alone.[97] Patients may experience mild erythema, edema, and desquamation lasting up to 48 hours after treatment. Therefore it is essential that the risk of a mild phototoxic reaction be discussed with patients prior to treatment. Rare, severe phototoxic reactions with intense erythema, edema, and crusting can be managed by cool compresses, oral analgesics, and topical corticosteroids (Fig. 13-9).

Nonablative Radiofrequency

A monopolar radiofrequency device (ThermaCool TC; Thermage Inc., Hayward, CA) has been studied for deep dermal heating with subsequent tightening of photodamaged skin. Unlike a laser in which light energy is converted into heat, the radiofrequency device generates electric current which produces heat through resistance in the dermis. The energy is delivered to the patient through a sophisticated handpiece and treatment tip with a coupling membrane which allows for uniform delivery of heat over the entire treatment area. Epidermal protection is provided by simultaneous cryogen cooling within the contact treatment tip. Using this technique, a reverse thermal gradient is generated. The depth of heat penetration is dependent upon the size and specifics of the detachable treatment tip and can be changed according to the clinical application. In a controlled study, investigators[101] demonstrated significant improvement in neck and cheek laxity in the majority of 50 patients treated with a monopolar radiofrequency device. Side effects were mild and limited to transient erythema, edema, and rare dysesthesia. No scarring or pigmentary alteration was

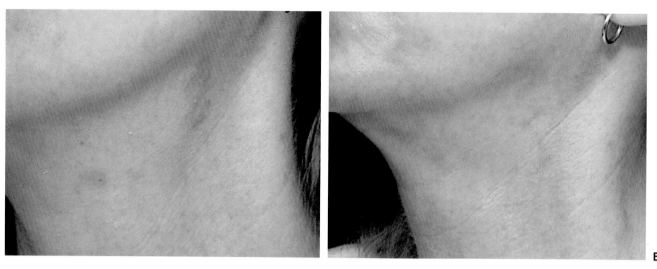

FIGURE 13-10. Erythematous papules lasting several days can be seen after radiofrequency treatment (A). Gentle skin care is indicated until the erythema resolves (B).

reported. Other groups have reported subtle, yet clinically significant improvement in facial and neck skin laxity with minimal adverse sequelae.[102–107]

A device that combines radiofrequency and diode laser energy has also been used for nonablative facial rejuvenation (Polaris WR; Syneron Medical LTD, Israel). This device delivers radiofrequency energy and optical energy in a sequential manner through a unique bipolar electrode tip. Thermoelectric cooling at 5°C provides epidermal protection throughout the pulse sequence. Investigators[108] demonstrated improvement in skin laxity in the majority of the 20 patients treated. Others[109] used bipolar radiofrequency combined with intense pulsed light energy (Aurora SR; Syneron Medical, Israel) for facial rejuvenation. In 108 patients, overall skin improvement was rated at 75% following a series of five treatments at 3-week intervals.

The side effects of nonablative radiofrequency devices are typically mild and transient. Most patients develop mild erythema as an acute clinical response. Erythematous papules lasting several days have been documented in a small percentage of patients and typically when higher energies had been applied to the skin (Fig. 13-10). Dysesthesia after radiofrequency treatment has also been reported and resolves without adverse sequelae several days following treatment. Blistering, crusting, dyspigmentation, scarring, and textural irregularities are rare. For both monopolar and bipolar radiofrequency systems, inadequate contact with the skin during treatment can lead to epidermal injury with focal erythema lasting days to weeks. Rare reports of permanent textural irregularities and fat necrosis may be associated with excessive treatment parameters or a pulse stacking technique.

Fractional Photothermolysis

An entirely novel treatment termed *fractional photothermolysis* was recently developed to address the limitations of currently available lasers and light sources used for skin photorejuvenation.[110] Although dramatic clinical improvement can be achieved with ablative laser skin resurfacing, patients are often hesitant to pursue this treatment option because of the extended postoperative recovery period and inherent risks of the procedure. On the other hand, nonablative lasers and light sources have demonstrated modest efficacy in the noninvasive treatment of mild facial rhytides and atrophic scarring, with minimal side effects. However, disadvantages of these nonablative treatments include the necessity for multiple therapeutic sessions, delayed clinical response, and inconsistent clinical results.

Fractional photothermolysis is based on the creation of microscopic thermal wounds with sparing of the surrounding tissue. Fractional resurfacing is performed using a 1550nm fiber laser (Fraxel; Reliant Technologies San Diego, CA) that targets water-containing tissue to photocoagulate small columns of tissue (microscopic thermal zones or MTZs) with a depth of 200 to 500μm delivered approximately 200 to 300μm apart. Histologic evaluation following treatment reveals thermal injury sharply confined to a small column of dermal collagen and lower epidermis in the MTZs. Microscopic epidermal necrotic debris (MEND) subsequently exfoliates several days to 2 weeks following treatment, depending on the density and intensity of the treatment parameters. The exfoliation process may give the treated skin a bronzed appearance for several days. The wound healing response differs from ablative techniques because the epidermal tissue that is spared

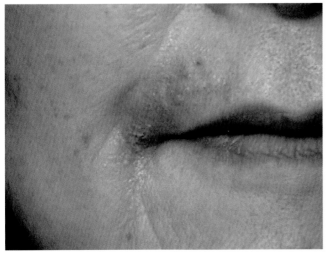
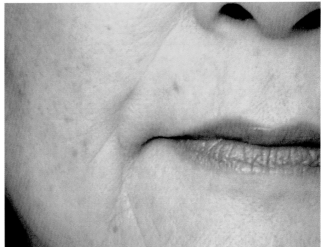

FIGURE 13-11. Aggressive fractional laser resurfacing techniques can result in erosions due to dense placement of microthermal treatment zones (A). Erosions can be managed with an open wound technique using cool compresses and healing ointment several times daily until reepithelialization is complete (B).

between treatment zones contains viable transient amplifying cells, capable of rapid reepilthelialization. Furthermore, because the stratum corneum has a low water content, it remains intact immediately after treatment. Therefore, the wound created by fractional resurfacing is unique and is not simply an ablative laser used to make "holes" in the skin. In addition, fractional resurfacing can provide an advantage over purely nonablative laser treatments due to the gradual exfoliation of the epidermis with resultant improvement in superficial dyspigmentation. Because only a fraction (17%–20%) of the skin is treated during each session, several fractional resurfacing treatments are typically required to effect the best clinical outcome.

In preliminary studies, investigators have shown fractional laser resurfacing to be safe and effective for a variety of indications.[110–112] Side effects of fractional resurfacing are typically mild and include erythema lasting up to 5 days, periocular edema, and a slight darkening of the skin (bronzing) as the MEND desquamates. Erosions are uncommon and can be managed by liberal application of healing ointment or plain petrolatum with cool water compresses every 2 to 3 hours (Fig. 13-11). Although the incidence of postinflammatory hyperpigmentation is lower than that seen after ablative laser skin resurfacing, topical bleaching agents and light glycolic acid peels can hasten its resolution. To date, permanent pigmentary alteration and scarring have not been reported. However, when an aggressive treatment protocol is used with a high density of MTZs placed, the risk of complete epidermal ablation is increased, along with the associated side effects and complications common to other ablative laser skin resurfacing procedures. Additional research is ongoing to determine optimal treatment parameters and the long-term consequences of this exciting new technology.

Conclusion

Modern laser and light-based systems that were developed based on the theory of selective photothermolysis are capable of destroying specific tissue targets whilst minimizing the risk of scarring and pigmentary changes. This is accomplished through the use of a wavelength and pulse duration that is best absorbed by a specific chromophore such as water or hemoglobin. Radiofrequency devices are also available for minimally invasive rejuvenation of skin laxity without the side effects and complications associated with surgical lifting procedures. Certainly, any laser, light-based, or radiofrequency device potentially can result in scarring and tissue damage when used incorrectly; therefore, adequate operator education and skill are essential. Side effects and complications that occur as a consequence of treatment can be significantly reduced if diagnosed and treated in an expeditious manner. In the future, as technology and techniques continue to evolve, patients will benefit from greater clinical improvement with fewer associated side effects and complications.

References

1. Tanzi EL, Lupton JR, Alster TS. Review of lasers in dermatology: four decades of progress. J Am Acad Dermatol 2003;49:1–31.
2. Lanzafame RJ, Naim JO, Rogers DW, Hinshaw JR. Comparisons of continuous-wave, chop wave, and superpulsed laser wounds. Lasers Surg Med 1988;8:119–124.
3. Alster TS, Lupton JR. An overview of cutaneous laser resurfacing. Clin Plast Surg 2001;28:37–52.
4. Anderson RR, Parrish JA. Selective photothermolysis: precise microsurgery by selective absorption of pulsed radiation. Science 1983;22:524–527.

5. Alster TS. Preoperative preparation for CO_2 laser resurfacing. In: Coleman WP, Lawrence N, eds. Skin resurfacing. Baltimore: Williams & Wilkins; 1998:171–179.

6. Alster TS. Cutaneous resurfacing with CO_2 and erbium: YAG lasers: preoperative, intraoperative, and postoperative consideration. Plast Reconstr Surg 1999;103:619–632.

7. Alster TS, Lupton JR. Prevention and treatment of side effects and complications of cutaneous laser resurfacing. Plast Reconstr Surg 2002;109:308–316.

8. Alster TS, Kauvar ANB, Geronemus RG. Histology of high-energy pulsed CO_2 laser resurfacing. Semin Cutan Med Surg 1996;15:189–193.

9. Alster TS, Garg S. Treatment of facial rhytides with a high-energy pulsed carbon dioxide laser. Plast Reconstr Surg 1996;98:791–794.

10. Alster TS, Nanni CA, Williams CM. Comparison of four carbon dioxide resurfacing lasers: a clinical and histopathologic evaluation. Dermatol Surg 1999;25:153–159.

11. Lowe NJ, Lask G, Griffin ME, et al. Skin resurfacing with the ultrapulse carbon dioxide laser: observations on 100 patients. Dermatol Surg 1995;21:1025–1029.

12. Alster TS. Comparison of two high-energy, pulsed carbon dioxide lasers in the treatment of periorbital rhytides. Dermatol Surg 1996;22:541–545.

13. Apfelberg DB. Ultrapulse carbon dioxide laser with CPG scanner for full-face resurfacing of rhytides, photoaging, and acne scars. Plast Reconstr Surg 1997;99:1817–1825.

14. Lask G, Keller G, Lowe NJ, et al. Laser skin resurfacing with the SilkTouch flashscanner for facial rhytides. Dermatol Surg 1995;21:1021–1024.

15. Waldorf HA, Kauvar ANB, Geronemus RG. Skin resurfacing of fine to deep rhytides using a char-free carbon dioxide laser in 47 patients. Dermatol Surg 1995;21:940–946.

16. Ratner D, Tse Y, Marchell N, et al. Cutaneous laser resurfacing. J Am Acad Dermatol 1999;41:365–389.

17. Walsh JT, Deutsch TF. Pulsed CO_2 laser tissue ablation: measurement of the ablation rate. Lasers Surg Med 1988; 8:264–275.

18. Fitzpatrick RE, Ruiz-Esparza J, Goldman MP. The depth of thermal necrosis using the CO_2 laser: a comparison of the superpulsed mode and conventional mode. J Dermatol Surg Oncol 1991;17:340–344.

19. Stuzin JM, Baker TJ, Baker TM, et al. Histologic effects of the high-energy pulsed CO_2 laser on photo-aged facial skin. Plast Reconstr Surg 1997;99:2036–2050.

20. Walsh JT, Flotte TJ, Anderson RR, et al. Pulsed CO_2 laser tissue ablation: effect of tissue type and pulse duration on thermal damage. Lasers Surg Med 1988;8:108–118.

21. Ruback BW, Schroenrock LD. Histological and clinical evaluation of facial resurfacing using a carbon dioxide laser with the computer pattern generator. Arch Otolaryngol Head Neck Surg 1997;123:929–934.

22. Bernstein LJ, Kauvar ANB, Grossman MC, et al. The short- and long-term side effects of carbon dioxide laser resurfacing. Dermatol Surg 1997;23:519–525.

23. Fitzpatrick RE, Smith SR, Sriprachya-anunt S. Depth of vaporization and the effect of pulse stacking with a high-energy, pulsed carbon dioxide laser. J Am Acad Dermatol 1999;40:615–622.

24. Walsh JT, Flotte TJ, Deutsch TF. Er:YAG laser ablation of tissue: effect of pulse duration and tissue type on thermal damage. Lasers Surg Med 1989;9:327–337.

25. Ross EV, Anderson RR. The erbium laser in skin resurfacing. In: Alster TS, Apfelberg DB, eds. Cosmetic laser surgery. 2nd ed. New York: Wiley; 1999:57–84.

26. Alster TS. Clinical and histologic evaluation of six erbium: YAG lasers for cutaneous resurfacing. Lasers Surg Med 1999;24:87–92.

27. Hibst R, Kaufmann R. Effects of laser parameters on pulsed Er:YAG laser ablation. Lasers Med Science 1991; 6:391–397.

28. Hohenleutner U, Hohenleutner S, Baumler W, et al. Fast and effective skin ablation with an Er:YAG laser: determination of ablation rates and thermal damage zones. Lasers Surg Med 1997;20:242–247.

29. Alster TS, Lupton JR. Erbium:YAG cutaneous laser resurfacing. Dermatol Clin 2001;19:453–466.

30. Khatri KA, Ross EV, Grevelink JM, et al. Comparison of erbium:YAG and carbon dioxide lasers in resurfacing of facial rhytides. Arch Dermatol 1999;135:391–397.

31. Goldman MP, Marchell N, Fitzpatrick RE. Laser skin resurfacing of the face with a combined CO_2/Er:YAG laser. Dermatol Surg 2000;26:102–104.

32. Sapijaszko MJA, Zachary CB. Er:YAG laser skin resurfacing. Dermatol Clin 2002;20:87–96.

33. Pozner JM, Goldberg DJ. Histologic effect of a variable pulsed Er:YAG laser. Dermatol Surg 2000;26:733–736.

34. Nanni CA, Alster TS. Complications of carbon dioxide laser resurfacing: an evaluation of 500 patients. Dermatol Surg 1998;24:315–320.

35. Tanzi EL, Alster TS. Side effects and complications of variable-pulsed erbium:yttrium-aluminum-garnet laser skin resurfacing: extended experience with 50 patients. Plast Reconstr Surg 2003;111:1524–1529.

36. David L, Ruiz-Esparza J. Fast healing after laser skin resurfacing: the minimal mechanical trauma technique. Dermatol Surg 1997;23:359–361.

37. Ruiz-Esparza J, Gomez JMB. Long-term effects of one general pass laser resurfacing: a look at dermal tightening and skin quality. Dermatol Surg 1999;25:169–174.

38. Alster TS, Hirsch RJ. Single-pass CO_2 laser skin resurfacing of light and dark skin: extended experience with 52 patients. J Cosmet Laser Ther 2003;5:39–42.

39. Tanzi EL, Alster TS. Single-pass carbon dioxide versus multiple-pass Er:YAG laser skin resurfacing: a comparison of postoperative wound healing and side-effect rates. Dermatol Surg 2003;29:80–84.

40. Newman JB, Lord JL, Ash K, et al. Variable pulse erbium: YAG laser skin resurfacing of perioral rhytides and side-by-side comparison with carbon dioxide laser. Lasers Surg Med 1998;24:1303–1307.

41. Fitzpatrick RE, Rostan EF, Marchell N. Collagen tightening induced by carbon dioxide laser versus erbium:YAG laser. Lasers Surg Med 2000;27:395–403.

42. Zachary CB. Modulating the Er:YAG laser. Lasers Surg Med 2002;26:223–226.

43. Rostan EF, Fitzpatrick RE, Goldman MP. Laser resurfacing with a long pulse erbium:YAG laser compared to the 950 ms pulsed CO_2 laser. Lasers Surg Med 2001;29:136–141.

44. Alster TS, Tanzi, EL. Laser skin resurfacing: ablative and non-ablative. In: Hanke CW, Sengelmann RD, Siegel DM, eds. Aesthetic surgical procedures. Philadelphia: Elsevier, Mosby; 2005:611–624.

45. Tanzi EL, Alster TS. Effect of a semiocclusive silicone-based dressing after ablative laser resurfacing of facial skin. Cosmetic Dermatol 2003;16:13–16.

46. Batra RS, Ort RJ, Jacob C, et al. Evaluation of a silicone occlusive dressing after laser skin resurfacing. Arch Dermatol 2001;137:1317–1321.

47. Horton S, Alster TS. Preoperative and postoperative considerations for cutaneous laser resurfacing. Cutis 1999;64: 399–406.

48. Sriprachya-anunt S, Fitzpatrick RE, Goldman MP, et al. Infections complicating pulsed carbon dioxide laser resurfacing for photo-aged facial skin. Dermatol Surg 1997; 23:527–536.

49. Fisher AA. Lasers and allergic contact dermatitis to topical antibiotics, with particular reference to bacitracin. Cutis 1996;58:252–254.

50. Alster TS, West TB. Effect of topical vitamin C on postoperative carbon dioxide resurfacing erythema. Dermatol Surg 1998;24:331–334.

51. McDaniel DH, Ash K, Lord J, et al. Accelerated laser resurfacing wound healing using a triad of topical antioxidants. Dermatol Surg 1998;24:661–664.

52. Alster TS, Nanni CA. Pulsed dye laser treatment of hypertrophic burn scars. Plast Reconstr Surg 1998;102:2190–2195.

53. Alster TS, Tanzi EL. Complications in laser and light surgery. In: Goldberg DB, ed. Laser skin surgery. Vol. 2. New York: Elsevier; 2005:103–118.

54. Walia S, Alster TS. Cutaneous CO$_2$ laser resurfacing infection rate with and without prophylactic antibiotics. Dermatol Surg 1999;25:857–861.

55. West TB, Alster TS. Effect of pretreatment on the incidence of hyperpigmentation following cutaneous CO$_2$ laser resurfacing. Dermatol Surg 1999;25:15–17.

56. Friedman PM, Geronemus RG. Use of the 308-nm excimer laser for postresurfacing leukoderma. Arch Dermatol 2001;137:824–825.

57. Grimes PE, Bhawan J, Kim J, et al. Laser resurfacing-induced hypopigmentation: histologic alteration and repigmentation with topical photochemotherapy. Dermatol Surg 2001;27:515–520.

58. Alster TS. Improvement of erythematous and hypertrophic scars by the 585 nm pulsed dye laser. Ann Plast Surg 1994;32:186–190.

59. Alster TS, Williams CM. Treatment of keloid sternotomy scars with 585 nm flashlamp pumped pulsed dye laser. Lancet 1995;345:1198–1200.

60. Alster TS. Laser scar revision: comparison study of 585-nm pulsed dye laser with and without intralesional corticosteroids. Dermatol Surg 2003;29:25–29.

61. Alster TS, Tanzi EL. Hypertrophic scars and keloids: a review of etiology and management. Am J Clin Dermatol 2003;4:235–243.

62. Hardaway CA, Ross EV. Nonablative laser skin remodeling. Dermatol Clin 2002;20:97–111.

63. Zelickson B, Kist D. Effect of pulse dye laser and intense pulsed light source on the dermal extracellular matrix remodeling. Lasers Surg Med 2000;12:68.

64. Bjerring P, Clement M, Heickendorff L, et al. Selective non-ablative wrinkle reduction by laser. J Cutan Laser Ther 2000;2:9–15.

65. Goldberg DJ, Cutler KB. Nonablative treatment of rhytids with intense pulsed light. Lasers Surg Med 2000;26:196–200.

66. Bitter PH. Noninvasive rejuvenation of photodamaged skin using serial, full-face intense pulsed light treatments. Dermatol Surg 2000;26:835–843.

67. Weiss RA, Weiss MA, Beasley KL. Rejuvenation of photoaged skin: 5 years results with intense pulsed light of the face, neck, and chest. Dermatol Surg 2002;28:1115–1119.

68. Fodor L, Peled IJ, Rissin Y, et al. Using intense pulsed light for cosmetic purposes: our experience. Plast Reconstr Surg 2004;113:1789–1795.

69. Goldberg DJ, Whitworth J. Laser skin resurfacing with the Q-switched Nd:YAG laser. Dermatol Surg 1997;23:903–906; discussion, 906–907.

70. Goldberg DJ, Metzler C. Skin resurfacing utilizing a low-fluence Nd:YAG laser. J Cutan Laser Ther 1999;1:23–27.

71. Lee MW. Combination visible and infrared lasers for skin rejuvenation. Semin Cutan Med Surg 2002;21:288–300.

72. Menaker GM, Wrone DA, Williams RM, et al. Treatment of facial rhytids with a nonablative laser: a clinical and histologic study. Dermatol Surg 1999;25:440–444.

73. Kelly KM, Nelson S, Lask GP, et al. Cryogen spray cooling in combination with nonablative laser treatment of facial rhytides. Arch Dermatol 1999;135:691–694.

74. Goldberg DJ. Nonablative subsurface remodeling: clinical and histologic evaluation of a 1320 nm Nd:YAG laser. J Cutan Laser Ther 1999;1:153–157.

75. Trelles MA, Allones I, Luna R. Facial rejuvenation with a nonablative 1320 nm Nd:YAG laser. A preliminary clinical and histologic evaluation. Dermatol Surg 2001;27:111–116.

76. Fatemi A, Weiss MA, Weiss RA. Short-term histologic effects of nonablative resurfacing: results with a dynamically cooled millisecond-domain 1320 nm Nd:YAG laser. Dermatol Surg 2002;28:172–176.

77. Goldberg DJ, Rogachefsky AS, Silapunt S. Nonablative laser treatment of facial rhytides: a comparison of 1450 nm diode laser treatment with dynamic cooling as opposed to treatment with dynamic cooling alone. Lasers Surg Med 2002;30:79–81.

78. Hardaway CA, Ross EV, Paithankar DY. Non-ablative cutaneous remodeling with a 1.45 micron mid-infrared diode laser: phase II. J Cosmet Laser Ther 2002;4:9–14.

79. Tanzi EL, Williams CM, Alster TS. Treatment of facial rhytides with a nonablative 1450-nm diode laser: a controlled clinical and histologic study. Dermatol Surg 2003;29: 124–129.

80. Tanzi EL, Alster TS. Comparson of a 1450 nm diode laser and a 1320 nm Nd:YAG laser in the treatment of atrophic facial scars: a prospective clinical and histologic study. Dermatol Surg 2004;30:152–157.

81. Itoh Y, Ninomiya Y, Tajima S, et al. Photodynamic therapy for acne vulgaris with topical aminolevulinic acid. Arch Dermatol 2000;136:1093–1095.

82. Hongcharu W, Taylor CR, Chang Y, Aghassi D, Suthamjariya K, Anderson RR. Topical ALA-photodynamic therapy for the treatment of acne vulgaris. J Invest Dermatol 2000;115:183–192.

83. Ibbotson S. Topical 5-aminolevulinic acid photodynamic therapy for the treatment of skin conditions other than non-melanoma skin cancer. Br J Dermatol 2002;146:178–188.

84. Svanberg K, Andersson T, Killander D, et al. Photodynamic therapy of non-melanoma malignant tumors of the skin using topical 5-aminolevulinic acid sensitization and laser irradiation. Br J Dermatol 1994;130:743–751.

85. Robinson D, Collins P, Stringer M, et al. Improved response of plaque psoriasis after multiple treatments with topical 5-aminolevulinic acid photodynamic therapy. Acta Dermatol Venereol 1999;79:451–455.

86. Stendar I-M, Na R, Fogh H, et al. Photodynamic therapy with 5-aminolevulinic acid or placebo for recalcitrant foot and hand warts: randomised double-blind trial. Lancet 2000;355:963–966.

87. Leman J, Dick D, Morton C. Topical 5-ALA photodynamic therapy for the treatment of cutaneous T-cell lymphoma. Clin Exp Dermatol 2002;27:516–518.

88. Fink-Puches R, Soyer HP, Hofer A, et al. Long-term follow-up and histological changes of superficial nonmelanoma skin cancers treated with topical δ-aminolevulinic acid photodynamic therapy. Arch Dermatol 1998;134:821–826.

89. Jeffes EW, McCullough JL, Weinstein GD, et al. Photodynamic therapy of actinic keratoses with topical aminolevulinic acid hydrochloride and fluorescent blue light. J Am Acad Dermatol 2001;45:96–104.

90. Alexiades-Armenakas MR, Geronemus RG. Laser-assisted photodynamic therapy of actinic keratoses. Arch Dermatol 2003;139:1313–1320.

91. Haller JC, Cairnduff F, Slack G, et al. Routine double treatments of superficial basal cell carcinomas using aminolevulinic acid-based photodynamic therapy. Br J Dermatol 2000;143:1270–1275.

92. Alster TS, Tanzi EL. Photodynamic therapy with topical aminolevulinic acid and pulsed dye laser irradiation for sebaceous hyperplasia. J Drugs Dermatol 2003;2:501–504.

93. Avram DK, Goldman MP. Effectiveness and safety of ALA-IPL in treating actinic keratoses and photodamage. J Drugs Dermatol 2004;3(Suppl 1):S36–S39.

94. Ruiz-Rodriguez R, Sanz-Sanchez T, Cordoba S. Photodynamic photorejuvenation. Dermatol Surg 2002;28:742–744.

95. Gold MH, Goldman MP. 5-Aminolevulinic acid photodynamic therapy: where we have been and where we are going. Dermatol Surg 2004;30:1077–1084.

96. Touma D, Yaar M, Whitehead S, et al. A trial of short incubation, broad-area photodynamic therapy for facial actinic keratoses and diffuse photodamage. Arch Dermatol 2004;140:33–40.

97. Alster TS, Tanzi EL, Welsh EC. Photorejuvenation of facial skin with topical 20% 5-aminolevulinic acid and intense pulsed light treatment: a split-face comparison study. J Drugs Dermatol 2005;4:35–38.

98. Alam M, Dover JS. Treatment of photoaging with topical aminolevulinic acid and light. Skin Ther Lett 2005;9:7–9.

99. Gold MH, Bradshaw VL, Boring MM, et al. The use of a novel intense pulsed light and heat source and ALA PDT in the treatment of moderate to severe inflammatory acne vulgaris. J Drugs Dermatol 2004;3:S15–S19.

100. Taub AF. Photodynamic therapy for the treatment of acne: a pilot study. J Drugs Dermatol 2004;3:S10–S14.

101. Alster TS, Tanzi EL. Improvement of neck and cheek laxity with a non-ablative radiofrequency device: a lifting experience. Dermatol Surg 2004;30:503–507.

102. Hsu TS, Kaminer MS. The use of nonablative radiofrequency technology to tighten the lower face and neck. Semin Cutan Med Surg 2003;22:115–123.

103. Fitzpatrick R, Geronemus R, Goldberg D, et al. Multi-center study of noninvasive radiofrequency for periorbital tissue tightening. Lasers Surg Med 2003;33:23–242.

104. Ruiz-Esparza J, Gomez JB. The medical face lift: a noninvasive, nonsurgical approach to tissue tightening in facial skin using nonablative radiofrequency. Dermatol Surg 2003;29:325–332.

105. Kushikata N, Negishi K, Tezuka Y, et al. Non-ablative skin tightening with radiofrequency in Asian skin. Lasers Surg Med 2005;36:92–97.

106. Nahm WK, Su TT, Rotunda AM, et al. Objective changes in brow position, superior palpebral crease, peak angle of the eyebrow, and jowl surface area after volumetric radiofrequency treatments to half of the face. Dermatol Surg 2004;30:922–928.

107. Fritz M, Counters JT, Zelickson BDE. Radiofrequency treatment for middle and lower face laxity. Arch Facial Plast Surg 2004;6:370–373.

108. Doshi SN, Alster TS. Combination radiofrequency and diode laser for treatment of facial rhytides and skin laxity. J Cosmet Laser Ther 2005;7:11–15.

109. Sadick NS, Alexiades-Armenakas M, Bitter P Jr, et al. Enhanced full-face skin rejuvenation using synchronous intense pulsed optical and conducted bipolar radiofrequency energy (ELOS): introducing selective radiophotothermolysis. J Drugs Dermatol 2005;4:181–186.

110. Manstein D, Herron S, Sink RK, et al. Fractional photothermolysis: a new concept for cutaneous remodeling using microscopic patterns of thermal injury. Lasers Surg Med 2004;34:426–438.

111. Wanner M, Tanzi EL, Alster TS. Fractional photothermolysis: treatment of facial and nonfacial cutaneous photodamage with a 1,550-nm erbium-doped fiber laser. Dermatol Surg 2007;33(1):23–28.

112. Alster TS, Tanzi EL, Lazarus M. The use of fractional laser photothermolysis for the treatment of atrophic scars. Dermatol Surg 2007;33(3):295–299.

14
Complications of Dermabrasion and Chemical Peeling Procedures

Chris Harmon and Betty Davis

Complications can occur with resurfacing procedures even with proper technique and appropriate patient selection. Physicians performing these techniques have an obligation to know the risks and benefits of the procedure as well as how to treat any side effect or complications that may arise. It is also important that patients receiving these procedures understand the risks and are willing to accept a complication if one does occur.

Preoperative Consultation

Informed Consent

To obtain informed consent, the risks, benefits, and alternatives of the procedure must be presented to the patient, who then acknowledges comprehension of this information and signs a consent verifying that they understand. Pictures of patients treated in the past, their postoperative course, and any side effects or complications that occurred can help the patient to understand the extensiveness of the procedure and what to expect in the postoperative period.

Education and Compliance

It is important to reinforce the extensiveness of any procedure, the timeline of healing, and obligations for postoperative wound care. Patients must have the capacity to complete postoperative care and attend postoperative appointments. An unreliable patient is at risk for complications. Proper wound care is needed after resurfacing techniques to reduce risk of infection and aid in healing. Patients will need to be able to follow a soaking and moisturizing regimen as well as be compliant taking their oral medications. Strict sun avoidance is critical for a period of 2 to 3 months following surgery. For some patients, these restrictions are more easily followed during the fall and winter months.

Photographs

Preoperative photographs should be standardized. Typically, a frontal view of the entire face, side views taken at 90° and 45° from each side, as well as close-up photographs of any defects or scars should provide a complete photographic record.

Realistic Expectations

The most important aspect of preoperative consultation is determining the patient's specific motivation for resurfacing and establishing realistic outcome expectations. Handing the patient a mirror and asking them to provide a list of what they would like to change in their appearance in order of importance is an excellent way that the patient can convey their desires to the physician in their own words. The patient must understand the ultimate goal for any resurfacing treatment should be an improvement rather than a complete eradication of the given defect being treated.

Patient Evaluation

The preoperative consultation should include a complete history specifically addressing herpes infections, impetigo, previous isotretinoin therapy, keloid or hypertrophic scarring, koebnerizing conditions, immunosuppression, bleeding disorders, and the skin type of the patient. Herpes infection prophylaxis is recommended for all patients, regardless of whether there is a previous history of herpetic episodes. A typical prophylactic regimen would be valacyclovir 500 mg taken twice daily for 10 to 14 days, beginning the day before the resurfacing procedure is performed. Because the herpes virus requires viable epidermal cells to establish infection, the patient is at greatest risk for a herpetic outbreak 7 to 10 days after surgery. Patients with a strong predisposition towards herpetic outbreaks, as well as breakthrough infections, should be treated with a higher dose of antiviral medication, such as that used to treat herpes zoster (e.g., famciclovir 500 mg taken 3 times daily for 7 days or valacyclovir 1 g taken 3 times daily for 7 days).

A history of impetigo warrants a nasal swab bacterial culture. These patients may be *Staphylococcus* carriers and should receive prophylactic antibiotics. However, typically, prophylactic antibiotics are not necessary for dermabrasive or chemical resurfacing procedures.

Isotretinoin therapy taken 6 to 12 months before resurfacing procedures has been found to cause an increased incidence of hypertrophic scarring and keloid formation. Consequently, resurfacing procedures should be preformed no sooner than 6 to 12 months after completing isotretinoin.[1-3]

Preoperative consultation should include a meticulous physical examination looking at the patient's skin type, any tendency towards hypertrophic or keloid scarring, the presence of facial telangiectasias, and the variation of pigmentation between cosmetic units of the face. If any asymmetries or dyspigmentation are noted, this should be discussed with the patient and documented. Smoking can lead to slower wound healing; consequently smoking cessation should be discussed. General skin care should also be reviewed with the patient so that the skin can be in its best possible condition before the procedure is performed as well as after the procedure has been completed. We recommend using a topical retinoid every day until 2 days prior to the procedure. Tretinoin used preoperatively has been shown to accelerate healing after trichloracetic acid chemical peels.[4]

Before surgery, laboratory studies should include a hepatitis panel, human immunodeficiency virus (HIV) antibody screening with informed consent, and a nasal swab for those with a history of impetigo.

Understanding Normal Postprocedure Findings

Dermabrasion

To understand potential complications, one must first understand and be able to recognize normal postprocedure findings. After the dermabrasive procedure, skin appears pink and pinpoint bleeding occurs; the papillary dermis is visible immediately after resurfacing (Fig. 14-1).[5] A compress with 1% lidocaine with epinephrine-soaked gauze applied for 5 to 10 minutes will decrease stinging and increase hemostasis. Afterwards, semipermeable dressings can be applied. Such semipermeable dressings are applied with telfa backing, gauze, paper tape, and Surgilast® net dressing. The use of these dressings for 3 to 5 days significantly decreases the time required for reepithelialization.[6,7] Kenalog (40 mg) intramuscularly

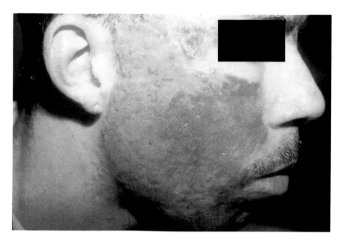

FIGURE 14-1. Three days following dermabrasion. Pinpoint bleeding produces a coagulum over the denuded surface and reepithelialization is partially complete.

will help reduce swelling around the eyes and throughout the face. A tapering oral prednisone dose pack can be substituted for the Kenalog.

By 3 to 5 days the epidermis is typically 30% to 50% reepithelialized.[5] An open technique of wound care can then be done using 0.25% vinegar soaks and Vaseline or Aquaphor for another 5 days until all oozing and crusting has ceased. Reepithelialization is usually complete within 7 to 10 days, at which time make-up application can be resumed. Concealing make-ups, especially those with green bases, are the most effective in camouflaging postoperative erythema. Bright redness fades to pink within 1 to 2 weeks. The pinkness may persist for 2 to 3 months. The texture of the skin should be smooth without any thickening.[5] Retinoic acid and hydroquinone creams can be started 3 to 4 weeks after surgery.[8] Alternating their usage every second or third day initially will decrease irritation. The most important postoperative precaution is strict sun avoidance during the 2 to 3 months of postoperative erythema. Intradermal postoperative swelling continues to improve for 3 months. As this swelling resolves 3 months after resurfacing, deep wrinkles and scars may appear to have returned. However, collagen remodeling continues for another 3 to 6 months. The remodeling phase of wound healing allows fibroblasts to lay down new collagen fibers, thereby filling in scars and rhytids.[5] Anticipating this 3-month lull during patient counseling sessions will be an encouragement to patients and will help avoid postoperative discouragement.

Medium and Deep Chemical Peels

The possibility of side effects and complications occurring after a peeling procedure are directly related to the depth of the peel. Superficial chemical peeling destroys the epidermis and invokes little inflammation. Further

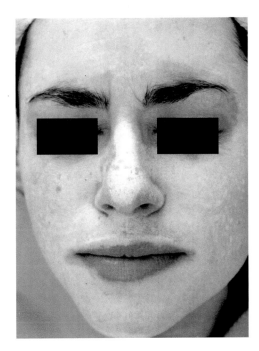

FIGURE 14-2. Medium-depth chemical peel with level III frosting.

destruction of the epidermis and induction of inflammation within the papillary dermis constitutes a medium-depth peel. When further inflammatory response in the deeper reticular dermis induces new collagen production and ground substances, a deep chemical peel is achieved.

Trichloracetic acid (TCA) is the gold standard in quantitating chemical peel strength and depth. The use of high concentrations of TCA has fallen out of favor due to its unreliability and higher incidence of pigmentary dyschromia, textural skin changes, and scarring. To reduce these risks, combination peels have been devised that produce medium-depth injury with a much lower risk of side effects. The combination peels include the following: solid CO_2 freezing followed by TCA,[9,10] Jessner's solution followed by 35% TCA,[11] and 80% glycolic acid followed by 35% TCA.[12]

Frosting of the skin is evident and serves as an end point during the peeling procedure. Level I frosting is erythema with a stringy or blotchy whitening of the skin, seen with light chemical peels. Level II frosting is defined as white-coated frosting with erythema showing through. A level III frosting, which is associated with penetration through the papillary dermis, is a solid white enamel frosting with little or no background of erythema (Fig. 14-2).[13] Most medium-depth peels use a level II frosting, especially over eyelids and areas of sensitive skin. Level III frosting can occur with multiple applications of solution in medium-depth peels or in deep chemical peels. Those areas with a greater tendency to scar, such as the

zygomatic arch, the bony prominences of the jawline, and chin, should only receive up to a level II frosting. The white frosting indicates keratocoagulation or protein denaturation of keratin, at which point the reaction is complete.

Postoperatively, edema, erythema, and desquamation are expected. As with dermabrasive procedures, intramuscular or oral steroids will lessen the erythema and edema. Soaking the peeled area and applying an emollient are necessary until desquamation is complete. Some physicians prefer to use a closed method of wound care for the first 2 to 3 days. The erythema intensifies as desquamation becomes complete within 1 week to 10 days. At the end of 1 week, the bright red color has begun to fade to pink and has the appearance of a sunburn. This redness can be covered by cosmetics and will fade within the next few weeks, typically 4 to 8 weeks for medium-depth peeling and 12 weeks for deep peeling are reasonable resolution times.[14] Patients with rosacea, atopy, or sensitive skin have a tendency to have slower fading of erythema. New collagen formation can occur for the next 3 to 4 months.

Complications

The complications of dermabrasive and chemical peeling procedures are similar (Table 14-1). A test spot can be performed before a full-face procedure is done. This may provide useful information about wound healing and the skin's response to resurfacing. However, a test spot is no guarantee that the rest of the face will react in the same manner.[15,16]

Pigmentary Changes

The most common complication following resurfacing procedures is pigmentary alteration. Typically, postoperative hyperpigmentation is transient, occurring 4 to 6 weeks following surgery (Fig. 14-3). This most commonly occurs on the malar prominence and upper cheeks. Strict sun avoidance and the use of typical hydroquinones will

TABLE 14-1. Complications.

Hyperpigmentation/hypopigmentation
Scars
Delayed wound healing
Infection
Allergic contact dermatitis
Pruritus
Textural skin changes
Acne/milia
Systemic reactions with phenol peeling
    Cardiac arrhythmias
    Laryngeal edema, hoarseness, tachypnea

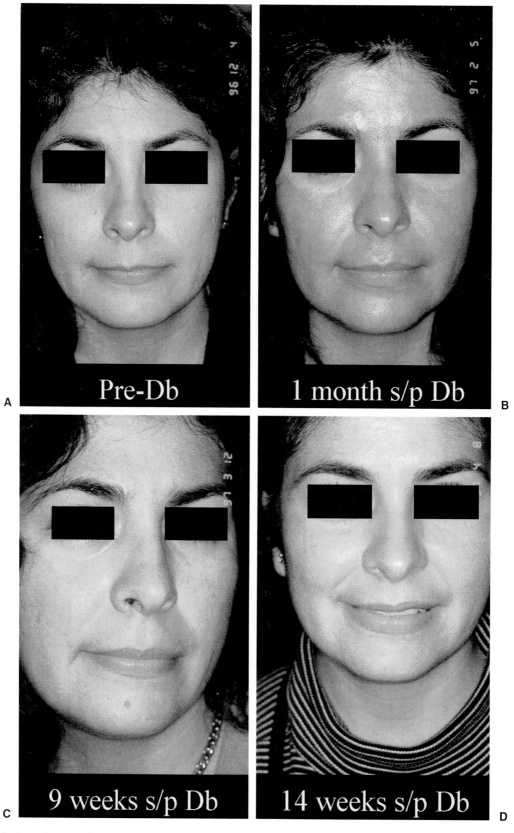

FIGURE 14-3. Patient with type 3 skin shows hyperpigmentation over the malar prominences 1 month following dermabrasion. The discoloration resolves after 6 to 8 weeks of topical retinoic acid and hydroquinone. (A) Preoperative photograph of a patient with type 3 skin. (B) One month after dermabrasion with hyperpigmentation over the malar prominences. (C) Nine weeks after dermabrasion. (D) Fourteen weeks after dermabrasion with resolution of discoloration after 6 to 8 weeks of topical retinoic acid and hydroquinone.

reduce this risk tremendously. The darkened areas, which will subside with treatment over 6 to 8 weeks, are more common in female patients taking estrogen.[11] Hypopigmentation, on the other hand, is usually a more permanent change and occurs after 10% to 20% of resurfacing procedures (Fig. 14-4). It is more common in medium skin tones, Fitzpatrick types III and IV, and tends to occur 12 to 18 months after surgery.[15,17-19] The excimer laser has shown some promising results with regards to the treatment of hypopigmentation following skin resurfacing. Raulin and colleagues noted repigmentation which was stable for 16 months in a patient treated with perioral leukoderma following CO_2 laser skin resurfacing after treatment with the excimer laser.[20,21]

The removal of lentigines and freckles in patients with Fitzpatrick skin types I and II will also produce lines of demarcation along the treatment and nontreatment zone. Feathering into the edges of adjacent cosmetic units will decrease the stark demarcation that can occur between treated and nontreated skin. When a peeling procedure is performed, feathering can be done by using a lower strength peeling agent on the neck and blending the stronger agent into the hairline. Treating the earlobes to a level I or II frost will also help to decrease the demarcation. Dermabrading to the submandibular area is warranted so that the transition zone between abraded and nonabraded skin is hidden beneath the mandible.

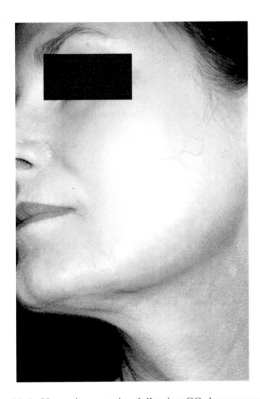

FIGURE 14-4. Hypopigmentation following CO_2 laser resurfacing.

When using Baker's phenol as a peeling agent, a small amount of pigment loss is an expected result and not a complication of the procedure. Phenol produces hypopigmentation by impairing melanin synthesis from melanocytes.[15] The porcelain or alabaster white color after peeling is most likely to occur in Fitzpatrick type I skin or in patients with only mild photodamage. Hypopigmentation is proportional to the amount of phenol applied to the skin and the subsequent depth of injury.

Scarring

It is unclear why scars develop in some patients; however risk factors for scarring after a resurfacing procedure are multifactorial and include a hereditary predisposition, the wound depth, and presence of a postprocedure infection. Previous chemical, laser, or abrasive resurfacing and isotretinoin use are also risk factors[1-3,22,23] (Fig. 14-5). With the advent of combination medium-depth peels, the risk of scarring using the lower strength TCA is less than 1%.[9,10,12] The incidence of scarring with the traditional Baker's phenol formula in a series of over 1000 patients peeled by Baker and Gordon is less than 1%, although the incidence of scarring may increase with deviations to the protocol.[15]

In general, a period of 1 to 3 months is recommended between a surgical facelifting procedure or blepharoplasty and a resurfacing procedure to aid in prevention of complications such as skin sloughing and ectropion. Extensive undermining, incisions, and the stress on tissue with repositioning can compromise blood flow so that an additional injury to the skin, such as a resurfacing procedure, cannot be tolerated and can lead to tissue necrosis, poor healing, or scarring.

Typically, a 6- to 12-month period of time is recommended to pass before a resurfacing procedure is performed on someone who has taken a course of isotretinoin due to the potential for slow healing with increased risk of hypertrophic scars or keloids. In a study done by Cruz and colleagues in which the effects of isotretinoin on the growth of keloid and embryonal human skin fibroblasts in vitro were studied, it was shown that isotretinoin significantly inhibited the growth of the fibroblasts.[24] Another study done by Hein and colleagues showed a decrease in syntheses of noncollagenous proteins and a decrease in production of both type I and type III collagen when retinoids were added to fibroblast cultures in vitro.[25] These inhibitory factors on fibroblasts may contribute to the increased tendency for scars to develop when a resurfacing procedure is done within 6 to 12 months following oral retinoid therapy.

Persisting erythema heralds the onset of a scar. Early scar recognition and aggressive management are essential in preventing permanent long-term sequelae. Topical steroid creams are useful in scar management only during

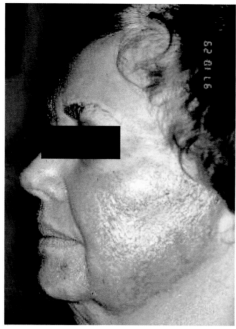
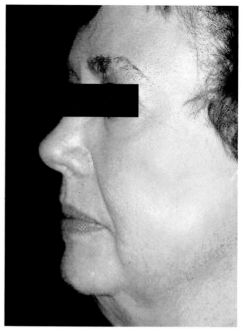

A   **B**

FIGURE 14-5. (A) Hypertrophic scarring following ablative resurfacing begins as hyperemia and progresses to indurated plaques. (B) Treatment with intralesional steroids and the pulsed dye laser can arrest this process and prevent permanent scars.

the initial phase of hyperemia. Once any papular quality or induration develops, intralesional steroids are more effective. The scar should be injected every 2 to 3 weeks. In addition, Cordran tape can be applied to the scar 4 to 5 nights a week. Telangiectasias may result from the aggressive use of steroids. However, steroid-induced telangiectasias may be treated with the KTP vascular laser. Pulsed dye lasers are helpful in treating the persisting erythema and induration of some scars. Aggressive management of hypertrophic scars will prevent hypopigmentation and contracture if begun early.

An idiosyncratic phenomenon of delayed wound healing has been noted after resurfacing procedures.[26–28] These patients give no indication during or prior to the procedure that they will have aberrant reepithialization. Friable, stellate, nonindurated, tender erosions with serous granulation tissue are present after reepithelialization should be complete. These areas can resemble infection and should be cultured and treated as such but will not respond to antibiotics. These lesions may heal with hypopigmented flat scars. Diligent wound care and topical or injected steroid preparations may be necessary. Studies have shown that a wound taking longer than 3 weeks to heal will have a 78% risk of scarring.[15]

Infection

A high index of suspicion for infection should occur with the onset of any pain or epidermal erosions and should be cultured and treated with zoster doses of antiviral medication, a broad spectrum antibiotic with excellent coverage of Gram-positive organisms and *Pseudomonas*, and anticandidal coverage (Fig. 14-6). Vinegar water soaks consisting of ¼% acetic acid should be continued 3 to 4 times daily followed by an ointment or cream.[29]

Because the herpes virus requires viable epidermal cells to establish infection, the patient is at greatest risk for herpetic outbreak 7 to 10 days after surgery. Toxic shock syndrome has been reported to occur after Baker's phenol peels.[30,31]

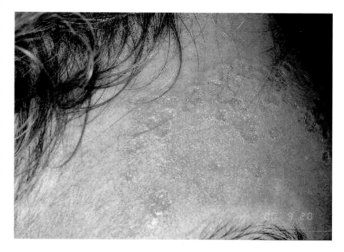

FIGURE 14-6. Secondary herpetic infections appear as punched-out ulcerations arising in reepithelialized areas.

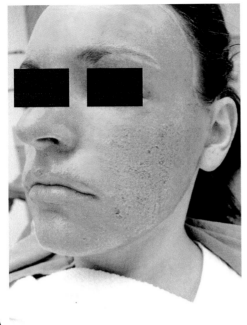
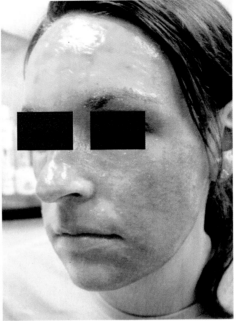

FIGURE 14-7. Three days following dermabrasion, this patient experienced increased pain with dressing changes and systemic symptoms consistent with toxic shock syndrome. Surgically treated areas showed no signs of infection and blood cultures did not reveal sepsis. Twenty-four hours after IV fluids and IV vancomycin, her symptoms resolved and the resurfaced areas healed without difficulty. (A) Postoperative day 3. (B) Postoperative day 5.

The authors encountered a healthy patient who was treated with a full-face CO$_2$ laser followed by dermabrasion performed over the bilateral cheeks for treatment of acne scars. She tolerated this procedure well and a Vigilon dressing was placed and changed daily. On day 3 postoperatively, the patient noted nausea, vomiting, general malaise, and fever and chills with a maximal temperature of 103.3°F. She experienced a marked increase of pain with dressing changes, which she had difficulty tolerating. There was no wound exudate or malodor and the skin appeared equivalent to a routine 3-day postoperative resurfacing procedure. The patient was hospitalized, given IV fluids and IV vancomycin. Valtrex was continued at zoster doses. Antistreptolysin O (ASO) titers, blood culture, and rapid viral culture for influenza A and B were obtained and remained negative. Wound culture revealed moderate growth of *Staphylococcus aureus*. The patient's untoward symptoms resolved in 24 hours and she was discharged from the hospital with no sequelae. Reepithelialization was complete in 7 days. The differential diagnosis included toxic shock syndrome, hemophilus influenza, and a culture-negative sepsis (Fig. 14-7).

Allergic Contact Dermatitis/Pruritus

Pruritus, a normal symptom of wound healing, can also signal an allergic contact dermatitis, especially when seen with an increase in erythema and small vesicles or pus-

tules. Oral antihistamines can be used to alleviate the normal pruritus of healing and if allergic contact dermatitis to a topical medicine (e.g., neosporin or polysporin) is present, a short course of topical corticosteroids can be used on the affected area in addition to antihistamines. Neosporin and polysporin can be substituted with Vaseline or Bactroban ointment.

Textural Changes

The appearance of enlarged pores, which may occur after any resurfacing procedure, tends to be temporary with chemical peeling without regard to peel depth. However, enlarged or wide-mouthed pores may be a permanent finding after dermabrasion.

Other textural changes include a blunted appearance of appendages in the skin usually in areas of hypopigmentation, with or without atrophy (Fig. 14-8). Telangiectasias, which typically remain unchanged after a peeling procedure, may become more apparent to the patient who has been pink for several weeks after the procedure. Dermabrasion decreases the number of telangiectasias by destroying blood vessels in the papillary dermis.

Acne/Milia

Milia can appear as part of the healing process and can be extracted by manual abrasion or by nicking the skin

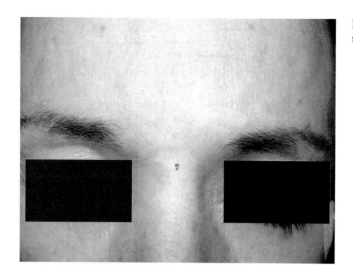

FIGURE 14-8. Prominent dilated pores produce a peau d'orange textural surface change in some patients.

with an #11 blade and extracting the cyst. If milia are beginning to form, switching from an ointment to a cream or lotion will also decrease their occurrence.

Acne flares, which can occur in many patients and may persist for 6 to 12 weeks, can be treated as any other acne outbreak. Usually these flares are temporary and will not produce new acne scars. In fact, after the postoperative flares, acne activity appears to subside over the long term.

Complications Occurring Exclusively from Deep Phenol Peels

Phenol is the only peeling agent that can cause systemic toxicity. The extent of cutaneous absorption depends more upon the total area of skin exposed to the chemical rather than concentration. Cardiac arrhythmias have been associated with full-face peeling. Typically tachycardia is first noted, followed by premature ventricular contractions, bigeminy, paroxysmal atrial tachycardia, and ventricular tachycardia. Diuresis with intravenous fluids promotes metabolism, excretion of phenol, and reduces arrhythmias. Cardiac abnormalities are reduced by waiting several minutes between applications of each cosmetic unit.[32–35] Laryngeal edema, hoarseness, and tachypnea developed within 24 hours of phenol peeling in 3 of 234 women. Each were smokers and their symptoms resolved within 48 hours with warm mist inhalation.[15,36]

Inherent Errors during the Procedure

When a peeling procedure is performed, special care should be taken around the periorbital area. While the peel is applied, a cotton swab is held at the medial and lateral canthi to absorb tears that may form, thus preventing the peeling agent from being wicked back into the eye. Peeling the periorbital area as the last cosmetic unit allows wet saline gauze to be applied quickly to help with the patient's discomfort. Also, when applying the solution, the authors gently advance a cotton swab with a counterclockwise motion in order to decrease potential exposure of the eye to the peeling solution. A syringe of saline should be immediately available if the peeling solution should enter the eye. Thirty-five percent TCA is not caustic enough to cause major corneal abrasions, but a burning sensation will be felt by the patient (Table 14-2).[15]

If phenol is spilled on skin, propylene glycol or glycerol should be used as a wash. If phenol is inadvertently placed in the eye, mineral oil can be used as a wash.

Manual dermabrasion performed with wet or dry sandpaper can produce a permanent or semipermanent carbon tattoo, which can be treated with bleaching agents and laser surgery. Carbon tattoos, like any other tattoo, can be difficult to remove. The wire brush is the most aggressive dermabrading head. Care must be taken when using a wire brush to not penetrate through the dermis. Particular attention to free skin edges such as the lip and nose must be made so that the brush does not grab and pull the tissue near these areas.

TABLE 14-2. Resurfacing tips.

When applying a peeling agent, hold cotton swabs at the medial and lateral canthi.
When applying a peeling agent to the lower lid, rotate the cotton tip away from the eye while advancing the cotton tip upward.
When using a wire brush, care must be taken due to its aggressive nature.

Conclusion

A complete understanding of normal postprocedure findings is key to recognition of complications if they may arise. Early recognition, treatment, and close monitoring with photographic documentation of postoperative complications can reduce long-term sequelae. By properly educating and selecting patients, one can alleviate many postoperative concerns and questions, build a better rapport with the patient, and help with the understanding of realistic expectations.

References

1. Katz BE, MacFarlane DE. Atypical facial scarring after isotretinoin therapy in a patient with previous dermabrasion. J Am Acad Dermatol 1994;30:852–853.
2. Rubenstein R, Roenigk HH Jr, Stegman SJ, Hanke CW. Atypical keloids after dermabrasion in patients taking isotretinoin. J Am Acad Dermatol 1986;15:280–285.
3. Moy RL, Moy LS, Bennett RB, et al. Systemic isotretinoin: effects on dermal wound healing in a rabbit ear model in vivo. J Dermatol Surg Oncol 1990;16:1142–1146.
4. Hevia O, Nemeth AJ, Taylor JR. Tretinoin accelerates healing after trichloroacetic acid chemical peel. Arch Dermatol 1991;127:678–682.
5. Harmon CB. How does skin respond to abrasive resurfacing. In: Colemen W, Lawrence N, eds. Skin resurfacing. Baltimore: Williams & Wilkins; 1998:89–96.
6. Collawn SS. Occlusion following laser resurfacing promotes reepithelialization and wound healing. Plast Reconstr Surg 2000;105:2180–2189.
7. Pinski JB. Dressings for dermabrasion: occlusive dressings and wound healing. Cutis 1986;37:471.
8. Mandy SH. Tretinoin in the preoperative and postoperative management of dermabrasion. J Am Acad Dermatol 1986;15:878–879.
9. Brody HJ. Variations and comparisons in medium depth chemical peeling. J Dermatol Surg Oncol 1989;25:953–936.
10. Brody HJ. Chemical peeling and resurfacing. St. Louis: Mosby; 1997:109–110.
11. Monheit GD. The Jessner's + TCA peel: a medium depth chemical peel. J Dermatol Surg Oncol 1989;15:945–950.
12. Coleman WP, Futrell JM. The glycolic and trichloroacetic acid peel. J Dermatol Surg Oncol 1994;20:76–80.
13. Rubin M. Manual of chemical peels. Philadelphia: Lippincott; 1995:120–121.
14. Monheit, GD. Medium-depth chemical peels. Dermatol Clin 2001;19:413–425.
15. Brody, HJ. Complications of chemical resurfacing. Dermatol Clin 2001;19:427–437.
16. Swinehart JM. Test spots in dermabrasion and chemical peeling. J Dermatol Surg Oncol 1990;16:557–563.
17. Ship AG, Weiss PR. Pigmentation after dermabrasion: an avoidable complication. Plast Reconstr Surg 1985;75:528–532.
18. Harmon CB. Dermabrasion. Dermatol Clin 2001;19:439–442.
19. Harmon CB. Dermabrasion. eMedicine. Available at: www.emedicine.com/derm/topic744.htm. Accessed August 16, 2007.
20. Raulin C, Greve B, Warncke Sh, Gundogan C. Excimer laser. Treatment of iatrogenic hypopigmentation following skin resurfacing. Hautarzt 2004;55:746–748.
21. Friedman PM, Geronemus RG. Use of the 308-nm excimer laser for postresurfacing leukoderma. Arch Dermatol 2001; 137:824–825.
22. Brackup AB. Combined cervicofacial rhytidectomy and laser skin resurfacing. Ophthal Plast Reconstr Surg 2002; 18:24–39.
23. Park GC, Wiseman JB, Hayes DK. The evaluation of rhytidectomy flap healing after CO2 laser resurfacing in a pig model. Otolaryngol Head Neck Surg 2001;125:590–592.
24. Cruz NI, Korchin L. Inhibition of human keloid fibroblast growth by isotretinoin and triamcinolone acetonide in vitro. Ann Plast Surg 1994;33:401–405.
25. Hein R, Mensing H, Muller PK, Braun-Falco O, Krieg T. Effect of vitamin A and its derivatives on collagen production and chemtactic response of fibroblasts. Br J Dermatol 1984;111:37–44.
26. Okan G, Nouri K, Trent JS, Barbarulo AM, Rendon M. Delayed wound healing after laser resurfacing. Dermatol Surg 2001;27:93–95.
27. Quaedvlieg PJ, Ostertag JU, Krekels GA, Neumann HA. Delayed wound healing after three different treatments for widespread actinic keratosis on the atrophic bald scalp. Dermatol Surg 2003;29:1052–1056.
28. Svedman C, Agner T, Esmann J. Delayed healing after CO2 laser resurfacing. J Cosmet Laser Ther 2003;5:183–184.
29. Milner SM. Acetic acid to treat Pseudomonas aeruginosa in superficial wounds and burns [letter]. Lancet 1992;340:61.
30. Dmytryshyn JR. Chemical face peel complicated by toxic shock syndrome. Arch Otolaryngol 1983;109:170.
31. LoVerme WE, Drapkin MS, Courtiss GH, et al. Toxic shock syndrome after chemical face peel. Plast Reconstr Surg 1987;80:115–118.
32. Botta SA, Straith RE, Goodvin HH. Cardiac arrhythmias in phenol face peeling: a suggested protocol for prevention. Aesthetic Plast Surg 1988;12:115–117.
33. Truppman F, Ellenberry J. The major electrocardiographic changes during chemical face peeling. Plast Reconstr Surg 1979;63:44.
34. Beeson WH. The importance of cardiac monitoring in superficial and deep chemical peeling. J Dermatol Surg Oncol 1987;13:949–950.
35. Litton C, Trinidad G. Complications of chemical face peeling as evaluated by a questionnaire. Plast Reconstr Surg 1981; 67:738–744.
36. Klein DR, Little JH. Laryngeal edema as a complication of chemical peel. Plast Reconstr Surg 1983;71:419–420.

15
Complications of Liposuction

J. Barton Sterling and C. William Hanke

In just a few decades since its first published description, the complication rates from liposuction have fallen considerably. Improvement in patient safety is largely due to the advent of tumescent liposuction, defined as liposuction performed solely using tumescent local anesthesia.

Tumescent liposuction eliminates the need for general anesthesia, which carries the increased risk of deep venous thrombosis, pulmonary thromboembolism, abdominal cavity perforation, iatrogenic intravenous fluid overloading, and compartmental fluid shifts. Further, because tumescent liposuction permits the use of smaller caliber cannulas, fewer blood vessels are transected, which results in less trauma and bleeding.

This chapter will focus on preventing, recognizing, and treating complications of liposuction. The risks of liposuction under general anesthesia, the tumescent technique, preoperative patient assessment, intraoperative patient monitoring, and postoperative care will be reviewed.

Liposuction under General Anesthesia

Until the 1990s, most physicians performed liposuction under general anesthesia. Today, many nondermatologists continue to perform liposuction under general anesthesia. Multiple complications may occur if liposuction is performed under general anesthesia.[1-8] First, the unconscious patient is unable to respond to injury and alert the physician if a cannula perforates the abdominal cavity or thorax. Diagnosis is then delayed, increasing the chances of infection and morbidity.

Second, physicians tend to remove excessive amounts of fat and perform multiple concurrent procedures in addition to liposuction when general anesthesia is used. This tendency towards exceeding the limits of safety holds true for semitumescent liposuction as well, in which both local anesthesia and general anesthesia or heavy intravenous (IV) sedation are employed. Morbidity and

mortality increase when multiple procedures are performed concurrently with liposuction. Recognizing this threat to patients, the Florida State Medical Board in 2001 banned the performance of liposuction with abdominoplasty or any procedure when greater than 1000 cc of fat is removed by liposuction. Potential complications of excessive surgical procedures include blood loss, hypovolemia, hypotension, pulmonary congestion, and hypothermia.

Third, patients often receive large volumes of IV fluid when liposuction is performed under general anesthesia. The intravenous fluid is usually given to compensate for third spacing that occurs when intravascular fluid shifts into the liposuctioned space. Large volumes of intravenous fluids may lead to electrolyte imbalances and pulmonary edema. There is no third space phenomenon and no need to administer intravascular fluids with tumescent liposuction because the tumescent fluid fills the liposuctioned space.

Fourth, the risk of thrombosis and embolism increases with general anesthesia, which may induce a hypercoagulable state. Pulmonary embolism is probably the leading cause of death with liposuction performed under general anesthesia or IV sedation.[4,9] Additional causes of death with liposuction under general anesthesia include abdomen or viscus perforation, anesthesia or sedative medication, fat embolism, cardiorespiratory failure, massive infection, and hemorrhage.[4,9]

Finally, the combination of local and general anesthesia increases the risk of drug interactions. Deaths reported from "tumescent anesthesia" have in fact occurred when the tumescent technique was combined with general anesthesia.[10] To date, there have been no reported fatalities from tumescent liposuction, defined as liposuction performed solely using tumescent local anesthesia.

In 2001, the Florida Board of Medicine also enacted the strictest outpatient surgery reporting requirements in the country. During the first 19 months of reporting, liposuction was the single most common cause of outpatient incidents and deaths. In total, there were nine complications from liposuction (eight under general anesthesia and one under deep IV sedation) and three deaths from liposuction under general anesthesia. There were no injuries or deaths reported from tumescent liposuction.[11]

In addition to general anesthesia, large caliber cannulas contribute to liposuction morbidity. Prior to the advent of the tumescent technique, large caliber cannulas with diameters of 6 to 10 mm were used to suction fat. These cannulas transect fibrous septae and their associated blood vessels, often leading to significant blood loss. Prior the 1990s, liposuction under general anesthesia was a leading cause of blood transfusions in the California. Today, cannulas 2 mm and less in diameter are used in tumescent liposuction. These smaller cannulas dissect between septae, causing less vessel transection.

Ultrasonic liposuction was another historical "innovation" in liposuction that led to a number of complications. The concept behind ultrasonic liposuction was that rapid vibrations and heat would facilitate removal of fat. Unfortunately, complications of ultrasonic liposuction include thermal burns, prolonged wound healing, and overly aggressive tissue trauma. Few physicians continue to use ultrasonic liposuction today.

Tumescent Local Anesthesia Liposuction and Lidocaine Toxicity

Tumescent liposuction performed solely under local anesthesia, first described by dermatologist Jeffery Klein,[12,13] revolutionized the practice of liposuction. Patients treated with tumescent liposuction are extremely comfortable, recover in a matter of several days, and consistently obtain excellent aesthetic results. Multiple studies have documented the superior safety record of tumescent liposuction compared with liposuction using general anesthesia or IV sedation.[14–17] Because the patient is conscious, tumescent liposuction can be performed in the office setting. Outpatient tumescent liposuction is associated with a higher safety record than any other form of liposuction.[18]

Tumescent liposuction uses large volumes of dilute concentrations of lidocaine and epinephrine, usually of 0.1% lidocaine, 1:1,000,000 epinephrine, and a sodium bicarbonate buffer. This technique permits liposuction by local anesthesia without general anesthesia or IV sedation. The dilute epinephrine produces widespread, prolonged vasoconstriction in the subcutaneous fat, resulting in minimal blood loss during the procedure. In general, specialty society guidelines recommend total lidocaine doses of less than 55 mg/kg, and total fat extraction volumes of less than 5 L.[19–21] The plastic surgery guidelines recommend a lower total lidocaine dose (35 mg/kg), presumably because of the frequent use of

general anesthesia or intravenous sedation as the primary method of anesthesia in combination with the tumescent solution.

Lidocaine toxicity may be avoided if physicians stay within the guidelines for maximum lidocaine doses. Nonetheless, physicians performing tumescent liposuction must be able to recognize and treat lidocaine toxicity, which may affect many organ systems. Initially, patients may experience confusion, dizziness, blurred vision, and nausea. Later symptoms, such as tinnitus and muscle twitching, may be a prelude to seizures, unconsciousness, and coma. Respiratory depression may occur as well, causing an acidosis that can worsen lidocaine toxicity.

Cardiovascular toxicity, the most dangerous complication of lidocaine toxicity, occurs at plasma lidocaine levels much higher than those that cause central nervous system toxicity. Symptoms of cardiac toxicity include bradycardia, vasodilation, depressed myocardial contractility, and depressed cardiac electrical conduction.

Ventilation and airway maintenance are the first steps in treating lidocaine toxicity. Midazolam, a benzodiazepine, is the treatment of choice for lidocaine-induced seizures. However, benzodiazepines should not be given as prophylaxis. For seizures, midazolam is given as a 5 to 7 mg oral bolus, followed by 1 to 2 mg doses until the seizure is controlled.

Precise documentation of surgical records is necessary to prevent lidocaine toxicity. The patient's weight in kilograms, the maximum lidocaine dose in milligrams per kilogram, the total milligrams per liter of solution, and the total amount of solution given must be recorded for each patient. Liposuction of multiple body areas during the same session should be avoided to prevent both the administration of excessive amounts of lidocaine and unnecessary trauma to the patient.

Preoperative Assessment

Laboratory tests that should be performed prior to liposuction include complete blood count (CBC), prothrombin time (PT), partial thromboplastin time (PTT), hepatitis B surface antigen, comprehensive metabolic panel, and an human immunodeficiency virus (HIV) test. All patients over the age of 50 years must obtain an electrocardiogram. Patients with multiple medical problems require medical clearance from their primary care physician. Medications that may interfere with lidocaine metabolism should be discontinued, despite the fact that this premise is based on theoretical data. Medications that may interfere with lidocaine metabolism are listed in Table 15-1.

Anticoagulants, platelet inhibitors, vitamin E, and herbal supplements, which may predispose to bleeding and hematoma formation, should also be stopped

TABLE 15-1. Medications that may interfere with lidocaine metabolism.

Amiodarone
Benzodiazepines (midazolam, triazolam)
Cimetidine
Clarithromycin
Chloramphenicol
Cyclosporine
Danazol
Dexamethasone
Diltiazam
Erythromycin
Fluconazole
Itraconazole
Isoniazid
Ketoconazole
Methadone
Methylprednisolone
Metronidazole
Miconazole
Nicardipine
Nifedipine
Pentoxyfylline
Propofol
Propranolol
Quinidine
Selective serotonin uptake inhibitors (sertraline)
Tetracycline
Terfenidine
Thyroxine
Verapamil
Antiseizure medications (carbamazepine)
Valproic acid
Verapamil

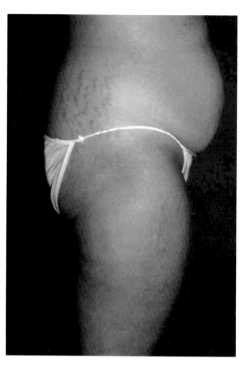

FIGURE 15-1. This 45-year-old woman has striae on the hips and abdomen. Striae are usually not improved by liposuction. (Used with permission, C. William Hanke, MD.)

preoperatively. Blood pressure, heart rate, respiratory rate, and blood oxygen levels should be monitored and recorded during the procedure.

During the preoperative assessment, patients should be screened to determine if they have realistic expectations and if they are ideal candidates for liposuction. Some patients may gain only minimal improvement with liposuction. For example, obese patients are typically poor candidates for liposuction because liposuction is intended for body contouring, not as a method of weight loss. The most appropriate candidate is in general good health, close to his or her ideal body weight, and has localized areas of fat resistant to diet and exercise. Many complications can be avoided by good patient selection.

For patients being evaluated for abdominal liposuction, the preoperative physical examination should always document the presence of a periumbilical or ventral hernia. An umbilical or periumbilical hernia may increase the risk of an accidental penetration of the peritoneal cavity during liposuction.

While the surgeon is examining the patient before surgery, superficial irregularities (e.g., waviness, rippling, and dimpling) already present in the skin should be pointed out to the patient and noted in the chart. These irregulari-

ties may not be improved by liposuction. Patients should be told that liposuction does not improve striae (Fig. 15-1) or contour in patients who suffer from diastasis recti, which requires surgical repair (Figs. 15-2, 15-3, and 15-4).

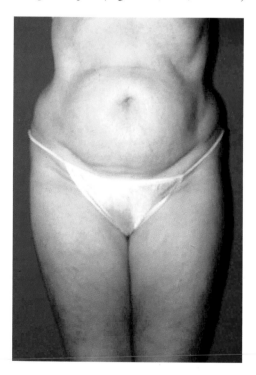

FIGURE 15-2. This 50-year-old woman has significant diastasis recti. (Used with permission, C. William Hanke, MD.)

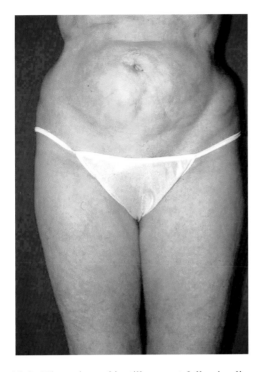

FIGURE 15-3. Diastasis recti is still present following liposuction of the upper and lower abdomen. Superficial liposuction (i.e., just under the dermis) has resulted in significant skin irregularity. (Used with permission, C. William Hanke, MD.)

Immediately before the procedure, it is important to preoperatively mark the patient in the anatomic position. Preoperative marking allows the surgeon to delineate areas that require liposuction and areas that should be avoided before the administration of large volumes of tumescent anesthesia, which can distort landmarks and potentially lead to excessive or inadequate amounts of liposuction. Focal excessive or inadequate liposuction can lead to asymmetry and contour irregularities.

Local Complications of Liposuction

The goal of liposuction is to sculpt the body and create a smooth, aesthetically pleasing contour. A moderate amount of fat on a female is aesthetically pleasing. Excess removal of fat may lead to a cadaveric or masculine appearance. It is always better to remove less fat and perform a touch-up procedure later than to remove too much fat during the initial procedure (Figs. 15-5, 15-6, and 15-7). Once an excess amount of fat is removed, all treatment options to improve the area, including autologous fat reinjection, are usually unsatisfactory.

A smooth, even appearance of the skin is also important. The lateral thighs are most prone to contour irregularities after liposuction. The use of micocannulas, multiple incision sites, deep placement of the cannula, pointing

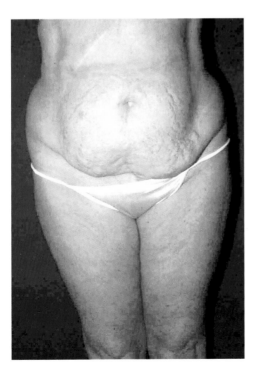

FIGURE 15-4. A 60-year-old woman has diastasis recti and striae on the abdomen. Although clothing would fit somewhat better following liposuction, the diastasis and striae would be unchanged. (Used with permission, C. William Hanke, MD.)

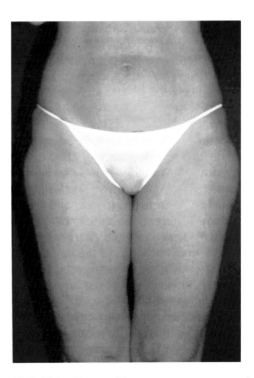

FIGURE 15-5. This 45-year-old woman was concerned about lateral thigh adiposities. (Used with permission, C. William Hanke, MD.)

a dusky blue discoloration. Later, anesthesia may replace pain, a sign that deeper nerves have been damaged. By the fourth or fifth day, skin may appear gangrenous. When suspecting necrotizing fascititis, cultures for aerobic and anaerobic bacteria should be obtained. The patient should be admitted to the intensive care unit, the affected area should immediately be surgically debrided, and appropriate antibiotics instituted. Magnetic resonance imagining may aid in delineating the extent of infection. Mortality is high even with appropriate therapy. Thus, early diagnosis is critical to survival.

Atypical mycobacterial infection should be suspected in a patient who has persistent inflammatory nodules for many months after liposuction surgery despite antibacterial treatment. The most common causative organisms are *Mycobacterium chelonei*, *M. fortuitum*, and *M. abscessus*. Lesions, which are slowly progressive and typically do not grow on routine cultures, should be biopsied and the pathologist alerted to the suspected diagnosis. Fresh tissue should also be sent for culture, smear, and antibiotic susceptibility testing. Infection may be a result of contaminated liposuction cannulas. Only steam autoclaving reliably kills atypical mycobacteria.

Conclusion

Physicians performing tumescent liposuction should be committed to maximizing patient safety. Tumescent liposuction has contributed greatly to patient safety by allowing liposuction to be performed with minimal complications and excellent results.

References

1. ASPRS Task Force on Lipoplasty. 1997 survey summary report. Arlington Heights, IL: American Society of Plastic and Reconstructive Surgeons; 1998.
2. Bruner JG, de Jong RH. Lipoplasty claims experience of U.S. insurance companies. Plast Reconstr Surg 2001;107: 1285–1291.
3. Dillerud E. Suction lipoplasty: a report on complications, undesired results, and patient satisfaction based on 3511 procedures. Plast Reconstr Surg 1991;88:239–246.
4. Grazer FM, de Jong RH. Fatal outcomes from liposuction: census survey of cosmetic surgeons. Plast Reconstr Surg 2000;105:436–446.
5. Hughes CE. Reduction of lipoplasty risks and mortality: an ASAPS survey. Aesthetic Surg J 2001;21:120–125.
6. Jackson RF, Dolsky RL. Liposuction and patient safety. Am J Cosmet Surg 1999;16:21–23.
7. Newman J, Dolsky RL. Evaluation of 5,458 cases of liposuction surgery. Am J Cosmet Surg 1984;1:25–80.
8. Teimourian B, Rogers WB. A national survey of complications associated with suction lipectomy: a comparative study. Plast Reconstr Surg 1989;84:628–631.
9. Teimourian B. Complications associated with suction lipectomy. Clin Plast Surg 1989;16:385–394.
10. Rao RB, Ely SF, Hoffman RS. Deaths related to liposuction. N Engl J Med 1999;340:1471–1475.
11. Coldiron B. Office surgical incidents: 19 months of Florida data. Dermatol Surg 2002;28:710–713.
12. Klein JA. The tumescent technique for liposuction. Am J Cosmet Surg 1987;4:263–267.
13. Klein JA. Tumescent technique for regional anesthesia permits lidocaine doses of 35 mg/kg for liposuction. J Dermatol Surg Oncol 1990;16:248–263.
14. Bernstein G, Hanke CW. Safety of liposuction: a review of 9478 cases performed by dermatologists. J Dermatol Surg Oncol 1988;14:1112–1114.
15. Coleman WP, Hanke CW, Lillis P, Bernstein G, Narins R. Does the location of the surgery or the specialty of the physician affect malpractice claims in liposuction? Dermatol Surg 1999;25:343–347.
16. Hanke CW, Bernstein G, Bullock S. Safety of tumescent liposuction in 15,336 patients. National survey results. Dermatol Surg 1995;21:459–462.
17. Hanke W, Cox SE, Kuznets N, Coleman WP. Tumescent liposuction report performance measurement initiative: national survey results. Dermatol Surg 2004;30:967–978.
18. Housman TS, Lawrence N, Mellen BG, et al. The safety of liposuction: results of a national survey. Dermatol Surg 2002;28:971–978.
19. Coleman WP, Glogau RG, Klein JK, et al. Guidelines of care for liposuction. J Am Acad Dermatol 2001;45:438–447.
20. Drake LA, Ceilley RI, Cornelison RL, et al. Guidelines of care for liposuction. Committee on Guidelines of Care. J Am Acad Dermatol 1991;24:489–494.
21. Lawrence N, Clark RE, Flynn TC, Coleman WP. American Society for Dermatologic Surgery guidelines of care for liposuction. Dermatol Surg 2000;26:265–269.
22. Ilouz YG. The fat cell "graft": a new technique to fill depressions. Plast Reconstr Surg 1986;78:122.
23. Teimourian B. Repair of soft tissue contour deficit by means of semiliquid fat graft. Plast Reconstr Surg 1986;78:123.
24. Gargon TJ, Courtiss EH. The risks of suction lipectomy: their prevention and treatment. Clin Plast Surg 1984;11: 457.
25. Courtiss EH, Mathias B. Skin sensation after suction lipectomy: a prospective study of 50 consecutive patients. Plast Reconstr Surg 1988;81:550.

16
Complications of Soft Tissue Fillers

Steven C. Bernstein

Soft tissue augmentation with filling agents (temporary, permanent, and semipermanent) has become one of the most requested interventions in facial aesthetic surgery. Fillers provide an opportunity to quickly correct certain defects that cannot be adequately treated with other modalities. The demand for fillers has created a strong incentive for industry to introduce newer and better products. Consequently, a burgeoning market has developed with multiple fillers possessing many of the attributes of the so-called ideal filler: an agent which is biocompatible, nonantigenic, noninflammatory, nontoxic, stable after injection, nonmigratory, long-lasting, natural looking and feeling, and not too expensive.

In this chapter, the reported complications associated with many of the currently available fillers will be discussed. Fillers will be categorized as temporary, permanent, or semipermanent based on their longevity in tissue. In general, complications caused by temporary fillers occur soon after the procedure, may resolve spontaneously, and usually are easy to treat. In contrast, complications caused by permanent or semipermanent fillers may appear long after the procedure and may be difficult to treat.

In addition, a review will be conducted of another group of fillers that elicit an active tissue reaction. Finally, some injectable facial implants and self-derived injectables will be discussed.

In order to objectively assess the complications associated with soft tissue fillers, it is important to differentiate complications due to injection technique (e.g., incorrect depth of injection, overcorrection, and undercorrection) from complications due to properties inherent in the individual filler. The success of soft tissue augmentation will depend on a marriage between safe, effective products and excellent delivery into the target tissue by the physician.

Temporary Fillers

Collagen-Based Products

Soft tissue augmentation with injectable fibrillar collagen began in 1976.[1] US Food and Drug Administration (FDA)

approval was obtained in 1981. Approximately 470,000 patients were treated with Zyderm or Zyplast collagen implants from 1981 through 1989.[2] Bovine collagen injections are specifically contraindicated in persons undergoing treatment with steroids or with a history of allergy to other bovine products or meat.[3] Additionally, patients with autoimmune disorders, especially collagen vascular disease, should not be treated.

There are three major types of adverse reactions to bovine collagen implants: immunologic, clinical, and histologic. Some authors have suggested that all patients will mount an immune response to collagen and it is only the severity of the response that varies. An allergy skin test is performed on all prospective patients to determine the risk of severe allergic reaction. Approximately 3% to 10% of persons tested will demonstrate a significant response to the test dose and should not be treated.[4] In addition, 1% to 2% of persons will develop or acquire allergy to bovine collagen despite initial nonreactivity of the test dose.[5] Thus, some physicians advocate double skin testing. One third of specimens from test site reactions show early, mild, normal, perivascular, periappendageal infiltrates. The other two thirds show either diffuse granulomas or pallisading foreign-body granulomas. Prolonged erythema, swelling, itching, and firmness of the injection sites may develop if allergy exists in a patient who undergoes treatment. Rare systemic complications, such as autoimmune syndromes, including inflammatory myositis, have been reported with bovine collagen.[6] Approximately 5 in 1000 patients may experience systemic reactions with flulike symptoms, paresthesias, or difficulty breathing.[7]

A localized hypersensitivity reaction, the most common adverse reaction to Zyderm, presents clinically as erythematous, frequently indurated, pruritic papules. The symptoms persist for an average of 3 to 5 months (Fig. 16-1A,B), but have been reported to occasionally last up to 24 months. During this time, patients will usually develop circulating antibodies to the bovine collagen implant.[8] Abscess formation, a serious manifestation of hypersensitivity to bovine collagen, has been reported in

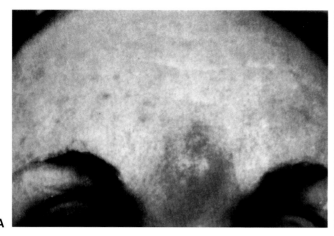
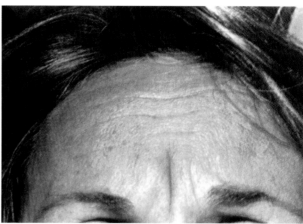

A   B

FIGURE 16-1. (A) Hypersensitivity reaction to Zyderm treatment site in the glabella. (B) Spontaneous resolution 4 months following treatment. (Reprinted from Stegman SJ, Chu S, Armstrong R, Adverse reactions to bovine collagen implants; clinical and histologic features. J Dermatol Surg Oncol, with permission from Blackwell Publishing.)

4 in 10,000 cases and typically occurs 8 to 12 weeks following treatment.[9] Treatment should be instituted by draining the abscesses with a #11 blade, a #15 blade, or a large-bore needle. Alternatively, intralesional steroid injections of triamcinolone acetonide (3–5 mg/cc) at weekly intervals can be considered. Resultant scar formation, if present, can be treated surgically by revision, dermabrasion, or laser resurfacing.

Another type of adverse reaction involves recurrent intermittent swelling of treatment sites for up to 3 years, occasionally accompanied by erythema and induration. This reaction can last from hours to weeks and can be triggered by any factor that induces peripheral vasodilatation.[10]

A different type of complication is the technique-dependent implantation of excessive volume of the filler too superficially in the dermis (Fig. 16-2). The implant will

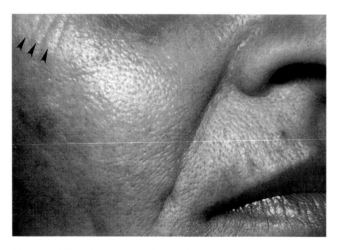

FIGURE 16-2. Linear ridges (arrows) resulting from overcorrection with Zyderm in a patient's crow's feet. (Reprinted from Stegman SJ, Chu S, Armstrong R, Adverse reactions to bovine collagen implants; clinical and histologic features. J Dermatol Surg Oncol, with permission from Blackwell Publishing.)

then be visible either as ridges in creases or wrinkles, or as opaque deposits at the base of scars. Overcorrection will resolve with time and requires no treatment.

A final category of complications are those that are mechanically induced. One example is bruising due to traumatic injection, which will cause minimal discomfort and resolve spontaneously. Localized tissue necrosis, which can develop in any patient, is very rare and completely unrelated to sensitivity to the product. It is considered to be the result of local vascular occlusion and occurs in 9 in 10,000 cases. Over 50% of cases of tissue necrosis following Zyplast occurred in the glabella, and its use is contraindicated in this area.[11] Symptoms of vascular occlusion, which include sudden pain, blanching, and transient cyanosis during or shortly after treatment, are reversible if the vessel is not completely blocked. However, there have been reports of vessel occlusion leading to partial blindness secondary to treatment of glabellar frown lines and occlusion by embolus of an ophthalmic vessel.[12] Because the majority of these events have occurred in the glabella area, only thinner fillers (e.g., Zyderm I, Cosmoderm, Fine Hylaform, and Restylane Touch) should be used in this site.[13] More viscous fillers, which usually need to be injected more deeply, may increase the risk of intra-arterial injection and tissue necrosis as a result of vascular occlusion.

If vascular compromise is suspected, injections should be discontinued immediately and the area massaged. Application of heat or nitroglycerine paste has also been reported to be effective. Good wound care should be instituted once necrosis has occurred. Fortunately, the reaction is limited to treatment sites. Pigmented or atrophic scars may form which, if necessary, can be addressed by surgical revision at a later date.

In March 2003, the FDA approved Cosmoplast and Cosmoderm, which are collagen-based injectables derived from human foreskin fibroblast culture. These two fillers are approved for filling facial wrinkles, acne scars, and soft tissue contour deficiencies. To date, the safety profile appears favorable. If injection is too deep the product will be absorbed too quickly; if placed too superficially, visible white bumps may form. Because this product is of human derivation, less allergenicity and immunogenicity are predicted than with bovine collagen implants. Swelling, bruising, and erythema with injection have been reported to be minimal with both products.

The final category of collagen-based products can be referred to as autologous. One such product is Autologen, which is an injectable collagen fibril material processed from the patient's skin. The disadvantages of this product include the limited supply, the length of time for preparation, and painful injections. However, there is virtually no risk of infection or allergy.

Dermologen is a suspension of human collagen processed from cadavers. Injections are difficult to perform and are reported to be painful. Moody and Sengelmann described a self-limited foreign-body reaction to a Dermologen test site.[14]

Cymetra, or micronized Alloderm, is another autologous collagen product. Clinical studies in 200 patients report no allergic or immunologic reactions. Adverse reactions include bruising, redness, swelling, and wrinkling of the skin. All of these complications resolve spontaneously and are reported to occur at a rate of 2.1%.[13]

Preserved particulate fascia lata, known as Fascian, is used for the correction acne scars and soft tissue augmentation. In one study, 81 patients with 109 injections were followed. No infections, allergic reactions or acute rejections were reported.[15]

Hyaluronic Acid Fillers

Hyaluronic acid fillers were first produced by extracting the substance from rooster combs. This product was introduced for cosmetic use in Europe in 1995 and commercialized under the name Hylaform™ (Genzyme; distributed by Innamed, FDA approved in 2004). In 1996, Q-Med formulated a non–animal stabilized hyaluronic acid from bacterial fermentation which was marketed under the same Restylane™ (Q-Med; distributed by Q-Med in Europe and Medicis in the USA, FDA approved in 2003). More recently, many other hyaluronic acid fillers have been introduced such as Juvederm, Hydrafill, and Rofilan, which are commercially available in Europe and Canada, but as of September 2005 are not yet FDA approved. A final group of products known as acrylic hydrogels (Dermadeep; Dermalive Lab. Biocrystal France, not FDA approved) are formulated with hyaluronic acid for injection purposes but strictly speaking are not hyaluronic acid fillers because they have a different mechanism of action and a different side-effect profile. Consequently, these fillers will be reviewed in a subsequent section.

Hyaluronic acids, along with collagen, are the two most widely used temporary fillers. Overall, resorbable hyaluronic acid fillers have an excellent safety profile and complications are usually rare and short-lived. However, complications can occur and should be recognized in order to institute timely treatment.

Reactions that may occur during injection or immediately thereafter include erythema, bleeding points at injection sites, edema, punctiform ecchymoses, mild pain, pruritus, or sensitivity at the injection sites. These reactions tend to resolve spontaneously within 1 to 36 hours. Erythema is so common and transient that it is largely considered a "normal" occurrence. Many of the other immediate side effects can be diminished or avoided with good injection technique. Bruising and bleeding complications can be minimized by discontinuation of anticoagulants, aspirin, anti-inflammatory drugs, vitamin E, and alcohol prior to treatment. Others have suggested the use of firm pressure, homeopathic arnica tablets, Vitamin K cream, or ice packs immediately following injections.[16]

When performing lip injections, edema and some sensitivity almost inevitably occur immediately and over the ensuing 12 hours, and can persist for 2 to 7 days. This is entirely a mechanical phenomenon and does not signify a delayed hypersensitivity reaction.[17]

The lips may also be at risk for bacterial and viral infection. Patients with recurrent dental, sinus, and herpetic infections may develop complications when these infections occur close to treated areas with any filler. Molecular mimicry, when bacterial and viral infections act synergistically to produce inflammatory and granulomatous complications, may explain this phenomenon.[17]

Faulty technique, either from inappropriate product selection or injecting the product too superficially or not smoothly, can lead to the formation papules, palpable visible nodules, or fine white lines the length of the wrinkle (Figs. 16-3 and 16-4). The best way to resolve this

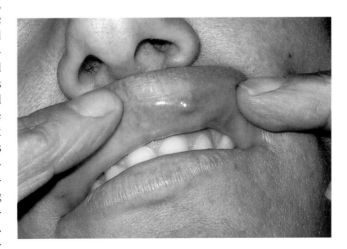

FIGURE 16-3. Lip nodule resulting from hyaluronic acid.

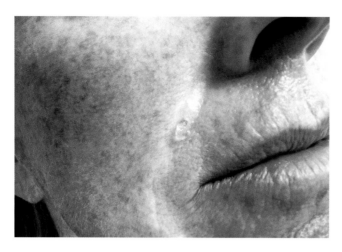

FIGURE 16-4. Superficial injection of hyaluronic acid leading to lumpy whitish or bluish lines the length of the wrinkle or fold. The hyaluronic acid can be extruded following large-bore needle puncture as seen above.

complication is with immediate vigorous massage, which can be repeated by the patient over the course of the few days following treatment.

Hyperpigmentation and a blue-gray linear pigmentation have also been described following hyaluronic acid injection. Typically this will resolve spontaneously in 3 to 6 months, but can last a year or more. Unfortunately, this complication is difficult to avoid because its mechanism is not fully understood. The bluish discoloration may be secondary to hemosiderin from vascular injury and/or visual distortion from light refraction to the filler through the skin.[18] Cosmetic products can be used to cover the affected area. Alternately, a puncture with a large-bore needle can be performed and the product expressed with bimanual pressure. This technique can often lead to bruising so the patient must be warned beforehand.

Complications that may occur within the first few days following injection include abscesses at the injection sites, hematomas, or facial asymmetry. Abscesses are usually due to inadequate disinfectant skin preparation. Bacterial infections associated with cosmetic procedures are usually caused by common skin pathogens such as *Streptococcus* and *Staphylococcus*. Patients usually present with one or more fluctuant, erythematous nodules which can be treated with appropriate antibiotics. However, the presence of a nodule more than 2 weeks after the initial procedure suggests the possibility of an atypical mycobacterial infection.[19]

Hematomas can form in the hours following treatment, especially in the perioral area, and can last up to a week. The best way to avoid hematoma formation is with immediate pressure and application of cold packs. Facial asymmetry, which may occur in the lip area following block anesthesia, will typically resolve spontaneously.

Complications that may occur 1 to 4 weeks following treatment include intense or indurated erythema, erythematous or violaceous granulomas, indurated folliculitis, and pseudocyst or nodule formation.[20] These reactions, which are similar to what can be observed with collagen based products,[21] may occur following the first or any subsequent session.

Treatment must be instituted as quickly as possible. Oral corticosteroid therapy for 14 days should be prescribed as soon as induration and erythema appear. Full recovery can be expected, but often requires months. Incision and drainage can be performed as well, but with a greater risk of scarring.

Delayed-type hypersensitivity reactions can be subdivided into two groups: immunologic and nonimmunologic. Immunologic delayed-type hypersensitivity reactions are mediated by antigen-specific T lymphocytes and can be caused by a foreign protein in the filler. The nonimmunologic reaction is a foreign-body–type granuloma which is mediated by cytokines produced by phagocytic cells and may occur after the implantation of any type of foreign material. These reactions are nonspecific and result in the formation of a granulomatous infiltrate around the implant composed of epithelioid cells surrounded by lymphocytes. The epithelioid cells often fuse to form multinucleated giant cells. Histologic examination is required to diagnose foreign-body granulomatous inflammation. Patients with granulomas usually present with nonfluctuant subcutaneous nodules in contrast to the fluctuant, erythematous nodules that may be a sign of infectious lesions. The rate of granuloma formation varies between 0.01% and 0.1% with collagen,[22] hyaluronic acid,[23] and particulate injectables.[24] Granulomas occur less frequently after injection of resorbable implants compared to more permanent products.

Permanent Fillers

Artefill/Artecoll

Artecoll, a permanent soft tissue filler which has been available worldwide (except in the United States) since 1994, has been used to treat over 200,000 patients. It is composed of a suspension of 25% polymethyl methacrylate (PMMA) microspheres, 30 to 40 microns in diameter, in 75% of 3.5% atelocollagen solution. The theory is that the atelocollagen serves as a vehicle that will be rapidly degraded and ultimately be replaced by natural collagen, which will encapsulate the PMMA microspheres. This product will bear the name Artefill when approved in the United States.

Due to its high viscosity and its permanence in tissue, Artecoll is subject to several complications, many of which are dependent on the injector. Artecoll's high viscosity can occasionally lead to an uneven distribution of the material in the form of a "string of pearls." This complication can be corrected by further injection to fill in the gaps between the "pearls." As a general rule, the more permanent a filler is, the more deeply it should be injected. However, if injected too deeply, Artecoll may be lost to the subcutaneous tissue and offer no clinical effect. If injected too superficially, it may cause streaks of erythema which can be thick and pruritic. Over aggressive injection may lead to irregularity or lumpiness. Hypertrophic scarring, granuloma formation, and necrosis of the tissue can also occur as a result of superficial injection. Topical corticosteroids or intralesional corticosteroid injections should be instituted initially. If unresponsive, nodules may be surgically excised.

Injector-independent complications of Artecoll include allergic reactions and delayed granuloma formation. The PMMA microspheres are considered to be nonallergenic. However, the collagen component of the mixture can lead either to systemic allergic reactions or delayed type IV allergic reactions as earlier described for collagen injections. The atelocollagen in Artecoll is considered to possess less allergenic potential than Zyderm or Zyplast and in Europe allergy testing is not recommended prior to treatment. In Canada, however, an allergy test solely to the collagen component is performed 4 weeks prior to treatment.

True granuloma formation has been reported to be a rare event, occuring in less than 0.01% of patients.[25] Granulomas typically occur 6 to 24 months following Artecoll treatment. However, the author has witnessed the formation of granulomas 4 or more years following treatment (Fig. 16-5). The etiology of these foreign-body granulomas remains unclear. Several hypotheses have been espoused, including injection that is too superficial, intramuscular injection, or injection into tissue that is

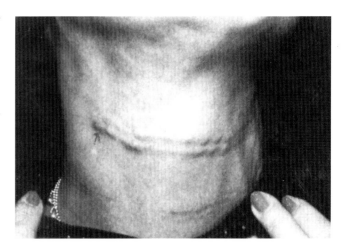

FIGURE 16-6. Artecoll-induced granulomas in the flaccid skin of the neck. (Reprinted from Kim KJ, Lee HW, Lee MW, et al., Artecoll granulomas: a rare adverse reaction induced by microimplant in the treatment of neck wrinkles. Dermatol Surg, with permission from Blackwell Publishing.)

active thereby extruding the PMMA particles, resulting in a foreign-body–type reaction.[25]

It has been suggested that areas subject to movement, such as the lips, be splinted with tape for 72 hours to prevent early migration of the implant secondary to facial animation. Hoffman and colleagues described nodule formation subsequent to lip injection that was unresponsive to intralesional corticosteroid injection and required surgical excision.[17] Kim and colleagues reported Artecoll-induced granulomas of the neck (Fig. 16-6), and concluded that implants into flaccid neck skin should be performed cautiously or be avoided altogether as these implants can be easily be inadvertently placed too shallow or too deep.[26] Most granulomas appear to improve with corticosteroid injection. Lemperle suggests a 1:1 mixture of lidocaine and triamcinolone acetonide up to 20 mg/mL injected directly into the nodule.[25] Surgical extirpation is, however, sometimes necessary if the nodules are not responsive to the intralesional corticosteroid treatment.

There is one case of blindness and total opthalmoplegia after Artecoll injection, presumably due to direct injection into a peripheral branch of the ophthalmic artery.[27]

Silicone

No chapter on soft tissue fillers would be complete without a discussion of silicone. There are presently two FDA-approved silicone products: Adatosil 5000 and Silikon 1000. Both products are medical-grade silicone and are approved for intraocular injection. Cosmetic use is currently off-label. The microdroplet technique of injection should be used as overcorrection can lead to visible lines and bumps. The permanence of the product

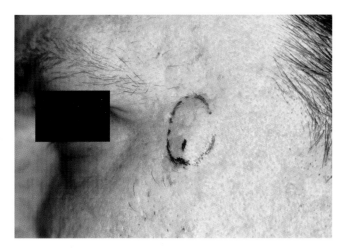

FIGURE 16-5. Foreign-body–type granuloma occurring 4 years following treatment.

probably permits more time for severe foreign-body reactions to occur. Silicone injections offer long-term benefit but may cause long-term complications. The most dreaded complications are granuloma formation and migration of the product to distant sites.

The incidence of granuloma formation with these newer formulations is not yet known. Silicone is unique in that complications may be delayed and patients may present with granulomatous reactions years after the initial procedure.[20] Among injectable products, silicone also has the unique ability to migrate to distant locations from the original treatment site. If inflammatory granulomas occur, oral or intralesional steroids are the treatments of choice. Senet and colleagues also reported successful treatment of two cases of cutaneous silicone granulomas with minocycline, likely related to the antibiotic's anti-inflammatory properties.[28] Surgery can be performed if the steroid injections are ineffective. The microdroplet technique may reduce nodular granulomas and migration of the injected product.

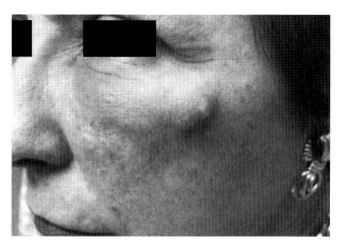

FIGURE 16-8. Large erythematous nodule at the site of previous polyacrylamide gel (PAAG) injection. (Reprinted from Amin SP, Marmur ES, Goldberg DJ, et al., Complications from injectable polyacrylamide, a new biodegradable soft tissue filler, Dermatol Surg, with permission from Blackwell Publishing.)

Semipermanent Fillers

A new filler, which has been commercially available in Europe since 1998 and in Canada since 2002, combines 60% hyaluronic acid and 40% acrylic hydrogel. This product, marketed as Dermalive or Dermadeep, is not yet FDA approved for use in the United States. The hyaluronic acid component is resorbed in the months following injection and the acrylic hydrogel particles are integrated into the tissue.

The only reported immediate side effects are pain following injection, redness, and edema.[18] These transitory, undesirable effects dissipate spontaneously within days. Of greater concern is a reaction to the foreign material, which may occur several months after the injection. One

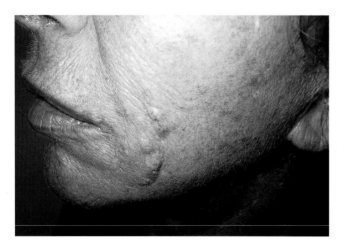

FIGURE 16-7. Granulomatous tissue response secondary to superficial placement of Dermalive.

group reported a complication rate of 1.2 per 1000,[18] with the development of nodules, swelling, and, sometimes, redness at the point of injection. The authors suggested that 60% of the complications were technique dependent, either due to superficial injection or overfill, or injecting in areas where other fillers (e.g., PMMA or silicone) were already present (Fig. 16-7). In 2004, Sidwell and colleagues reported a marked local reaction to the injection of Dermalive in the nasolabial fold developing 4 months postoperatively with histological confirmation of a granulomatous response.[29] Treatment with intralesional corticosteroid injections was usually curative, although occasionally surgical excision of the nodule was necessary.

Polyacrylamide gels (PAAGs) are another new generation, long-acting fillers that have been commercially marketed in Europe since 2001 under the name Aquamid, which is currently unavailable in North America. Aquamid contains 2.5% PAAGs and 97.5% water. There is no pretest required for use and the product is said to be biocompatible, nontoxic, and nonmigratory. Slight redness or a temporary swelling was found directly after injection with duration of less than 36 hours.[30] The symptoms typically disappear without treatment. To date, only 28 cases of postinjection infections have occurred in over 20,000 treatments. The infections are normally diagnosed 8 to 10 days following treatment.

In 2004, Amin and colleagues reported a patient who presented with an 8-week history of erythematous facial nodules at the site of previous PAAG injection (Fig. 16-8).[31] The nodules were entirely unresponsive to two courses of oral antibiotics, but resolved completely with intralesional corticosteroid injections and did not recur.

Poly-L-lactic acid has been in use for cosmetic treatments in Europe since 1999. In Europe it is known as Nu-Fill, while in North America it has the name Sculptra. In the United States, it is FDA approved only for volume restoration in human immunodeficiency virus (HIV) patients with lipoatrophy, with cosmetic use being an off-label indication. Poly-L-lactic acid is a synthetic biocompatible, biodegradable, absorbable polymer and allergy testing is not required. The implant itself is broken down and it is the collagen produced in response to the implant that leads to a progressive correction. The cosmetic effect of Sculptra is estimated to last 18 to 24 months.

Side effects of Sculptra include erythema, tenderness, and edema which usually resolve within 2 to 3 days. Valantin and colleagues, in a study of severe HIV lipoatrophy, reported 44% of patients noticed palpable but nonvisible and nonbothersome subdermal papules, spontaneously resolving in 12% by week 96.[32] In a study by Burgess and colleagues, only 2 of 61 patients developed clinically palpable and occasionally visible intradermal papules in the infraorbital region as a result of the placement of 4cc of reconstituted Sculptra.[33] There were no incidents of swelling, edema, allergic reactions, infection, erythema, or clinical evidence of adverse reaction.

Radiance is a new injectable filler compound composed of calcium hydroxylapatite (Caha) microspheres suspended in an aqueous gel carrier. The Caha microspheres stimulate innate collagen formation. The cosmetic effect is said to last for 2 to 5 years. This product is FDA approved for use in the United States for injection laryngoplasty and correction of craniofacial defects. Cosmetic use is presently off-label.

Short-term side effects of Radiance include bruising, pain, and erythema at the injection sites. If the product is injected too superficially (e.g., intradermally), white nodules may appear in the mid- or superficial dermis.[34] These nodules should be punctured with a needle and expressed immediately. Overfilling must be avoided as the material may be long-lasting. The Radiance implant is much denser than normal soft tissue and therefore remains palpable for 2 to 3 months. It should not, however, be visible. An occasional patient may experience erythema for 4 to 8 weeks, which can be camouflaged with makeup. Visible or palpable nodules can be treated with intralesional steroids at a concentration of 40mg/cc. Superficial nodules which are not expressed immediately may become very firm and subsequently require surgical excision.

Fillers permit instant patient gratification with minimum down time and risk. They have an important niche in the treatment of a variety of cosmetic problems that cannot be effectively improved by other modalities. However, the introduction of a foreign substance into the dermis or subcutaneous tissue may lead to complications. In general, the less durable products cause transient complications, whereas more permanent fillers may lead to permanent complications. Patients should be informed thoroughly of potential adverse reactions, particularly with permanent fillers, so that they may weigh the consequences of their decision to undergo an elective cosmetic procedure.

Finally, it is important to distinguish between adverse reactions due to the nature of the filler, or those that arise from poor technique. To minimize the former, stringent testing with long-term follow-up should be required for each product. The prevalence of injector-dependent complications underscores the need for proper training of physicians and the utilization of these procedures in appropriate medical facilities instead.

References

1. Knapp TE, Kaplan EN, Daniels JR, et al. Injectable collagen for soft tissue augmentation. Plast Reconstr Surg 1997; 60:398–405.
2. Hanke CW. Injectable collagen implants. Arch Dermatol 1983;119:533–534.
3. Burgess CP, Goode RC. Injectable collagen. Facial Plastic Surg 1992;8:176–182.
4. Pollack SV. Silicone, Fibrel, and collagen implantation for facial lines and wrinkles. J Dermatol Surg Oncol 1990;16: 957–961.
5. DeLustra F, Smith ST, Sundsmo J, et al. Reaction to injectable collagen in human subjects. J Dermatol Surg Oncol 1998;14(Suppl 1):49.
6. Hochberg MC. Cosmetic surgical procedures and connective tissue disease: the Cleopatra syndrome revisited. Ann Intern Med 1993;118:981–982.
7. Douglas RS, Dansoff I, Cook T, et al. Collagen fillers in facial aesthetic surgery. Facial Plast Surg 2004;2:117–123.
8. Ellingsworth CR, Delustra F, Brennan SE, et al. The human immune response to reconstructive bovine collagen. J Immunol 1986;136:877–887.
9. Hanke CW, Hingley R, Jolivette DM, et al. Abscess formation and local necrosis after treatment with Zyderm or Zyplast collagen implant. J Am Acad Dermatol 1991;25: 319–326.
10. Stegman SJ, Chu S, Armstrong R. Adverse reactions to bovine collagen implants; clinical and histologic features. J Dermatol Surg Oncol 1998;14:39–48.
11. Hanke CW. Adverse reactions to bovine collagen. In: Klein A, ed. Augmentation in clinical practice: procedures and techniques. New York: Marcel Dekker; 1998:145.
12. McGrew F, Wilson RS, Havener W, et al. Sudden blindness secondary to injections of common drugs in the head and neck, part 1: clinical experiences. Otolaryngology 1978;86: 147–151.
13. Klein AW. Collagen substances. Facial Plast Surg Clin North Am 2001;9:205–218.
14. Moody BR, Sengelmann RD. Self limited adverse reaction to human derived collagen injectible product. Dermatol Surg 2000;26:936–938.
15. Cheng JT, Perkins SW, Hamilton AM, et al. Collagen and injectable fillers. Otolaryngol Clin North Am 2002;35:73–85.

16. Ascher B, Cerceau M, Baspeyras M, et al. Soft tissue filling with hyaluronic acid. Ann de Chir Plast Esth 2004;49:465–485.
17. Hoffman C, Schuller-Petrovic, Soyer HP, Kerl H. Adverse reactions after cosmetic lip augmentation with permanent biologically inert implant materials. J Am Acad Dermatol 1999;40:100–102.
18. Bergeret-Galley B, Latouche X, Illouz Y-G. The value of a new filler material in corrective and cosmetic surgery: Dermalive and Dermadeep. Aesthetic Plast Surg 2001;25:249–255.
19. Toy BR, Frank PJ. Outbreak of *Mycobacterium abscessus* infection after soft tissue augmentation. Dermatol Surg 2003;29:971–973.
20. Bergeret-Galley C. Comparison of absorbable soft-tissue fillers. J Aesthetic Surg 2004;24:33–46.
21. Barr R. Stegman SJ. Delayed skin test reaction to injectable collagen implant (Zyderm). The histopathologic comparative study. J Am Acad Dermatol 1984;10:652–658.
22. Lemperle G, Morheim V, Charrier U. Human histology and persistence of various injectable filler substances for soft tissue augmentation. Aesthetic Plast Surg 2003;27:354–366.
23. Lowe NJ, Maxwell CA, Lowe P, et al. Hyaluronic acid skin fillers: adverse reactions and skin testing. J Am Acad Dermatol 2001;45:930–933.
24. Cotran RS, Kumar V, Robins SL. Pathologic basis of disease. 5th ed. Philadelphia: Saunders; 1994.
25. Lemperle G, Romano JJ, Busso M. Soft tissue augmentation with Artecoll: 10-year history, indications, techniques, and complications. Dermatol Surg 2003;29:573–587.
26. Kim KJ, Lee HW, Lee MW, et al. Artecoll granulomas: a rare adverse reaction induced by microimplant in the treatment of neck wrinkles. Dermatol Surg 2004;30:545–547.
27. Silva MT, Curi AL. Blindness and total opthalmoplagia after aesthetic polymethyl methacrylate injection. Arq Neuropsiquiatr 2004;62:873–874.
28. Senet P, Backclez H, Ollivaud L. Minocycline for the treatment of cutaneous silicone granulomas. Br J Dermatol 1999;140:985–987.
29. Sidwell RV, Dhillon AP, Butler PE, et al. Localized granulamotous reaction to a semi-permanent hyaluronic acid and acrylic hydrogel cosmetic filler. Clin Exp Dermatology 2004;29:630–637.
30. De Cassia Novaes W, Berg A. Experiences with a new non-biodegradable hydrogel (Aquamid): a pilot study. Aesthetic Plast Surg 2003;27:376–380.
31. Amin SP, Marmur ES, Goldberg DJ, et al. Complications from injectable polyacrylamide, a new biodegradable soft tissue filler. Dermatol Surg 2004;30:1507–1509.
32. Valantin MA, Aubron-Olivier C, Ghosn J, et al. Polylactic acid implants (New-Fill) to correct facial lipoatrophy in HIV-infected patients: results of the open label study VEGA. AIDS 2003;17:2471–2477.
33. Burgess CM, Quiroga RA. Assessment of the safety and efficacy of poly-L-Lactic acid for the treatment of HIV-associated facial lipoatrophy. J Am Acad Dermatol 2005;52:232–239.
34. Flaherty P. Radiance. Facial Plast Surg 2004;20:165–169.

17
Complications of Botulinum Toxin

Deborshi Roy and Neil S. Sadick

Botulinum toxin is a powerful medication that has been used to treat various conditions for over two decades. In the last few years, there has been an explosion in the use of this drug for cosmetic purposes. While millions have benefited from the therapeutic effects of botulinum toxin, many have experienced complications. For the neophyte clinician or casual user, technique-related complications are more common. For those who treat a large number of patients or use large volumes, systemic reactions can become more common. In this chapter, the mechanisms, treatment options, and strategies for avoiding the complications of botulinum toxin therapy will be discussed.

Mechanism of Therapeutic Action

The mechanism of action of botulinum toxin (BTX) has been well established.[1-4] Protein interactions of BTX at the neuromuscular junction prevent the release of acetylcholine. There are eight known antigenically distinct types of BTX (A–G). The most widely used and studied is botulinum toxin type A (BTX-A). This protein irreversibly binds and cleaves the SNAP-25 protein. There are currently two available preparations of BTX-A on the market, Botox (Allergan, Irvine, CA) and Dysport (Ipsen, United Kingdom). A third preparation, Reloxin (Inamed Corp., Santa Barbara, CA), will be available in the near future. Botulinum toxin type B (BTX-B), which binds to synaptobrevin, is available commercially as Myobloc (Solstice Neurosciences, San Francisco, CA). The temporary nature of therapeutic BTX therapy is a result of axonal sprouting at the motor endplate of the neuromuscular junction and the development of extrajunctional acetylcholine receptors,[5] which both occur over the course of several months after BTX therapy.

Mechanisms of Complications

BTX-A is currently approved by the US Food and Drug Administration (FDA) for the treatment of blepharospasm, strabismus, and glabellar frown lines. BTX-B is cleared for the treatment of cervical dystonia. Both are used off-label by physicians for the treatment of other facial and cervical rhytides, migraine headaches, and hyperhidrosis.

Complications can be divided into two main categories: local and systemic. Diffusion of toxin and misplacement of toxin are the two most common mechanisms of local complications. Asymmetry is the most common local complication and can be easily corrected. When adjacent muscles are inadvertently paralyzed, aesthetic as well as functional problems may arise. Brow ptosis can result from the treatment of horizontal forehead rhytides, especially with laterally placed injections. Upper eyelid ptosis and diplopia can result from periorbital injections, most often when injecting near the orbital rim. Oral incompetence can occur when injecting the perioral musculature. Problems with neck movements and dysphagia can occur with treatment of cervical dystonia or neck rhytides.

The exact mechanism of systemic complications is unknown. It has been postulated that a small amount of BTX can be absorbed into the bloodstream or undergo retrograde axonal transport and exert an effect on distant sites. There have been anecdotal descriptions as well as published reports problems ranging from headache, facial pain, transient numbness, flulike syndrome, nausea, dysphagia, diarrhea, muscle weakness, and skin rashes to exacerbation of neuromuscular diseases. Studies have also demonstrated subclinical electromyographic (EMG) changes in muscles distant from the injection sites.[6-10]

Immunoresistance is another entity that has been clinically described in select patients (especially those injected with large doses in multiple treatment sessions). Again, the exact mechanism is unknown, but it is postulated that immune complexes present in the BTX preparations induce blocking antibodies.[11] Other immune-mediated reactions are possible, especially those involving hypersensitivity to BTX.

Avoiding Complications

The technique-related complications are the easiest to avoid. Thorough knowledge of detailed facial anatomy coupled with skilled injection should yield a low complication rate for most practitioners. Facial muscle assessment is critical. Only by assessing the muscle activity prior to injection can one decide upon the appropriate dose of BTX to use (Fig. 17-1). Also, careful inspection of the dynamic and static effects of the facial muscles is

a key part of understanding which areas of the face to treat for the desired effect. After the assessment, patient preparation is the next step. The authors utilize a clean technique and prepare the skin with alcohol swabs prior to injection. Patient positioning varies from physician to physician — most prefer to keep the patient partially reclined. The best position is one where both the patient and the physician are most comfortable. The authors do not use topical or local anesthetics. Instead, a Zimmer Cryo 5 skin-cooling device (Zimmer Medizinsystems, Irvine, CA) is utilized (Fig. 17-2).

Pain can also be minimized by using a preservative-containing saline solution to dilute the BTX-A. Although the package insert recommends using preservative-free saline solution, Sarifakioglu has found that using the preservative-containing saline significantly reduces pain without compromising efficacy.[12]

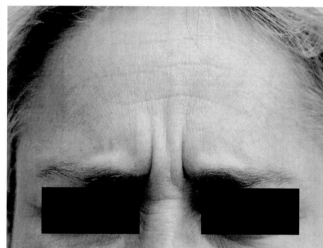

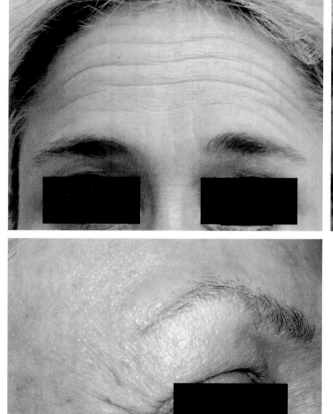

FIGURE 17-1. Assessment of the (A) frontalis muscle, (B) corrugator muscle group, and (C) lateral orbicularis oculi muscle.

The next step, which is crucial, is the actual injection. Precise injection of highly concentrated, small volumes is the best way to avoid widespread diffusion of the toxin into adjacent musculature. A bimanual technique, with digital pressure on bony landmarks, is another maneuver that decreases the chances of diffusion of BTX to unintended areas. Brow ptosis, which is more common in the elderly and in men, often occurs because of overtreatment of the frontalis muscle. Brow ptosis can be avoided by reducing the amount of BTX injected into the frontalis muscle, especially the lateral segments. Caution should be used in treating the forehead in individuals over 60 years of age, who depend on the frontalis muscle to elevate the brow in order to improve peripheral vision.

Eyelid ptosis, which typically presents 2 to 10 days after BTX treatment, can be avoided by injecting at least 1 cm above the orbital rim. When injecting the glabella, placing the fingertip of the noninjecting hand along the orbital rim minimizes diffusion of BTX beyond that bony landmark. Fortunately, eyelid ptosis usually does not last as long as the full effect of BTX at the intended treatment site, an average of 2 to 3 weeks.

Diplopia may occur after the injection of crow's feet (lateral orbital rhytides) when BTX is injected inside the orbital margin. When injecting crow's feet, the physician should inject no closer to the eye than 1 cm lateral to the orbital rim or 1.5 cm lateral to the lateral canthus. Digital pressure with the noninjecting hand along the orbital rim also minimizes the chances of this complication.

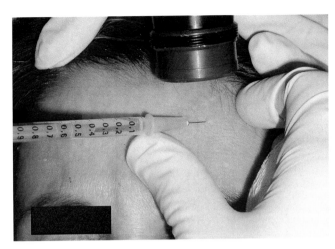

FIGURE 17-3. Bimanual injection technique with simultaneous skin cooling.

Lateral orbital lines often extend medially and inferiorly onto the lower eyelid–malar complex. When treating this area with BTX, it is important not to inject too inferiorly or deeply because the zygomaticus major and minor muscles can be weakened, causing an asymmetric smile or lateral mouth drooping.

The risk of bruising can be minimized by avoiding forehead and periorbital vessels, utilizing a small (30-gauge) needle, and applying gentle digital pressure after each injection (Fig. 17-3). Ice packs are applied after the injections to minimize local tissue edema and ecchymosis. Patients are only instructed to avoid massaging the area for 48 hours. All other light activity is permitted. In the past, most physicians counseled their patients not to lie down flat for several hours following BTX injections. There is no scientific evidence that body position effects diffusion of the toxin. We no longer recommend this to our patients.

Absolute contraindications to BTX treatments include pregnancy, neuromuscular disorders (e.g., myasthenia gravis), current facial infection, and known hypersensitivity reactions. Relative contraindications include an upper respiratory infection or other viral syndrome and recent surgery or trauma in the area to be injected. Caution must be exercised with patients who have experienced severe side effects or idiosyncratic reactions with previous injections. A detailed history followed by extensive discussion with the patient is important to alleviate the anxiety associated with an adverse outcome.

Treating Complications

It is very important to recognize a complication once it arises. Only after a proper diagnosis can the complication be treated. Often, treatment may only consist of assuring

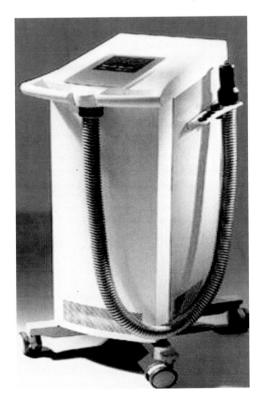

FIGURE 17-2. The Zimmer Cryo 5 skin cooling device.

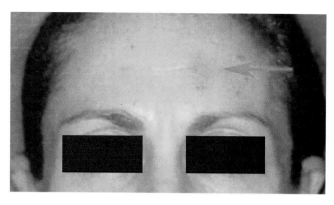

FIGURE 17-4. A patient with ecchymosis of the forehead following BTX treatment (*arrow*).

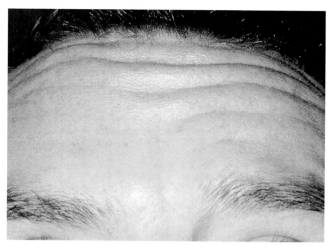

FIGURE 17-5. Forehead asymmetry after BTX treatment.

the patient that the complication is temporary and will soon resolve. In other instances, there are specific methods of treating individual complications.

1. **Ecchymosis** (Fig. 17-4). This problem may be avoided by carefully screening patients. Patients who bruise easily and those on prescription anticoagulant therapy that cannot be interrupted should be prepared for bruising. Bruising can be minimized but usually not eliminated with application of ice packs before and after the injections. Cessation of daily aspirin, nonsteroidal anti-inflammatory drug therapy, or Vitamin E supplements 2 weeks prior to any injections will also minimize the risks of bruising. Some practitioners use topical vitamin K and Arnica Montana preparations directly on areas with eccyhmoses.

2. **Asymmetry**. All preexisting asymmetries should be documented and pointed out to the patient prior to any injections. Most patients are not aware of asymmetry before treatment, but may notice them after injections. It is important to discuss these asymmetries and whether or not they will be improved or exacerbated with the BTX injections. Asymmetry after BTX treatment is most commonly seen in the forehead, but may occur anywhere (Fig. 17-5). When asymmetry occurs, it may be remedied with well-placed touch-up injections.

3. **Brow ptosis** (Fig. 17-6). It is crucial to recognize brow ptosis and make the patient aware of this condition if it exists prior to injection. If brow ptosis occurs after BTX treatment of lateral forehead rhytides, it is treated with injection of BTX into the depressor muscles of the brow (i.e., the depressor supercilii medially and the lateral portion of the orbicularis oculi laterally). By paralyzing the brow depressors, there is a slight lifting of the brow due to the unopposed resting tone of the brow elevator (frontalis).

4. **Cocked eyebrow** (Fig. 17-7). Cocked eyebrow occurs due to the paralysis of the brow depressors with unopposed resting tone of the brow elevators laterally, usually

secondary to the injections being placed in too medial a location. Small injections weakening the lateral frontalis muscle can diminish this problem. One must avoid too much weakening of the lateral frontalis, which will lead to ptosis of the lateral brow.

5. **Upper eyelid ptosis**. Again, if this condition exists prior to injection, it should be documented and pointed out to the patient (Fig. 17-8). If lid ptosis occurs after periorbital BTX treatment, it is due to diffusion of the toxin into the levator palpebrae superioris muscle. This condition is temporary, and usually does not last as long as the overall effect of the BTX in the intentionally treated areas. Apraclonidine 0.5% ophthalmic drops can be used up to three times a day to temporarily relieve the ptosis through its sympathomimetic action.

6. **Decreased tearing**. This condition, which often occurs secondary to injection of the pretarsal portion of the orbicularis oculi, is treated with ocular lubricants.

7. **Muscle twitching**. If this condition exists prior to treatment, it can often be relieved after the injections. If twitching starts after an injection, it is best to wait 7 to 10

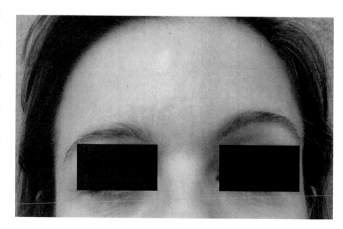

FIGURE 17-6. Brow ptosis after BTX treatment.

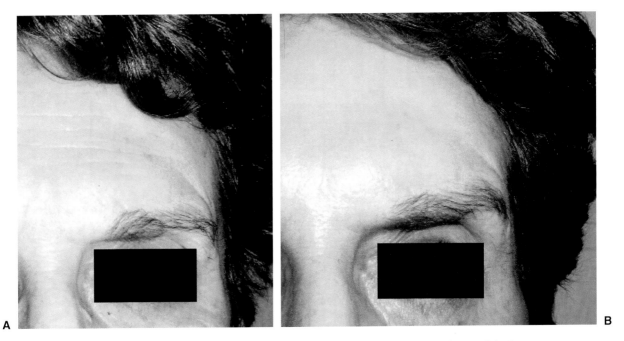

FIGURE 17-7. Patient (A) before and (B) after BTX treatment; note the shape of the brow.

days to see if it subsides. If not, then adding a few more units of BTX to the area usually resolves the issue.

8. **Infection**. Preventing an infection with clean technique is best. If an infection does occur, it should be treated promptly with the appropriate antibiotics. Viral infections, especially around the mouth, should be treated with antiviral therapy.

Systemic reactions such as malaise and flulike symptoms should be treated with supportive care. Gastrointestinal symptoms can be treated individually as they occur. Headache, depending on the type and the severity, should be treated with the advice of a physician. Usually the above symptoms last for 24 to 48 hours following BTX therapy. However, there are case reports of intractable headache

following BTX treatment lasting for several weeks.[13] Unusual reactions should be thoroughly investigated, and consultations with specialists may be necessary.

Conclusion

Complications will become more prevalent as the cosmetic use of Botulinum toxin increases. The majority of patients undergo BTX treatments without complications. With proper patient education, meticulous technique, and careful follow-up, complications rates can be minimized and patients can be treated effectively. Botulinum toxin plays a vital role in facial rejuvenation and should be utilized carefully, respectfully, and safely.

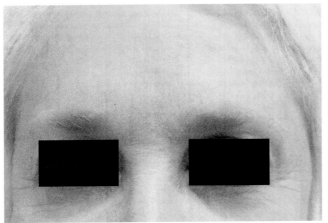
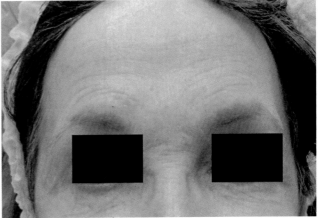

FIGURE 17-8. (A, B) Two patients with upper eyelid ptosis after BTX treatment.

References

1. Sakaguchi G. Clostridium botulinum toxins. Pharmacol Ther 1983;19:165–194.
2. Carruthers JDA, Carruthers JA. Treatment of glabellar frown lines with C botulinum-A exotoxin. J Dermatol Surg Oncol 1992;18:17–21.
3. Keen M, Blitzer A, Aviv J, et al. Botulinum toxin A therapy for hyperkinetic facial lines: results of a double-blind, placebo-controlled study. Plast Reconstr Surg 1994;94:94–99.
4. Hambleton P. Clostridium botulinum toxins: a general review of involvement in disease, structure, mode of action and preparation for clinical use. J Neurol 1992;239:16–20.
5. de Paiva A, Meunier FA, et al. Functional repair of motor endplates after botulinum neurotoxin type A poisoning: biphasic switch of synaptic activity between nerve sprouts and their parent terminals. Proc Natl Acad Sci U S A 1999;96:3200–3205.
6. Bhatia KP, et al. Generalised muscular weakness after botulinum toxin injections for dystonia: a report of three cases. J Neurol Neurosurg Psych 1999;67:90–93.
7. Lange DH, Brin MF, Warner CL, et al. Distal effects of locally injected botulinum toxin: incidences and effects. Adv Neurol 1988;50:609.
8. Tugnoli Y, Eleopra R, Quatrale R, et al. Botulism-like syndrome after BTX-A for local hyperhidrosis. Br J Dermatol 2002;147:8080.
9. Klein A. Botulinum toxin complications. Dermatol Surg 2002;29:5:549–556.
10. Goschel H, Wohlfaqrth K, Frevert J, et al. Botulinum A toxin therapy: neutralizing and non-neutralizing antibodies: therapeutic consequences . Exp Neurol 1997;147:96–102.
11. Jankovic J, Schwartz K. Response and immunoresistance to botulinum toxin injections. Neurology 1995;45:1743–1746.
12. Sarifakioglu N, Sarifakioglu E. Evaluating effects of preservative-containing saline solutions on pain perception during botulinum toxin type-a injections at different locations: a prospective, single-blinded, randomized controlled trial. Aesthetic Plast Surg 2005;29:113–115.
13. Alam M, Arndt KA, Dover JS. Severe, intractable headache after injection with botulinum. J Am Acad Dermatol 2002; 46:62–65.

18
Complications of Sclerotherapy

Girish S. Munavalli and Robert A. Weiss

Sclerotherapy is the systematic, targeted elimination of intracutaneous and subcutaneous varicose, reticular telangiectasias by the injection of a locally irritating chemical substance, called a sclerosant. Physicians practicing phlebology (the study and science of diagnosis and treatment of veins) rely heavily on the use of sclerotherapy to rid the body of diseased veins. Sclerosants work by direct mechanisms to provoke marked damage of the endothelium of the vessels and possibly transmural wall damage. Subsequently, a local thrombus is generated and, in the long term, damaged veins will be transformed into a fibrous cord, a process referred to as *sclerosis*. The purpose of sclerotherapy is not just a thrombosis of the vessel, but the definite transformation into a fibrous cord which is impossible to recanalize.[1] In essence, the endpoint of this process is functionally analogous to surgical removal of a vein.

Unlike the symptomatology associated with reflux in the larger leg veins, telangiectatic lesions more often present as a cosmetic concern and represent the most common target of sclerotherapy. The term *telangiectasias*, which are more commonly referred to as spider veins on the leg, was first used in the early 1800s to describe a superficial vessel of the skin visible to the human eye.[2] They typically measure 0.1 to 1mm in diameter and can represent either a distended arteriole or venule. Varicose veins most likely lead to the formation of telangiectasias through either associated venous hypertension with resulting angiogenesis or vascular dilation. These varicose veins may or may not be clinically evident at the time of the presentation of telangiectasias, but should trigger the systematic proximal to distal vein evaluation of the affected extremity in efforts to unmask subclinical venous disease.

Three major advances in sclerotherapy in recent years have greatly benefited physicians practicing phlebology: (1) the ability to target veins of a given size with different sclerosing agents in order to maximize treatment, (2) the development of foaming techniques to rapidly mix room air with detergent sclerosants (e.g., sodium tetradecyl sulfate and polidocanol) to create a foam which enhances the sclerosant's potency and efficacy, and (3) the advent of duplex guidance to percutaneously visualize and treat subdermal varicosities.[3]

Sclerotherapy has known contraindications with which all phlebologists should be intimately familiar (Table 18-1).[3,4] The simplest way to minimize problems is to avoid treating patients who have predisposed contraindicating factors. However, despite the best intentions, complications can and will occur with enough sclerotherapy treatments. Complications resulting from sclerotherapy can be divided into the following categories for ease of explanation: (1) frequent but temporary, (2) rare but self-limited, and (3) rare but major complications (Table 18-2).[5] The category of frequent but temporary complications makes up the largest number of adverse reactions occurring postsclerotherapy. Chief among these are post-treatment hyperpigmentation and telangiectatic matting. Fortunately, meticulous technique can reduce the incidence and severity of these problems to a very low level. This chapter will focus on the incidence of complications in sclerotherapy, review the most common complications observed, and discuss how the aforementioned advances in sclerotherapy treatment have lessened the likelihood of complications.

Frequent but Temporary Complications

Postsclerotherapy Hyperpigmentation

Postsclerotherapy pigmentation refers to persistent pigmentation (usually brown) along the course of a treated vein (Fig. 18-1). Pigmentation occurs in 10% to 30% of patients, is usually is noticed within 3 to 4 weeks after sclerotherapy, and can last from 6 to 12 months in spite of attempts at therapy.[6] Although spontaneous resolution occurs in 70% of patients at 6 months, pigmentation may persist longer than 1 year in up to 10% of patients (Fig. 18-2).[7]

TABLE 18-1. Absolute and relative contraindications for performing sclerotherapy.

Absolute contraindications	Relative contraindications
Known allergy to the sclerosant	Longstanding history of leg edema
Allergy to disulfuram (if using chromated glycerine)	Hypercoagulabilty disorder
Acute superficial or deep vein thrombosis	Diabetic late-stage complications
Local infection in the area of sclerotherapy or severe generalized infection	Allergic diathesis
Immobility/bedridden state	Thrombophilia with history of deep vein thrombosis
Advanced peripheral arterial occlusive disease	Bronchial asthma
Hyperthyroidism (in the case of sclerosants containing iodine)	Chronic renal insufficiency (if using glycerin)
Pregnancy in the first trimester and after the 36th week of gestation	Extreme needle phobia

Source: Modified from Rabe et al.[4] and Guex.[3]

The incidence of hyperpigmentation depends primarily on the size of the treated vessel, the type of sclerosing agent, and the concentration of the sclerosant. In general, the incidence of hyperpigmentation is higher when treating larger veins (greater than 1 mm) as opposed to smaller veins and venules. Additionally, there is a direct correlation between the incidence of hyperpigmentation and an increasing strength of concentration of any given sclerosing agent. However, amongst the three most commonly used agents, the incidence can vary widely.

The incidences of hyperpigmentation of various sclerosants are 10% to 30% (hypertonic saline), 11% to 30% (polidocanol), and 11% to 80% (sotradecol, sodium tetradecyl sulfate). Postsclerotherapy pigmentation can occur anywhere on the leg, but appears most commonly in vessels below the thighs, particularly around the medial and lateral knees and malleolar area. This probably is the result of a combination of factors including increased capillary fragility, increased intravascular pressure, and the difficulty of obtaining constant compression over these irregular and mobile surfaces.[8–15]

It is important to note that in certain patients lower extremity hyperpigmentation may already be present along the course of superficial varicosities and telangiectasias before any therapy is performed, especially if reflux is longstanding or stasis dermatitis has occurred. Discussion with the patient, along with careful preoperative documentation including photographs, is essential to avoid confusion during follow-up patient visits.

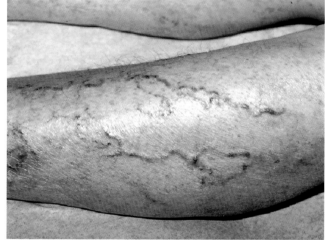

A

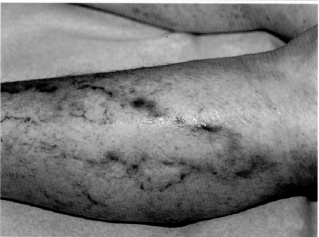

B

FIGURE 18-1. (A) Reticular and varicose veins prior to treatment. (B) Posttreatment hyperpigmentation following the use of 0.5% sodium tetradecyl sulfate for sclerotherapy.

TABLE 18-2. Categorization of sclerotherapy complications.

Frequent but temporary complications
Postsclerotherapy pigmentation (10%–30%)
Telangiectatic matting (10%–30%)
Pain with injection (hypertonic saline)
Urtication postinjection (worse with polidocanol)
Formation of intravascular microthrombus/intravascular hematoma
Bruising at injection site (especially reticular veins)

Rare but self-limited complications
Cutaneous necrosis
Superficial thrombophlebitis
Nerve damage (saphenous, sural)
Transient visual disturbances, especially in migraine patients,
Hematuria (using foam sclerotherapy and using chromated glycerin)

Rare but major complications
Arterial injection
Anaphylaxis
Deep venous thrombosis, pulmonary embolism

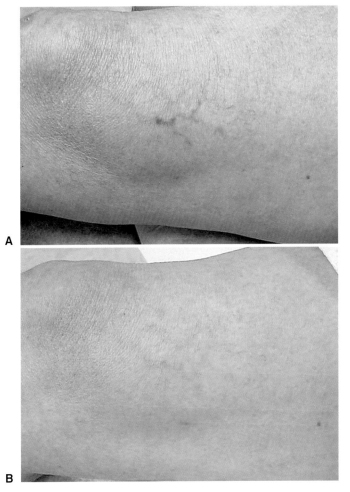

FIGURE 18-2. (A) Posttreatment hyperpigmentation following the use of 0.2% sodium tetradecyl sulfate for sclerotherapy. (B) Hyperpigmentation resolves spontaneously after 2 to 3 months following treatment.

The etiology of this pigmentation most likely occurs from a combination of postinflammatory hyperpigmentation as well as direct hemosiderin deposition.[5,6] Initially, histological examination shows hemosiderin that is present regardless of the type of sclerosing solution or baseline pigmentation of the patient.[12] Hemosiderin is an indigestible residue of hemoglobin degraded from red blood cells, which enters the dermis by extravasation after the rupture of treated vessels. Spontaneous hemosiderin pigmentation is also common in patients with chronic venous insufficiency.[20] Red cells also enter the dermal layer by erythrocyte diapedesis, which is triggered by phlebitis and other inflammatory states. Phagocytosis and digestion of red blood cells result in the deposition of hemosiderin in the form of aggregates up to $100\mu m$ in diameter that may contain iron in several forms.[21] In its most insoluble form, iron hydroxide may take years to be eliminated from the dermis.

The risk of hyperpigmentation depends on many factors, including general health, skin type, the size and depth of vessels to be treated, the location of vessels on the body, other medications being taken, and the type and concentration of sclerosant used. It has been suggested to use an individual's response to chromated glycerin injection as a test for susceptibility to pigmentation, because those patients that pigment with this mild sclerosing solution should be treated with only the mildest of solutions so that inflammatory reactions are kept to a minimum.[22]

Patient factors play an important role in determining the potential for developing hyperpigmentation after sclerotherapy. Total body iron stores, vessel fragility, increased sensitivity to histamines, elevated ferritin levels, and defects in iron transport have all been associated with an increased risk of postsclerotherapy pigmentation.[23] Hyperpigmentation is more common and more pronounced in patients with dark hair and dark-toned skin, such as Asian and African-American patients. Hyperpigmentation in dark skin may occur even with the mildest of sclerosing solutions. Patients with type IV, V, and VI skin are forewarned about the likelihood of temporary and possibly permanent hyperpigmentation. These patients need at least 4 to 6 months from the last treatment before hyperpigmentation begins to resolve.

Superficial veins are more likely to exhibit postsclerotherapy hyperpigmentation than deeper ones for several reasons. Reabsorption of extravasated heme is more efficient in the deeper dermis and deeper vessels have a more robust perivascular environment that limits extravasation. Hemosiderin pigment is also less visible when it is deposited lower in the dermis. However, the larger the vessel treated, the greater is the potential volume of trapped red blood cells and the greater capacity for hemosiderin deposition. In the authors' experience, hyperpigmentation is rare in vessels less than 1 mm in diameter.

Physician treatment technique can also play a role in the development of hyperpigmentation. For example, excessive intravascular pressure from too-rapid injection may cause vessel rupture. This is particularly true of smaller venules composed essentially of endothelial cells with a thin muscular coat. When an excessive volume is injected too rapidly, the venule walls expand beyond capacity and rupture, leading to the escape of red blood cells. Therefore, it is essential to control the rate of injection and to inject the tiniest veins as slowly as possible. Experienced phlebologists choose syringe types and sizes to suit their personal preferences. As a practical matter, the authors prefer smaller 3 cc or 1 cc syringes for injection of the smallest veins to most easily control the flow rate.

Lastly, the incidence of hyperpigmentation can depend on the degree of endothelial destruction, which is directly correlated with type and concentration of the sclerosing solution used for treatment. Excessive vascular injury allows greater extravasation of red blood cells and causes an increase in hyperpigmentation. The minimum effective concentration of the weakest effective sclerosant will minimize the likelihood of hyperpigmentation. Lower flow rates are also less likely to cause vessel rupture, so that minimal thumb pressure is recommended.

There is some disagreement as to which sclerosing agents are most likely to cause hyperpigmentation. Polidocanol (POL) has been reported to have a high incidence of pigmentation when high concentrations are used, but a lower incidence when low concentrations are used.[24] Although chromated glycerin (CG) often is said to have an extremely low incidence of hyperpigmentation, one author reports hyperpigmentation in 8% of CG-treated patients and in none of POL-treated patients.[22] In a more recent study, authors compared 72% glycerin with 0.25% sodium tetradecyl sulfate, and found a significantly lower incidence of posttreatment dyschromia with glycerin treated vessels.[25]

The choice of sclerosing solution probably is less important than the concentration of that solution used for a specific vessel. There is a threefold increase in pigmentation in telangiectasias treated with 1% POL compared with 0.5% POL.[26] A solution that is too concentrated for small vessels causes too much wall damage and perivascular inflammation, with excessive red blood cell leakage and cutaneous deposition.

The treatment of established hyperpigmentation is not very effective. Thus, the utilization of techniques for prevention is of prime importance. Hyperpigmentation depends on leakage of blood cells out of the treated vessels. Risk reduction is accomplished by keeping vessel wall damage to the minimum necessary for effective sclerosis, reducing the volume of blood trapped within treated vessels, and reducing the intravascular pressure experienced by treated vessels during treatment and in the postsclerosis period. A guiding principle to help minimize the intravascular pressure is to identify and treat proximal reflux points before treating smaller distal veins, and to identify and treat reticular feeding veins before treating smaller telangiectasias.

Another important fundamental principle is the proper use of graduated compression to help minimize the amount of intravascular coagulum that remains trapped within a vessel. Although most patients do not like to wear compression stockings for extended periods of time posttreatment, the literature shows a definite reduced incidence of hyperpigmentation with the use of compression following sclerotherapy.[27]

To minimize the risk of pigmentation and to hasten vessel fibrosis, intravascular coagulum can be removed by puncture extraction using an 18-gauge needle and a 3cc

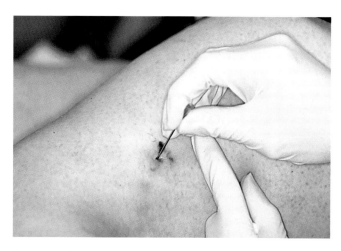

FIGURE 18-3. An 18-gauge needle is utilized to express trapped coagulum within 2 weeks following treatment. The overlying area was numbed with local anesthesia prior to needle insertion.

syringe, followed by manual expression of any residual material within the vein. Many patients require local anesthesia with lidocaine for this procedure. Smaller deposits of coagulum can be removed after a 22-gauge needle puncture (Fig. 18-3). Always remind patients to return for evaluation and possible coagulum removal if they notice any firm, brown lumps in the treated areas that persist after 2 weeks.

Hyperpigmentation can be reduced more rapidly if incision and draining of coagulum is performed within 2 months of treatment. The physician should stress the importance of wearing the compression hose. These patients should be added to the schedule within a week of their call for their quick check for a potential "vein nicking," a no-charge visit in the authors' practice. There is no highly effective method for treating postsclerotherapy hyperpigmentation. Treatments that may have some value include exfoliation with mild peeling agents and laser therapy. Most patients will have spontaneous resolution of hyperpigmentation within 1 year. Watchful waiting with periodic photographic documentation of the pigmentation is satisfactory in most cases.

Exfoliants such as trichloroacetic acid can reduce hemosiderin staining, but carry the risk of scarring, permanent hypopigmentation, and postinflammatory hyperpigmentation. Traditional bleaching agents such as hydroquinones are ineffective because they work by affecting melanocyte function, while postsclerotherapy pigmentation is composed predominantly of hemosiderin.

Postsclerotherapy pigmentation is similar to tattooing with hemosiderin, thus it is not surprising that lasers may offer a reasonably effective therapy. It is believed that laser treatment causes physical fragmentation of hemosiderin granules that are later removed by phagocytosis. A quality-switched (QS) laser with nanosecond pulses should theoretically be effective to break hemosiderin particles with a 1064 nm wavelength reaching to the depth of hemosiderin. Hemosiderin has an absorption spectrum throughout the visible range, with major peaks at 410 to 415 nm. Utilization of the QS-694 laser has been described in this regard.[9] The authors' experience has been promising utilizing a blended QS 532 nm and 1064 nm laser (Palomar Q Yag 5™; Palomar Medical Technologies, Burlington, MA) to break apart the pigment with several treatments. The authors typically use low fluences (4–7 J/cm²), making several passes to achieve faint peri-pigment erythema as an endpoint.

Telangiectatic Matting

Telangiectatic matting (TM) refers to appearance of tiny new red (occasionally violaceous) telangiectasias that appear in patients after sclerotherapy or surgical removal of varicose veins or venulectasia. Telangiectatic matting presents as "blush type" regions containing large numbers of "new" blood vessels less than 0.2 mm in diameter, located in and around the site of treatment (Fig. 18-4). Telangiectatic matting is often seen on the medial and lateral thighs, medial ankle, and medial and lateral calves. The inner thigh just above the knee is the most common

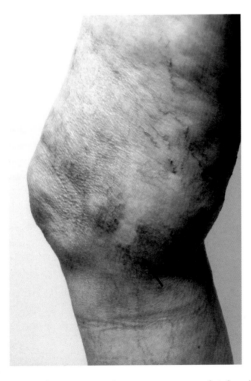

FIGURE 18-4. The arrow points to an area of telangiectatic matting appearing at the site of an old injection.

site of telangiectatic matting,[28,29] possibly due to movement at the knee causing rapid fluctuations in venous pressure or to relative skin anoxia during sleep when the opposite knee in the lateral position compresses this area. Microvessels that remain after treatment of larger telangiectasias can be confused with early telangiectatic matting. Photographs taken before treatment are helpful in distinguishing the two.

The incidence of TM is between 15% and 24%.[30] It is predominantly seen in women, but can also occur in men. Telangiectatic matting may occasionally be associated with intolerable burning pain and leg edema. TM usually resolves spontaneously in 3 to 12 months but occasionally can be permanent, and pretreatment patient information should make this explicitly clear.[5,26,30]

The precise cause of telangiectatic matting remains unknown, and it is not even certain whether the tiny vessels that make up the blush are dilated vessels that already existed, or whether they are new vessels that have grown into the area. One possibility holds that angiogenic and inflammatory processes cause preexisting subclinical blood vessels to dilate as they carry collateral flow from arteriovenous anastomoses. Another maintains that matting represents angiogenesis: new blood vessels grow as a natural reaction to the sclerotic obstruction of existing vessels and to meet increased metabolic demands caused by perivascular inflammation after sclerotherapy.[31]

Disruption of endothelial continuity and obstruction of outflow from a vessel (the results of sclerotherapy) are physical factors that are known to trigger angiogenesis. Regardless of the mechanism, it is clear that phlebologists walk an "angiogenic" tightrope every time sclerotherapy is performed and must be prepared to deal with the eventuality of encountering matting.[29]

Risk factors for TM have been a subject of great debate in the sclerotherapy literature. It is widely believed, although unsubstantiated, that TM is more common when higher infusion pressures, larger volumes, and higher concentrations of sclerosant are used. The authors have observed that when increased infusion pressure is utilized, resulting in blanching of the entire capillary network of the skin, TM is more likely to occur. Patient factors associated with an increased risk of TM include excessive body weight, a family history of telangiectasias, and longer duration of spider veins.[30]

Exogenous and endogenous increases in estrogen may be an important risk factor for matting, but the mechanism for this is not clear. Estrogen is recognized as a receptor-mediated angiogenic factor in a variety of tumors, but conflicting reports of estrogen and progesterone receptors in telangiectasias make the role of hormones in TM uncertain.[30]

Efforts to minimize TM are especially important because treatment efforts other than waiting are often not successful. In the authors' opinion, the three most important recommendations are to use the minimal effective concentration of sclerosant for a given vessel, the lowest possible volume of sclerosant to flush the vessel, and the lowest possible infusion pressure to deliver the sclerosant. When a patient who is taking exogenous estrogens demonstrates a tendency toward telangiectatic matting, she may wish to temporarily stop the estrogen during the period of treatment.

The most important first step in treating this complication is to repeat the clinical evaluation of the patient, looking for any previously unrecognized sources of increased hydrostatic pressure. Percutaneous transillumination may help locate a previously unseen reticular vein. At the minimum, Doppler examination of the problem areas should be done to listen for unresolved reflux. Much more information can be gained from a duplex ultrasound examination. The duplex study should be performed in the standing position, because previously unrecognized high-pressure reflux from an intermittently incompetent (clinically unapparent) saphenous vein may be the culprit. When the saphenous vein itself is competent, duplex often reveals failed perforators and an unsuspected reticular feeding vessel lying below the subcutaneous tissues. Treatment of this vessel by sclerotherapy or by phlebectomy usually causes resolution of the overlying telangiectatic mats.

Instead of succumbing to the immediate urge for multiple treatments with stronger liquid sclerosants, often simple reassurance and passage of time is all that is required to resolve matting. The patient is given a mild anti-inflammatory cream to apply to the area, and photographs are taken of the area at 6- to 8-week intervals until resolution occurs. Patients can be reassured that even the worst matting can resolve completely over time, and patients are much more tolerant of this waiting period when they have been suitably informed before start of treatment that TM may occur.

If there is no identifiable feeding vessel and if the matting does not resolve within a reasonable time, then the vessels that make up telangiectatic mats can themselves be treated by sclerotherapy. Disposable insulin syringes and 33-gauge needles can facilitate cannulation of these extremely small vessels. In some patients the effort is successful, but in other patients the tiny vessels seem impervious to sclerosing agents. Treatment with the 595 nm or the 1064 nm laser with pulse durations of 5 to 20 ms can also be of utility if the vessels are too small to cannulate with a 30- or 33-gauge needle.

Pain with Injection

Postinjection pain is mostly experienced with usage of the osmotically active sclerosant, hypertonic saline (HS). The pain with HS is typically described as burning or stinging and is more intense with injection into reticular veins than spider veins. Pain is typically minimal following injection with sodium tetradecyl sulfate, polidocanol, or 72% nonchromated glycerin (off-label indication for sclerotherapy). For this reason, the authors discontinued the use hypertonic saline many years ago in favor of other aforementioned sclerosants.

Urtication

Urtication is common following sclerotherapy and most likely represents a localized histamine response to vascular injury. Edema and erythema in a perivascular pattern typically manifest within minutes of treatment (Fig. 18-5). Patients should be reassured that itching and redness with fade in 4 to 24 hours. Patients with a known history of dermatographism and urtication may be prophylactically treated with a nonsedating antihistamine medication to minimize this reaction.

Purpura

Purpura results most commonly after sclerotherapy of reticular veins, as opposed to spider veins. Venous pressure in large, especially bulging, reticular veins can be enough to result in bleeding into the skin after injection. The purpura is transient and typically lasts 1 to 2 weeks in contrast to postinflammatory hyperpigmentation, which can last 3 to 6 months (Fig. 18-6). Patients on nonsteroidal anti-inflammatory medications and blood thinning agents are most prone to purpura. If medically prudent, encourage patients discontinue nonvital over-the-counter anticoagulation medications 10 to 14 days prior to sclerotherapy sessions.

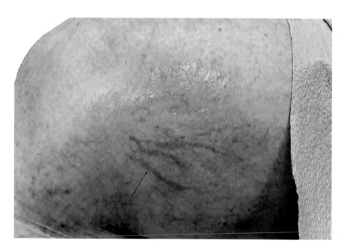

FIGURE 18-5. Typical urticarial response following sclerotherapy.

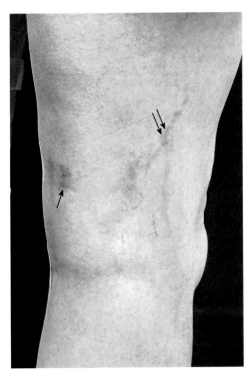

FIGURE 18-6. Focal purpura 3 days following sclerotherapy (*single arrow*) in comparison with postinflammatory hyperpigmentation present for 2 months (*double arrows*).

Rare but Self-Limited Complications

Cutaneous Necrosis

Cutaneous tissue necrosis refers to the localized superficial tissue damage which can occur around the treatment area as a direct result of sclerotherapy treatment (Fig. 18-7). There are several causes for cutaneous necrosis. The most common cause is the extravasation of sclerosant into perivascular tissues.

Extravasation necrosis is most common with hypertonic saline, seen with some regularity with most other agents, but is rare with polidocanol. Extravasation necrosis is rare in experienced hands, but is relatively common when a practitioner with little experience performs treatment. Signs which herald the possible evolution of extravasation "chemical" necrosis are immediate localized pain, petechia, and prolonged blanching.[30]

A second type of cutaneous necrosis does not come from extravasation, but rather from back-flow of sclerosant through an unsuspected cutaneous arteriovenous malformation, to produce sclerosis of an end-arteriole with subsequent necrosis of the cutaneous tissues depending on that arteriole. This type of necrosis can occur with the injection of any sclerosing agent even under ideal circumstances and does not necessarily represent physician error. Arteriolar spasm is believed to play a role in

many of these cases. The histological presence of arteriovenous (AV) microshunts has been proposed as an implicating factor.[32] Cutaneous necrosis may also result from excessive local compression or from excessive traction on the skin (usually due to tape). Another cause for necrosis, direct intra-arterial injection, should be avoidable by proper technique. One should cease injection immediately if a patient complains of sudden severe pain, as arterial puncture is much more painful than venipuncture. This chapter will focus on extravasation, the most common cause of necrosis.

During injection of an abnormal vein or telangiectasias, even the most adept physician may inadvertently inject a small quantity of sclerosing solution into the perivascular tissue. In some cases, sclerosant may flow back out of the vein when the needle is withdrawn. In others, vascular spasm causes the needle tip to pass completely through the small vessel, allowing sclerosant to be deposited in the deep perivenous tissues. Fragile veins may tear during needle placement, allowing immediate leakage during injection. The advent of duplex-guided techniques have greatly lessened the likelihood of extravasation of more concentrated solutions, especially when injecting deeper reticular veins and refluxing axial branches. Additionally, extravasation into deeper tissues seems to be better tolerated, possibly because of more rich blood supply in those areas.

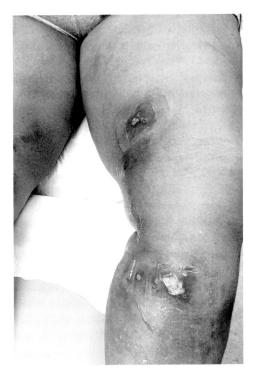

FIGURE 18-7. Cutaneous necrosis in two sites following sclerotherapy for bulging varicosities in the medial aspect of the left lower leg.

and immediate blanching. The etiology of the pain should be determined immediately if possible. Unfortunately, some patients will have no complaint of immediate pain and will only demonstrate a mild, sharply demarcated erythema which becomes dusky and cyanotic after a few hours to days.[40]

If sodium tetradecyl sulfate is injected into an artery the affected area may be infiltrated with procaine, which forms a complex with sodium tetradecyl sulfate and renders it inactive. The ischemic, blanched area should be cooled with ice packs to minimize tissue anoxia by decreasing tissue metabolism. However, cooling may also cause undesirable local vasoconstriction. Immediate heparinization with low-molecular-weight subcutaneous heparin should be administered and continued for 6 days. Administration of low-molecular-weight dextran at a rate of 10 mL/kg for 3 days may be attempted. In severe cases, arteriography and installation of vasodilators may be indicated. Thrombolytic agent may also be beneficial. Finally, use of oral prazosin, hydralazine, or nifedipine for 30 days should be considered.[40]

In conclusion, sclerotherapy is a remarkably safe and effective procedure that can provide both physicians and their patients with a great deal of satisfaction for a job well done. Being cognizant about the most common complications helps the physician to prepare treatment plans, reassure patients, and minimize discomfort after treatment.

References

1. Guex JJ, Allaert FA, Gillet JL, et al. Immediate and midterm complications of sclerotherapy: report of a prospective multicenter registry of 12,173 sclerotherapy sessions. Dermatol Surg 2005;31:123–128.
2. Goldman MP. Sclerotherapy: treatment of varicose and telangiectatic leg veins. Baltimore: Mosby; 1991.
3. Guex JJ. Contraindications of sclerotherapy, update 2005. J Mal Vasc 2005;30:144–149.
4. Rabe E, Pannier-Fischer F, Gerlach H, et al. Abstract: guidelines for sclerotherapy of varicose veins (ICD 10: I83.0, I83.1, I83.2, and I83.9). Dermatol Surg 2004;30:687–693.
5. Weiss RA, Feied CF, Weiss MA. Vein diagnosis and treatment: a comprehensive approach. New York: McGraw-Hill; 2001.
6. Goldman MP, Kaplan RP, Duffy DM. Postsclerotherapy hyperpigmentation: a histologic evaluation. J Dermatol Surg Oncol 1987;13:547–550.
7. Georgiev M. Postsclerotherapy hyperpigmentations: a one-year follow-up. J Dermatol Surg Oncol 1990;16:608–610.
8. Weiss MA, Weiss RA. Efficacy and side effects of 0.1% sodium tetradecyl sulfate in compression sclerotherapy of telangiectasias: comparison to 1% polidocanol and hypertonic saline. J Dermatol Surg Oncol 1991;17:90–91.
9. Tafazzoli A, Rostan EF, Goldman MP. Q-switched ruby laser treatment for postsclerotherapy hyperpigmentation. Dermatol Surg 2000;26:653–656.
10. Chatard H. Post-sclerotherapy pigmentation. Phlebol 1976;29:211–216.
11. Duffy DM. Small vessel sclerotherapy: an overview. Adv Dermatol 1988;3:221–242.
12. Weiss RA, Weiss MA. Incidence of side effects in the treatment of telangiectasias by compression sclerotherapy: hypertonic saline vs. polidocanol. J Dermatol Surg Oncol 1990;16:800–804.
13. Alderman DB. Surgery and sclerotherapy in the treatment of varicose veins. Conn Med 1975;39:467–471.
14. Weiss RA, Weiss MA. Resolution of pain associated with varicose and telangiectatic leg veins after compression sclerotherapy. J Dermatol Surg Oncol 1990;16:333–336.
15. Bodian EL. Techniques of sclerotherapy for sunburst venous blemishes. J Dermatol Surg Oncol 1985;11:696–704.
16. Alderman DB. Therapy for essential cutaneous telangiectasias. Postgrad Med 1977;61:91–95.
17. Goldman PM. Sclerotherapy for superficial venules and telangiectasias of the lower extremities. Dermatol Clin 1987;5:369–379.
18. Tournay PR. Traitment sclerosant des tres fines varicosites intra ou saous dermiques. [Sclerosing treatment of very fine intra or subdermal varicosities]. Soc Fran de Phlebol 1966;19:235–241.
19. Tretbar LL. Spider angiomata: treatment with sclerosant injections. J Kansas Med Soc 1978;79:198–200.
20. Cuttell PJ, Fox JA. The etiology and treatment of varicose pigmentation. Phlebol 1982;35:387–389.
21. Richter GW. The nature of storage iron in idiopathic hemochromatosis and in hemosiderosis. J Exp Med 1960;11:551–569.
22. Georgiev M. Postsclerotherapy hyperpigmentations. Chromated glycerin as a screen for patients at risk (a retrospective study). J Dermatol Surg Oncol 1993;19:649–652.
23. Thibault PK, Wlodarczyk J. Correlation of serum ferritin levels and postsclerotherapy pigmentation — a prospective study. J Dermatol Surg Oncol 1994;20:684–686.
24. McCoy S, Evans A, Spurrier N. Sclerotherapy for leg telangiectasia — a blinded comparative trial of polidocanol and hypertonic saline. Dermatol Surg 1999;25:381–385.
25. Leach BC, Goldman MP. Comparative trial between sodium tetradecyl sulfate and glycerin in the treatment of telangiectatic leg veins. Dermatol Surg 2003;29:612–615.
26. Norris MJ, Carlin MC, Ratz JL. Treatment of essential telangiectasia: effects of increasing concentrations of polidocanol. J Am Acad Dermatol 1989;20:643–649.
27. Weiss RA, Sadick NS, Goldman MP, Weiss MA. Postsclerotherapy compression: controlled comparative study of duration of compression and its effects on clinical outcome. Dermatol Surg 1999;25:105–108.
28. Duffy DM. Small vessel sclerotherapy: an overview. Adv Dermatol 1988;3:221–242.
29. Duffy DM. Sclerotherapy. In: Alam M, Nguyen TH, eds. Treatment of leg veins. Philadelphia: 2006.
30. Davis LT, Duffy DM. Determination of incidence and risk factors for postsclerotherapy telangiectatic matting of the lower extremity, a retrospective analysis. J Dermatol Surg Oncol 1990;16:327–330.

31. Barnhill RL, Wolfe JE Jr. Angiogenesis and the skin. J Am Acad Dermatol 1987;16:1226–1229.

32. Bihari I, Magyar E. Reasons for ulceration after injection treatment of telangiectasia. Dermatol Surg 2001;27:133–136.

33. Shields JL, Jansen GT. Therapy for superficial telangiectasias of the lower extremities. J Dermatol Surg Oncol 1982; 8:857–860.

34. Zimmet SE. The prevention of cutaneous necrosis following extravasation of hypertonic saline and sodium tetradecyl sulfate. J Dermatol Surg Oncol 1993;19:641–646.

35. Breu FX, Guggenbichler S. European Consensus Meeting on Foam Sclerotherapy, April 4–6, 2003, Tegernsee, Germany. Dermatol Surg 2004;30:709–717.

36. Forlee MV, Grouden M, Moore DJ, Shanik GD. Stroke after varicose vein foam injection sclerotherapy. J Vasc Surg 2006;43:162–164.

37. Meier B, Lock JE. Contemporary management of patent foramen ovale. Circulation 2003;107:5–9.

38. Feied CF, Jackson JJ, Bren TS, et al. Allergic reactions to polidocanol for vein sclerosis. Two case reports. Dermatol Surg Oncol 1994;20:466–468.

39. Bergan J, Pascarella L, Mekenas LJ. Venous disorders: treatment with sclerosant foam. Cardiovasc Surg (Torino) 2006; 47:9–18.

40. Bergan JJ, Weiss RA, Goldman MP. Extensive tissue necrosis following high-concentration sclerotherapy for varicose veins. Dermatol Surg 2000;26:535–541.

19
Complications of Facelifting Procedures

Greg S. Morganroth, Hayes B. Gladstone, and Isaac M. Neuhaus

Surgical facelifting procedures remain popular despite the recent introduction of laser, light source, and radiofrequency devices as facial rejuvenation alternatives. In recent years, facelift surgery has remained one of the most popular cosmetic procedures in the United States.[1] Its popularity persists because of the reproducible surgical rejuvenation with many years duration and minimal risk in experienced hands. Recent innovations with shorter scars, supra-SMAS (superficial musculoaponeurotic system) dissection, the addition of liposuction as a concomitant procedure, and less undermining provide comparable surgical outcomes to traditional techniques with less risk and downtime.[2-4] While other specialties have contributed novel ideas,[5] cutaneous surgeons have been innovators of a number of less aggressive lifting procedures that can be performed under local anesthesia and consequently eliminate the complications associated with general anesthesia and minimize the complications associated with deep plane or composite lifts.[6-14] Ongoing innovations in less aggressive techniques will allow facelifting procedures to continue to rise in popularity as patients seek facial rejuvenation with less risk, scarring, and downtime.

Facelifts Are Cutaneous Surgery

The facelifting procedures performed by cutaneous surgeons primarily involve supra-SMAS dissection and plication of the SMAS for resuspension of facial support structures. The anatomy, surgical instrumentation, undermining, tissue mobilization, and suturing techniques are the same as used in the routine facial skin excision and reconstruction procedures commonly performed by cutaneous surgeons.[15] Therefore, the complication profile of facelifting procedures closely mirrors that of reconstructive surgery. However, the elective cosmetic nature of these lifting procedures creates a lower acceptance for complications by the surgeon, lower threshold for patient dissatisfaction, and higher potential for incomplete realization of patient expectations.

As with all cutaneous procedures, complications will arise no matter the level of expertise or breadth of experience of the surgeon. The cutaneous surgeon must be well versed in patient selection and education, setting realistic patient expectations, anticipating potential complications, developing sound technique, instructing postoperative care, and, finally, the management of all potential complications.

Preoperative Phase — Minimizing Complications

Consultation and Preoperative Appointments

The preoperative phase of the facelift procedure involves the patient consultation and preoperative appointments. During these visits, the patient's goals and expectations are discussed and matched with a procedure list to provide a treatment plan to achieve the outcome that matches the expectations of both physician and patient. A complete patient history and examination are performed to evaluate the presence of a medical or social history that may impact the procedure outcome. Patients at a higher risk for complications include those with a history of diabetes, chronic obstructive pulmonary disease (COPD), uncontrolled hypertension, alcohol abuse, bleeding disorder, keloids, or smoking history. Patients taking anticoagulants, platelet inhibitors, isotretinoin, or dietary supplements that impact coagulation are also at risk for complications.

The patient should discontinue any medication that inhibits platelets, such as aspirin or nonsteroidal anti-inflammatory drugs (NSAIDS), 4 weeks before the operation.[16] A list of medications that should be avoided should be given to the patient at the preoperative consultation. If there is any history of a bleeding disorder, coagulation studies should be performed to evaluate the underlying etiology.[17]

Smoking decreases tissue perfusion and can increase the risk of flap necrosis. Patients who smoke should be counseled to stop smoking at least 1 week prior to surgery and for at least 1 week after surgery.[18,19] Additional strategies to increase tissue perfusion in smokers include creating a thicker flap with a short scar incision with limited undermining.

Patients over the age of 55 or with underlying medical conditions should undergo a preoperative examination, including electrocardiogram and laboratory studies, by their primary care physician for surgical clearance.

Finally, patient education at the preoperative visits regarding proper wound care supplies, bandaging techniques, wound care details, avoidance of anticoagulants, appropriate activity level, and importance of routine follow-up is critical for the minimization of complications.

Operative Phase

Day of Surgery — Minimizing Surgical Complications

An understanding of anatomy is critical for obtaining a good result without serious complications. The location and anatomical relationships and variations of the facial and neck sensory and motor nerves are critical. The great auricular, lesser occipital, and temporal, buccal, and marginal mandibular branches of the facial nerve are at risk and can be avoided by remaining in the subcutaneous plane at all times.[20]

Accurate planning of incisions, marking out undermining and liposuction zones, and noting nerve danger zones will also decrease the risk of potential complications. Male patients should have the preauricular incision within the preauricular crease to prevent lateral displacement of hair-bearing skin over the tragus.[21] High temporal hairlines require modification of the incision to avoid displacing the hairline even higher. Placement of buried sutures during closure of the incision will minimize scar spread and hypertrophy, localized alopecia, distortion of the earlobe position, and premature sagging. The addition of postauricular buried sutures anchored to the underlying mastoid fascia will minimize scar movement and distortion of the earlobe.

One of the most important surgical techniques that has minimized complications is the use of tumescent anesthesia, the injection of large, dilute volumes of lidocaine with epinephrine.[22,23] Tumescent anesthesia enables face- and necklifting without general anesthesia and reduces the associated postoperative nausea and vomiting. Although tumescent anesthesia has not been shown to decrease the risk of postoperative hematoma, it does reduce the rate

of skin necrosis, alopecia, hypertrophic scars, spread scars, and scar revision.[23] The infiltrated tumescent fluid induces vasoconstriction to minimize intraoperative bleeding and expands the subcutaneous compartment to facilitate dissection and minimize the risk of injury to nerves. Postoperatively, the authors believe tumescent anesthesia lowers the risk of bleeding, bruising, hematoma, and pain, although there is no data to support this claim. Using small, blunt-tipped cannulae (2 mm to 16 gauge) for neck and facial liposuction will reduce trauma and minimize skin irregularity due to uneven fat removal.

Creation of the subcutaneous flap, especially in the fibrous areas of the cheeks and pre- and postauricular regions, can be facilitated by undermining prior to dissection with a 2 mm spatula cannula without suction. The pre-undermining with the cannula creates multiple tunnels that can be easily connected by spreading the undermining scissors and will reduce the risk of skin perforation, nerve injury, parotid gland injury, and bleeding. Flap creation and elevation is also facilitated by using dual overhead surgical lights to provide transillumination of the flap, fiberoptic headlamps or retractors for direct visualization of the tissue plane, and countertraction by nursing staff. Suction coagulation is helpful for hemostasis, especially deep in the neck. Dissecting with the scissor tips up and in a vertical orientation will also maintain the correct plane. Plication is considered safer than imbrication (excision of SMAS prior to suturing)[5] and should be performed with a vertical vector of lift, rather than in a horizontal direction, to provide a natural rejuvenation and prevent the "wind tunnel" effect. Plication sutures can be absorbable or nonabsorbable. Absorbable sutures may result in a delayed foreign-body reaction and permanent sutures may be palpable if care is not taken to bury the knots after the postoperative edema resolves.

Complications

Intraoperative Complications

Bleeding

Bleeding and subsequent hematomas are the most frequent complications of rhytidectomy, with an incidence of 0% to 9.6% in studies published in the past decade.[23–33] A higher incidence in men is attributed to the sebaceous nature of the skin and increased density of hair follicles and associated vascularity.

Prevention of intraoperative bleeding is facilitated by preoperative screening blood tests, discontinuation of medications and over-the-counter products that impact coagulation at least 4 weeks prior to surgery, avoidance of alcohol at least 1 week preoperatively, and ensuring proper control of hypertension. Tumescent anesthesia

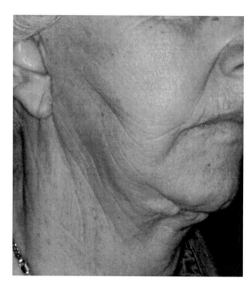

FIGURE 19-1. Contour irregularities from an anterior suture suspension lift and inadequate undermining of the neck in a patient seeking facelift revision by the author. (Courtesy of Greg S. Morganroth, MD.)

orientation during spreading will provide a less traumatic dissection.

Intraoperative bleeding is managed by a combination of electrocoagulation and pressure. Obtaining hemostasis is facilitated by good visualization with fiberoptic light sources, retraction of the flap by assistants, and long cotton-tipped applicators or gauze. Suction-assisted coagulation will increase visualization and prevent nonspecific tissue trauma. The use of temporary drains is optional with tumescent anesthesia unless there is excessive bleeding intraoperatively or the patient is male, where an increased risk of postoperative hematoma exists. Following surgery, proper compression dressing placement is critical.[34] The risk of bleeding can be minimized in the immediate postoperative phase of the procedure by ensuring that patients continue their antihypertension medications, providing adequate pain medications, and minimizing nausea.

containing epinephrine 1:500,000 is highly effective at vasoconstriction and decreasing intraoperative bleeding. Minimizing patient pain is critical because pain-induced hypertension will result in intraoperative bleeding despite the vasoconstriction of tumescent anesthesia. Meticulous hemostasis and visualization while maintaining dissection in the subcutaneous plane will reduce bleeding, especially in the distal aspects of the flap. In addition, vertical scissor

Alterations in Contour

Contour irregularities on the face and neck occur primarily as a result of poor intraoperative technique (Fig. 19-1) and may be temporary or permanent. The most common causes of contour irregularities are uneven fat removal with liposuction, inadequate undermining, especially of the neck overlying the sternocleidomastoid muscle, plication sutures (Fig. 19-2A,B), and resolving hematomas and seromas. Occasionally, irregularities in contour result from improper compression garment placement.

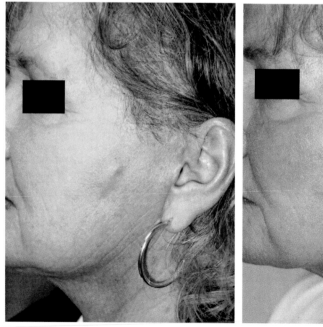
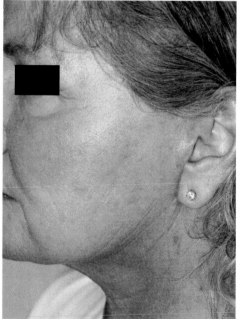

FIGURE 19-2. (A) Linear scar from plication suture reaction. (B) Two weeks following intralesional kenalog injection. (Courtesy of Greg S. Morganroth, MD.)

The prevention of skin irregularities during liposuction and undermining is facilitated by using small, blunt-tipped cannulas and even, fanlike movements that cover the entire cosmetic unit. Palpation and massage of the skin will help to determine the thickness of the adipose layer. Undermining should be performed following plication to release areas of tension and ensure the formation of a smooth pocket, especially during dissection over the medial cheek and inferior neck over the sternocleidomastoid muscle. Plication sutures should be buried and placed in a symmetrical manner with even tension.[5] Palpation of plication sutures through the skin will ensure a smooth surface. Occasionally, the vertically elevated SMAS creates a fullness of the superior cheek, which can be gently reshaped by scissor excision. The SMAS fullness superior to the plication may need to be surgically reduced to minimize focal fullness and create better symmetry. An untreated hematoma or seroma may also cause long-term skin irregularity. The use of a cervical collar postoperatively helps to position the neck and prevent movement of the garment or folding of the skin.

Prevention is the best management for irregularities from uneven fat removal. In some cases, touch-up mini-liposuction procedures or microlipoinjection can be used for significant cases. For most other causes of irregularity, frequent massage and patient reassurance will induce resolution of most of the contour issues with time.

Perforation of the Skin Flap (Button Holing)

Perforation of skin during elevation of the flap is most common at the medial cheek, the bound down skin of the postauricular region, and skin overlying the sternocleidomastoid muscle in thin patients. This complication occurs during undermining and results from an excessively superficial dissection.

Skin perforation is a preventable complication with good technique and the assistance of the nursing staff. Direct visualization with fiberoptic lighting, transillumination of the flap, and countertraction by surgical assistants are important technical components of flap formation. Surgical assistants should be trained to alert the surgeon if the instruments appear too close to the skin surface. Alternating between a vertical and horizontal spreading technique after pre-undermining with a cannula is critical to minimize thinning of the flap.

If flap perforation should occur, the tear should be repaired immediately. The defect should be released distally by restarting the undermining proximal to the perforation and undermining deeper below and beyond the tear. The perforation should be repaired with multiple 6.0 vicryl buried sutures from the underside of the flap to reapproximate the skin edges. Interrupted 6.0 nylon or fast-absorbing gut sutures are used to reappose the skin

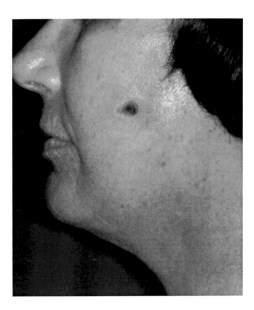

FIGURE 19-3. Full-thickness injury to flap from electrocoagulation injury during effort to obtain hemostasis. (Courtesy of Andrew B. Menkes, MD.)

edges externally. For smaller injuries, this approach will result in minimal to no significant scarring. In rare cases where the injury creates a large gap, a skin graft or granulation followed by a delayed scar revision should be considered.

On rare occasions, a burn injury from aggressive electrocoagulation of a vessel on the skin flap may result in a full-thickness skin heat injury (Fig. 19-3). These thermal injuries often heal with puckered and contracted scars, but the scars tend to be smaller than the original injury zone. Postoperative management consists of topical wound care similar to that of a granulating wound. Excision of these contracted scars with broad undermining and release of adjacent scarring followed by a layered repair is performed as soon as possible.

Nerve Injury

Nerve injury, either motor or sensory, is the most concerning complication of facelift surgery for both patients and physicians. The deficit is usually temporary but it may take up to 1 year for the patient to regain full function. If using tumescent anesthesia, most patients will experience a temporary weakness of a single or all facial nerve branches that resolves within 8 hours. If weakness persists beyond the first postoperative day without intraoperative indications of nerve injury, the patient should be reassured that loss of motor function is temporary and typically resolves slowly over weeks to months. Complete loss of function postoperatively suggests a more significant injury, yet return of function may be possible if the nerve has multiple branches.

Prevention of nerve injury is accomplished by meticulous technique guided by a thorough knowledge of the facial anatomy and the course of the facial nerve, the great auricular and lesser occipital nerves, and the spinal accessory nerve. Although less likely with expansion of the adipose layer with tumescent solution, nerve injury may result from inadvertent trauma from the liposuction cannula, nerve sheath edema from manipulation, overzealous use of electrosurgery, nerve entrapment with plication sutures, infection, hematoma and seroma, or complete division during scissor dissection. If the surgeon recognizes that there has been a nerve transection and can visualize the nerve endings, an effort should be made to repair the injury. Typically, this intervention requires the assistance of an otolaryngology/head and neck surgeon experienced in microsurgery.

Sensory Nerves

The most common nerve injured during a facelift is the great auricular nerve, which is damaged in up to 7% of procedures.[35] This nerve courses deep to the platysma along the sternocleidomastoid muscle fascia approximately 6.5 cm below the earlobe.[36,37] The nerve courses posterior to the external jugular vein and injury often occurs while attempting to obtain hemostasis after inadvertent injury to the external jugular vein during undermining of the postauricular portion of the flap as the dissection advances into the neck over the mid-portion of the sternocleidomastoid muscle.[38] Injury to the great auricular nerve creates a sensory deficit of the lower two thirds of the ear and the periauricular skin, which is particularly concerning for women because it results in complete loss of earlobe sensation and difficulty in inserting a pierced earring. It is not unusual to have temporary numbness of this area 2 to 6 weeks postoperatively from

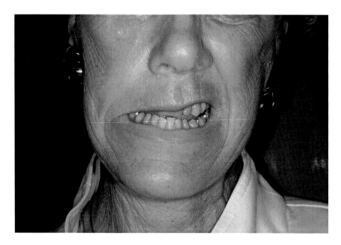

FIGURE 19-4. Temporary injury to buccal nerve during undermining of medial cheek during facelift. (Courtesy of Andrew B. Menkes, MD.)

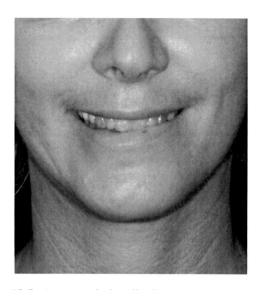

FIGURE 19-5. Asymmetrical smile due to temporary injury to marginal mandibular nerve during facelift and chin implant. (Courtesy of Andrew B. Menkes, MD.)

disruption of small sensory nerves following a facelift. In contrast, the sensory deficit from transection injury to the great auricular nerve is usually permanent; however the anesthetic area typically decreases with time. Occasionally, painful neuromas may result following great auricular nerve transection.[39]

Motor Nerves

In supra-SMAS rhytidectomies, it is estimated that motor nerve injury occurs in up to 3.1% of patients based on a review of recent studies (Fig. 19-4).[23,27,29,30,33,40–42] The risk of motor nerve injury is higher for deep plane or composite facelifts where sub-SMAS dissection increases the exposure to motor nerve fibers. Of the five branches of the facial nerve, the temporal, marginal mandibular, and buccal branches have the highest chance for damage.[42,43]

The marginal mandibular nerve is the most commonly injured facial nerve branch, followed by the temporal and buccal nerves. After exiting the parotid gland, the marginal mandibular nerve courses beneath the SMAS as it approaches the angle of the mandible. It then passes deep to the platysma and superficial to the facial artery and vein approximately 2 to 3 cm below the mandible prior to heading more superiorly toward the oral commissure and terminating in the perioral depressor muscles. Permanent damage to the marginal mandibular has serious consequences. The patient will not only have an asymmetric smile, but may drool on the affected side (Fig. 19-5).

The marginal mandibular nerve is most susceptible to injury anterior to the angle of the mandible during liposuction and undermining. It is important to use blunt dissection with vertical undermining to ensure a thin flap.

When performing liposuction, it is important to always visualize the tip of the cannula and lift the skin to prevent rasping the mandible. Injury may also occur during undermining lateral to the oral commissure or while attempting to obtain hemostasis after inadvertent injury to the facial vein.

The temporal branch of the facial nerve exits the parotid gland deep to the SMAS as it approaches the zygomatic arch. After crossing superficially over the middle portion of the zygomatic arch, the nerve travels in the temporoparietal fascia in the temporal fossa and exits along the deep side of the frontalis muscle. The nerve is most susceptible to injury during undermining over the zygomatic arch. Care must be taken to stay in the adipose layer using vertical dissection, countertraction, transillumination, and fiberoptic lighting.

Injury to the temporal branch which innervates the frontalis muscle will result in ipsilateral brow ptosis and inability to raise the eyebrow (Fig. 19-6A). Consequently, the patient will complain of both brow and lid heaviness and possibly some decrease in peripheral vision. A direct or endoscopic browlift will provide elevation of the eyebrow and alleviate this condition (Fig. 19-6B).

The buccal branch exits the parotid gland and courses deep to the SMAS. The buccal branches can also be injured in the preparotid area during sub-SMAS procedures, but the risk is less than for the temporal or marginal mandibular nerves. Unlike the temporal or marginal mandibular nerves, the buccal branches have many anastomoses including connections with the zygomatic branches so permanent injury is less likely.

Because of redundancy similar to the buccal branches, injury to the cervical branches typically will not cause the same degree of morbidity as injury to the temporal or marginal mandibular branches. Because the platysma is thin, the cervical branches are at risk for injury during postauricular undermining. Because the cervical branches also innervate the perioral depressor muscles, transection will cause some loss of depressor function. This pseudo-paralysis of the marginal mandibular nerve due to a cervical branch injury has an incidence of 1.7%. This injury can be distinguished from true marginal mandibular nerve damage because the patient will be able to evert the lower lip as the result of a functioning mentalis muscle. In addition, full recovery may occur in less than a month, and usually no more than 6 months.

The spinal accessory nerve, which crosses the posterior inferior portion of the sternocleidomastoid muscle (SCM), is less commonly injured.[44,45] This nerve innervates the trapezius muscle and injury results in pain and winging of the scapula. Unfortunately, physical therapy provides only partial improvement.

If a motor nerve deficit persists following resolution of the local anesthesia, patient education and reassurance should be instituted. Referral to a surgeon specializing in nerve injury and repair will reinforce the typical temporary nature of these deficits and allow the patient to understand the surgical options and when they are indicated. Fortunately, transient paralysis is more likely than permanent deficits. If a motor nerve is transected during surgery, immediate microscopic neurorrhaphy is indicated by an experienced surgeon.[46]

Postoperative Complications

Hematoma

Hematomas represent one of the most common facelift complications with an incidence as high as 9.6%.[33] The majority of small-to-medium hematomas (<20 cc) occur in the first 24 hours after surgery (Fig. 19-7). Risk factors for hematoma include a preoperative history of

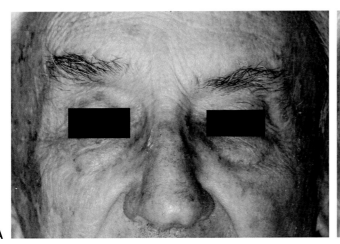
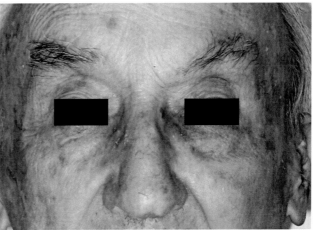

A   B

FIGURE 19-6. (A) Permanent injury to left temporal branch of the facial nerve resulting from Mohs surgery for recurrent basal cell carcinoma. (B) Result following direct browlift by author to elevate brow for symmetry. (Courtesy of Greg S. Morganroth, MD.)

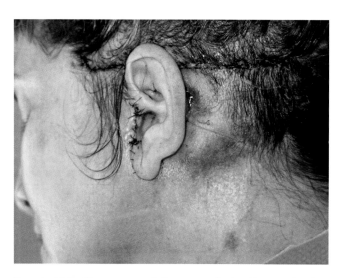

FIGURE 19-7. Hematoma of the postauricular flap on the first postoperative day. (Courtesy of Greg S. Morganroth, MD.)

hypertension, bleeding abnormality, antiplatelet medication use, an intraoperative technical problem, use of propofol, blood loss, postoperative hypertension, coughing, retching, and agitation. Hematomas increase the risk of skin necrosis, infection, delayed healing, scarring, and skin irregularity. Hematomas do not appear to be associated with age and no studies have been done to assess whether there is a difference in the risk of hematoma after full rhytidectomy compared to the S-lift or other short scar lifts.

Tumescent anesthesia has not been shown to decrease the risk of hematoma. A recent retrospective study suggested that lidocaine without epinephrine may decrease the risk of postoperative hematoma, presumably due to the epinephrine-induced vasoconstriction which reverses with vasodilatation several hours following surgery.[47] Despite the findings of this study, the authors believe that epinephrine has a positive effect and have empirically found that an increase in concentration of epinephrine to a dilution of 1:500,000 from 1:1,000,000 decreased intraoperative bleeding and postoperative hematomas. Although the authors do not routinely place drains because of the effectiveness of tumescent anesthesia, males and patients with excessive intraoperative bleeding may benefit from the insertion of a drain for 24 hours.

Expanding hematomas represent one of the most feared complications of SMAS rhytidectomies. Unilateral, painful swelling and bruising warrants immediate attention to minimize the risk of flap necrosis, infection, and nerve compression. Despite quick intervention, delayed healing with fibrosis, discoloration, and skin irregularity will need to be managed with patient reassurance, intralesional steroids, and massage.

Management of the hematoma involves evacuation of the blood clot and restoration of hemostasis. Expanding

hematomas require aspiration. Rebandaging will rarely solve the problem because the hematoma will reaccumulate and continue to threaten flap viability. Take down of the flap is necessary to visualize the underside of the flap and surface of the SMAS and obtain hemostasis. Irrigation with saline will help to remove clot fragments and increase visibility, which aids in obtaining hemostasis. Repeated daily visits for aspiration of residual serosanguinous fluid is required to assist in healing. A drain may be placed if desired and monitored over the next few days.

For the patients with small, stable hematomas that develop shortly after surgery, aspiration may be attempted first prior to flap take down. Aspiration may be achieved with a liposuction cannula connected to a vacuum device followed by serial needle aspiration as needed. A 12-gauge or 3 mm liposuction cannula with a single or double port can be inserted between sutures without suture removal. The clot is gently massaged toward the open port of the cannula that is placed sideways to prevent suction trauma to the skin or underlying tissue. Repeat daily visits for 3 to 5 days are still required to assess for reaccumulation of blood and to aspirate the serosanguinous fluid.

Seromas

Seromas can occur secondary to generalized inflammation, in the resolution phase of a hematoma, or following injury to the parotid gland. Frequent needle aspirations are necessary and often a drain may need to be placed for several weeks if the seroma overlies the parotid gland.[48] Similar to a hematoma, seromas can compromise the flap in the early postoperative period, increase the risk for infection, and potentially result in an uneven surface contour. The best way to prevent a seroma is to minimize the risk for hematoma formation, remain in the proper plane of dissection above the parotid gland, and avoid injuring the parotid gland when placing plication sutures.

Infection

Infections following facelifts are rare and range from 0% to 1% in recent studies.[27,29,30,33,41,49] Factors that minimize the risk of infection include the use of sterile technique, a healthier patient population due to the elective nature of the procedure, patient education of proper wound care, the standard protocol of preoperative prophylactic antibiotics, and the excellent vascularity of the face and neck. Presdisposing conditions for infection include diabetes, immunosuppression, and systemic illness. Postoperative risk factors include undetected hematoma or seroma, buried suture reactions, and wound contamination. Steam autoclave sterilization of instrumentation will minimize the recently reported mycobacterial infections seen in offices using cold sterilization techniques.[50,51]

If an infection is suspected, a bacterial culture should be obtained for pathogen identification and antibiotic sensitivities. The patient should be seen daily to prevent progression of the infection that might compromise the flap. In the case of a rapidly progressive infection or antibiotic-resistant pathogens, consultation with an infectious disease specialist and hospital admission for intravenous antibiotics would be indicated. Diabetic patients are at higher risk for an ear chondritis and should be treated with oral ciprofloxacin.

Flap Necrosis and Slough

Skin slough and full-thickness necrosis result from vascular compromise and may be secondary to an excessively superficial dissection, excessive skin tension on the flap, hematoma or seroma, or electrosurgery injury. The flap region most susceptible to superficial dissection is the bound down skin overlying the fascia of the sternocleidomastoid muscle and postauricular region, especially in thin women with minimal adipose tissue. Care should be taken to minimize tension on the flap during skin excision, placement of anchor sutures, and suturing skin edges. However, the temporal incision and postauricular incision will contain the highest level of tension in vertical vector lifts and be furthest from the cutaneous blood supply.

A large or expanding blood or fluid collection can also compromise the flap's perfusion pressure. If a hematoma of seroma forms, drainage and close follow-up to prevent reaccumulation are necessary to prevent flap loss and infection. Aggressive laser resurfacing or chemical peeling of flap skin may also increase the risk of flap failure.

Compromised flap skin will appear to have venous congestion — a bluish-purple hue — before evolving to pallor and epidermolysis within the first few days. Over the next few days, blisters evolve into erosions and finally an eschar. As the wound heals there is shrinkage of the violaceous skin color because of perfusion from the periphery. Therefore, the ulceration is typically much smaller than the original zone of violaceous discoloration (Fig. 19-8A,B).

The patient should be seen within the first 24 hours to inspect the skin and be certain that the pressure dressing is not compromising blood flow. If an area of vascular compromise is noted, hematoma and seroma must be ruled out. Wound care consisting of daily cleansing, topical antibiotics, and nonstick bandages should by instituted with daily follow-up, patient reassurance, and monitoring for the possibility of infection.

Most sloughs are small and localized in the postauricular region out of direct view. Partial-thickness sloughs may heal with minimally visible scarring (Fig. 19-9), especially when it is hidden by the ear and hair. In more significant sloughs, the granulation phase may be followed by the development of a hypertrophic scar. Aggressive scar management with intralesional steroids (3–10 mg/cc triamcinolone acetonide), vascular laser, frequent massage, and silicone gel sheeting are helpful.

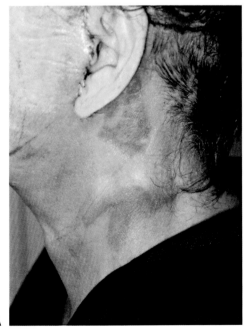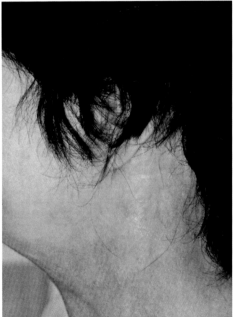

FIGURE 19-8. (A) Thin flap from superficial dissection of bound-down skin over the sternocleidomastoid muscle on postoperative day 1. (B) At 6 weeks postoperatively, there is a pink scar much smaller than original area of vascular compromise. (Courtesy of Greg S. Morganroth, MD.)

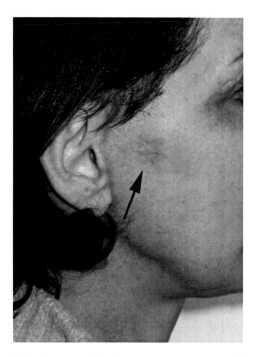

FIGURE 19-9. Scar resulting from superficial slough. (Courtesy of Greg S. Morganroth, MD.)

Despite treatment, the patient should be counseled of the possibility of persistent texture change, discoloration, and, in severe cases, a permanent uneven contour. Scar revision can be performed following healing of the flap for locations amenable to excision and repair.

The best method for addressing necrosis and slough is prevention and patient education. Gentle handling of tissue, minimal manipulation of the flap, selective vessel cauterization, careful undermining with vertical spreading, direct visualization and transillumination to ensure a generous layer of fat underneath the flap, accurate skin trimming under minimal tension, and a two-layered closure will reduce the risk of flap necrosis. In diabetics, smokers, and transplant patients, preexisting vascular compromise increases the risk of skin slough.

Alteration of Hair Density and Distribution

The incidence of alopecia following rhytidectomy has been reported to be up to 8.4%.[52] Temporary hair loss is more common and is related to trauma and tension along the incision line in the pre- and postauricular incisions. Permanent hair loss results from transection of follicles during the incision, direct trauma or transection of follicles during underming of a hair-bearing skin flap, or electrocoagulation injury. Misalignment of the postauricular hairline creates a step-off deformity that is obvious when the patient wears their hair back. Preauricular incisions in men should be made in the preauricular crease to prevent displacement of beard hair onto the tragus. Patients with high temporal hairlines require modifica-

tion of the temporal incision to prevent superior displacement of non–hair-bearing skin (Fig. 19-10).

Techniques to prevent injury to hair follicles include gentle tissue handling technique, careful undermining beneath the hair follicles, minimizing electrocoagulation of the flap underside, using a trichophytic incision which is created parallel to the hair follicles, and minimizing tension on the flap. Careful planning of incisions will minimize the chance of postauricular hairline misalignment or preauricular displacement in men (Fig. 19-11).[53] For women with high temporal hairlines, a pretrichal incision will prevent elevation of the hairline but may leave a visible scar with certain hair styles. For patients undergoing revision facelift who seek correction of the high temporal hairline, an anterior-based transposition flap has been described to provide hair coverage.[54] In some patients, the prophylactic use of topical minoxidil in the perioperative period may decrease the risk of alopecia.[55] Permanent alopecia can be corrected with hair transplantation, hair extensions, or local flaps.[56,57]

Allergic and Irritant Contact Dermatitis

Contact dermatitis is a common complication in cutaneous surgery and presents as a pruritic, dermatitic patch or plaque often with a shape or pattern corresponding to the contactant. Allergens and irritants include adhesive tape, topical antibiotics, skin disinfectants, and over-the-counter topical products.[58–62] Most commonly, contact dermatitis is a minor

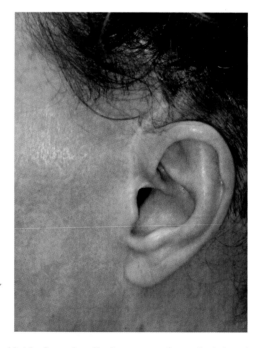

FIGURE 19-10. Superior displacement of non–hair-bearing skin in the temporal incision in a patient who had a traditional facelift and sought scar revision. (Courtesy of Greg S. Morganroth, MD, from author.)

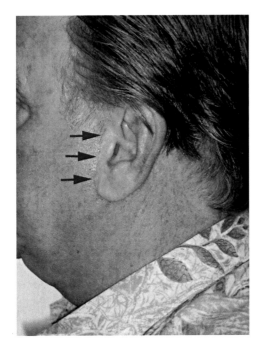

FIGURE 19-11. In men, incision is placed in preauricular crease to prevent displacement of hair onto tragus. (Courtesy of Greg S. Morganroth, MD.)

postoperative complication. If left untreated, progressive inflammation or patient scratching can result in infection, delayed healing, wound dehiscence, and scarring.

A history of known allergies should be taken prior to surgery to document allergies to iodine, neomycin, disinfectants, adhesives, and tape. Hypoallergenic paper tape and avoidance of neomycin will reduce the incidence of contact dermatitis. Changing the bandage on a daily basis may also diminish the risk of contact dermatitis. Discontinuation of all topical medications and treatment with a low-potency topical corticosteroid, level VI to VII, applied twice daily should be initiated to decrease the inflammation. Topical antibiotics can be substituted with petrolatum ointment.

Hypertrophic and Keloid Scars

Despite care and attention to detail, hypertrophic and keloid scars may be unavoidable. Hypertrophic scars typically appear approximately 1 month after surgery and resolve within the first year, whereas keloid scars may be permanent and tend to be treatment resistant.[63] The most common cause of these scars is high wound tension and/or inadequate suturing techniques resulting in incision spread. This phenomenon is most common in areas of high tension, such as the postauricular flap, and in areas of partial slough or necrosis. Predisposing factors for keloids include race, ethnicity, skin type, and family history.[64]

Treatment options to reduce scar thickness include frequent daily massage, daily application of silicone gel

sheeting, intralesional steroids every 3 to 4 weeks, and Imiquimod cream.[65–68] Pulsed dye laser and other vascular lasers have been shown to be effective for decreasing scar erythema and thickness.[69] Intralesional kenalog injections can range from 3 mg/cc to 10 mg/cc and must be carefully injected to prevent steroid atrophy in surrounding normal skin. Hypertrophic scars related to early scar spread from inadequate suturing technique can be reexcised and closed in a layered fashion. Keloids are difficult to treat and may grow beyond the footprint of the original incision scar. Keloids are treated with the same therapies as hypertrophic scars, but their response to treatment is poor.

Prevention of thickened scars is best achieved by obtaining a good medical history during the consultation appointment. Patients found to have a personal or family history of keloids should be counseled regarding the high risk of abnormal scarring and alternative noninvasive options for facial rejuvenation.

Prevention of scar spread can be minimized by careful excision of excess skin without causing excess tension and then closing the incision with a layered closure of buried absorbable sutures and permanent surface sutures. Incision closures consisting of a single layer of superficial sutures or staples are at higher risk of scar spread because there is limited wound support 7 to 10 days after surgery. At this time, there is less than 5% tensile strength, therefore the placement of buried sutures is critical to provide optimal wound healing and minimize scarring (Fig. 19-12).[70]

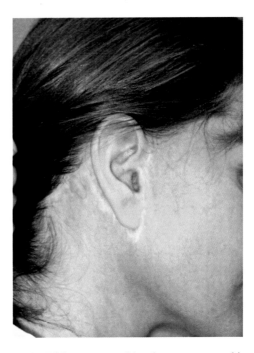

FIGURE 19-12. White scars resulting from scar spread in patient who underwent traditional facelift without using buried sutures in closure. (Courtesy of Greg S. Morganroth, MD.)

An additional tool to minimize scar spread, especially in the pre- and postauricular crease, is passing the buried sutures from flap edge, through the mastoid fascia or cartilage, and back to skin edge to provide fixation to an immobile structure. In order to maximize the anchoring of these sutures,[71] the incision must be made in the postauricular crease. The incision placement and suturing technique differs from the traditional facelift incision closure, where the postauricular incision is carried approximately 1 cm medially onto the posterior conchal cartilage. The traditional technique employs a single layer of sutures and allows for approximately 1 cm of flap stretch-back that will reposition the posterior ear incision from the conchal cartilage into the less visible postauricular crease. Because of the incision placement over the conchal cartilage, it is not possible to take a bite of mastoid fascia without causing excessive tension and distortion of the ear shape.

Alteration of Ear Shape

Alteration of ear shape may present as inferior displacement of the earlobe (pixie ear deformity) or displacement of the tragus (Fig. 19-13). These changes are due to excessive tension on the closure, poor incision placement, and asymmetrical vectors of tightening.[53,72,73] Treatment requires a revision facelift in which the skin is elevated, resuspended, and redraped without tension.

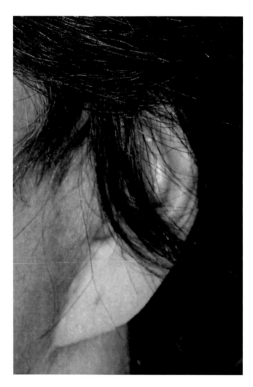

FIGURE 19-13. Pixie ear deformity resulting from inferior displacement of the earlobe due to tension on incision. (Courtesy of Greg S. Morganroth, MD, from traditional facelift.)

Prevention of ear distortion is based on accurate incision placement, tension-free skin redraping, and meticulous layered suturing of the incision. The preauricular incision should be made just medial or along the edge of the tragus to prevent tragal displacement and blunting of the acute angle of the cartilage. To avoid injuring the tragus cartilage at the beginning of flap elevation, a second incision 6 to 8 mm medial to the edge of the tragal incision will allow for elevation of skin off of the tragus from medial to lateral. To prevent the pixie ear deformity, the cartilage and mastoid fascia retention sutures described for the prevention of incision spread will also create points of fixation to reduce inferior displacement and rotation of the earlobe.[74]

Short- and Long-Term Pain

All patients will experience some degree of discomfort in the immediate postoperative period that improves within a few days of surgery and gradually resolves over 2 to 4 weeks. Pain is typically localized to the postauricular region where the ear is under the most tension. Severe pain beyond the immediate postoperative period is unusual and may indicate the development of a complication. An expanding hematoma will present as increasing, unilateral pain in the first day after surgery and infection will present as increasing pain associated with erythema and swelling.

For the rare instance of severe and prolonged pain in the absence of hematoma or infection, one should consider a neuroma resulting from nerve transection or nerve entrapment by a plication suture.[39] Neuroma-induced pain is difficult to treat but may be helped by intralesional steroids, nerve blocks, or referral to a pain specialist. Nerve entrapment from a plication suture can be treated with a suture release. If no obvious cause for the pain can be elucidated, evaluation of underlying psychological reasons should be considered.[75,76]

Facial Asymmetry and Premature Sagging

Asymmetry is an uncommon complication and must be distinguished from preoperative baseline asymmetry on preoperative photos. Asymmetry and premature sagging can be caused by surgery and may be related to uneven SMAS plication, poor liposuction technique, differences in plication vectors, premature resorption or rupture of plication sutures, dehiscence of incisions, hematoma, seroma, trauma, infection, or asymmetrical pressure garment placement.

These concerns may be prevented by good preoperative photographs and patient education to clarify preexisting asymmetry or contour irregularities and accurately informing the patient about limitations of the technique and anticipated stretch back after the first few months after surgery. An important component of the consultation is high resolution digital preoperative photography that can be used to illustrate to the patient preexisting asymmetry or contour issues. Prevention of asymmetry is dependent on good surgical technique and intraoperative recognition of contour differences. Asymmetry or premature sagging warranting revision typically requires a revision facelift to allow for undermining and redraping of the skin.

Conclusion

Facelifting procedures mirror the surgical technique subset and risk profile of facial flap reconstruction routinely performed by dermatologic surgeons. Conscientious patient education and selection, surgical planning and execution, and postoperative management will minimize the risk of potential complications and effectively treat complications that arise. Facelift procedures provide reproducible results and remain the gold standard for facial rejuvenation despite the numerous minimally invasive procedures presently available.

References

1. Rohrich RJ. The increasing popularity of cosmetic surgery procedures: a look at statistics in plastic surgery. Plast Reconstr Surg 2000;106:1363–1365.
2. Baker DC. Minimal incision rhytidectomy (short scar face lift) with lateral SMASectomy: evolution and application. Aesthetic Surg 2001;2:14.
3. Massiha H. Short-scar face lift with extended SMAS platysma dissection and lifting and limited skin undermining. Plast Reconstr Surg 2003;112:663–669.
4. Tonnard PL, Verpaele A, Monstrey S, et al. Minimal access cranial suspension lift: a modified S-lift. Plast Reconstr Surg 2002;109:2074–2086.
5. Webster RC, Smith RC, Papsidero MJ, et al. Comparison of SMAS plication with SMAS imbrication in facelifting. Laryngoscope 1982;92:901.
6. Coleman WP 3rd, Hanke CW, Orentreich N, Kurtin SB, Brody H, Bennett R. A history of dermatologic surgery in the United States. Dermatol Surg 2000;26:5–11.
7. Warmuth IP, Bader R, Scarborough D, Bisaccia E. Dermatologic surgery into the next millennium: part I. Cutis 1999;64:245–248.
8. Hancox JG, Venkat AP, Coldiron B, Feldman SR, Williford PM. The safety of office-based surgery: review of recent literature from several disciplines. Arch Dermatol 2004;140:1379–1382.
9. Chrisman BB, Field LM. Facelift surgery update: suction assisted rhytidectomy and other improvements. J Dermatol Surg Oncol 1984;10:544–548.
10. Asken S. Cervicofacial rhytidectomy. In: Coleman WP, Hanke CW, Alt TH, Asken S, eds. Cosmetic surgery of the skin. St. Louis: Mosby; 1997:428–452.
11. Fulton JE, Saylan Z, Helton P, et al. The S-lift facelift featuring the U-suture and O-suture combined with skin resurfacing. Dermatol Surg 2001;27:18–22.
12. Brandy DA. A method of augmenting the cheek area through SMAS, sub SMAS and subcutaneous tissue recruitment during facelift surgery. Dermatol Surg 2003;29:265–271.
13. Bisaccia E, Khan AJ, Scarborough DA. Anterior face-lift for correction of middle face aging utilizing a minimally invasive technique. Dermatol Surg 2004;30:769–776.
14. Alster TS, Doshi SN, Hopping SB. Combination surgical lifting with ablative laser skin resurfacing of facial skin: a retrospective analysis. Dermatol Surg 2004;30:1191–1195.
15. Cook JL, Perone JB. A prospective evaluation of the incidence of complications associated with Mohs micrographic surgery. Arch Dermatol 2003;139:143–152.
16. Kargi E, Babuccu O, Hosnuter M, Babuccu B, Altinyazar C. Complications of minor cutaneous surgery in patients under anticoagulant treatment. Aesthetic Plast Surg 2002;26:483–485.
17. Borud LJ, Matarasso A, Spaccavento CM, Hanzlik RM. Factor XI deficiency: implications for management of patients undergoing aesthetic surgery. Plast Reconstr Surg 1999;104:1907–1913.
18. Akoz T, Akan M, Yildirim S. If you continue to smoke, we may have a problem: smoking's effects on plastic surgery. Aesthetic Plast Surg 2002;26:477–482.
19. Krueger JK, Rohrich RJ. Clearing the smoke: the scientific rationale for tobacco abstention with plastic surgery. Plast Reconstr Surg 2001;108:1063–1073; discussion, 1074–1077.
20. Larrabee WF, Makielski KH, ed. Surgical anatomy of the face. New York: Raven Press; 1993:41–48.
21. De Castro CC. Preauricular and sideburns operating procedures for a natural look in facelifts. Aesthetic Plast Surg 1991;15:149–153.
22. Klein JA. Tumescent technique chronicles. Local anesthesia, liposuction and beyond. Dermatol Surg 1995;21:449–457.
23. Jones BM, Grover R. Reducing complications in cervicofacial rhytidectomy by tumescent infiltration: a comparative trial evaluating 678 consecutive face lifts. Plast Reconstr Surg 2004;113:398–403.
24. Seify H, Jones G, Bostwick J, Hester TR. Endoscopic-assisted face lift: review of 200 cases. Ann Plast Surg 2004;52:234–239.
25. Grover R, Jones BM, Waterhouse N. The prevention of haematoma following rhytidectomy: a review of 1078 consecutive facelifts. Br J Plast Surg 2001;54:481–486.
26. Kamer FM, Song AU. Hematoma formation in deep plane rhytidectomy. Arch Facial Plast Surg 2000;2:240–242.
27. Sullivan CA, Masin J, Maniglia AJ, Stepnick DW. Complications of rhytidectomy in an otolaryngology training program. Laryngoscope 1999;109:198–203.
28. Perkins SW, Williams JD, Macdonald K, Robinson EB. Prevention of seromas and hematomas after face-lift surgery with the use of postoperative vacuum drains. Arch Otolaryngol Head Neck Surg 1997;123:743–745.
29. Pina DP. Aesthetic and safety considerations in composite rhytidectomy: a review of 145 patients over a 3-year period. Plast Reconstr Surg 1997;99:670–678; discussion, 679.

30. Jones BM. Facelifting: an initial eight year experience. Br J Plast Surg 1995;48:203–211.

31. Rees TD, Barone CM, Valauri FA, Ginsberg GD, Nolan WB 3rd. Hematomas requiring surgical evacuation following face lift surgery. Plast Reconstr Surg 1994;93:1185–1190.

32. Marchac D, Sandor G. Face lifts and sprayed fibrin glue: an outcome analysis of 200 patients. Br J Plast Surg 1994; 47:306–309.

33. Lawson W, Naidu RK. The male facelift. An analysis of 115 cases. Arch Otolaryngol Head Neck Surg 1993;119:535–539.

34. Alt T. Facelift surgery. In: Ratz JL, ed. Dermatologic surgery. Philadelphia: Lippincott; 1998:245–311.

35. Kaye BL, Kurse JC. General anesthesia for rhytidectomy. Plast Reconstr Surg 1977;60:747–751.

36. Izquierdo R, Parry SW, Boydell CL, Almand J. The great auricular nerve revisited: pertinent anatomy for SMAS-platysma rhytidectomy. Ann Plast Surg 1991;27:44–48.

37. McKinney P, Gottlieb J. The relationship of the great auricular nerve to the superficial musculoaponeurotic system. Ann Plast Surg 1985;14:310–314.

38. McKinney P, Katrana DJ. Prevention of injury to the great auricular nerve during rhytidectomy. Plast Reconstr Surg 1980;66:675–679.

39. de Chalain T, Nahai F. Amputation neuromas of the great auricular nerve after rhytidectomy. Ann Plast Surg 1995; 35:297–299.

40. Daane SP, Owsley JQ. Incidence of cervical branch injury with "marginal mandibular nerve pseudo-paralysis" in patients undergoing face lift. Plast Reconstr Surg 2003; 111:2414–2418.

41. Kamer FM, Damiani J, Churukian M. 512 rhytidectomies. A retrospective study. Arch Otolaryngol 1984;110:368–370.

42. Baker DC. Complications of cervicofacial rhytidectomy. Clin Plast Surg 1983;10:543–562.

43. Zani R, Fadul R Jr, Da Rocha MA, Santos RA, Alves MC, Ferreira LM. Facial nerve in rhytidoplasty: anatomic study of its trajectory in the overlying skin and the most common sites of injury. Ann Plast Surg 2003;51:236–242.

44. MacGregor MW, Greenberg RL. Rhytidectomy. In: Goldwyn RM, ed. The unfavorable result in plastic surgery. Boston: Little Brown; 1972:335–349.

45. Sarala PK. Accessory nerve palsy: an uncommon etiology. Arch Phys Med Rehab 1982;63:445–446.

46. Piza-Katzer H, Balogh B, Muzika-Herczeg E, Gardetto A. Secondary end to end repair of extensive facial nerve defects: surgical technique and postoperative functional results. Head Neck 2004;9:770–777.

47. Jones BM, Grover R. Avoiding hematoma in cervicofacial rhytidectomy: a personal 8-year quest. Reviewing 910 patients. Plast Reconstr Surg 2004;113:381–387.

48. Perkins SW, Williams JD, Macdonald K, Robinson EB. Prevention of seromas and hematomas after facelift surgery with the use of postoperative vaccum drains. Arch Otolaryngol Head Neck Surg 1997;123:743–745.

49. LeRoy JL Jr, Rees TD, Nolan WB 3rd. Infections requiring hospital readmission following face lift surgery: incidence, treatment, and sequelae. Plast Reconstr Surg 1994;93:533–536.

50. Akers JO, Mascaro JR, Baker SM. Mycobacterium abscessus infection after facelift surgery: a case report. Oral Maxillofac Surg 2000;58:572–574; discussion, 574–575.

51. Pennekamp A, Pfyffer GE, Wuest J, George CA, Ruef C. Mycobacterium smegmatis infection in a healthy woman following a facelift: case report and review of the literature. Ann Plast Surg 1997;39:80–83.

52. Knuttel R, Torabian SZ, Fung M. Hair loss after rhytidectomy. Dermatol Surg 2004;30:1041–1042.

53. Kridel RW, Liu ES. Techniques for creating inconspicuous face-lift scars: avoiding visible incisions and loss of temporal hair. Arch Facial Plast Surg 2003;5:325–333.

54. Brennan HG, Toft KM, Dunham BO, Goode RL, Koch RJ. Prevention and correction of temporal hair loss in rhytidectomy. Plast Reconstr Surg 1999;104:2219–2225.

55. Eremia S, Umar SH, Li CY. Prevention of temporal alopecia following rhytidectomy: the prophylactic use of minoxidil. A study of 60 patients. Dermatol Surg 2002;28:66–74.

56. Nordstrom RE, Greco M, Vitagliano T. Correction of sideburn defects after facelift operations. Aesthetic Plast Surg 2000;24:429–432.

57. Parkes ML, Kamer FM, Bassilios MI. Treatment of alopecia in temporal region following rhytidectomy procedures. Laryngoscope 1977;87:1011–1014.

58. Marks JG Jr, Rainey MA. Cutaneous reactions to surgical preparations and dressings. Contact Dermatitis 1984;10:1–5.

59. Sood A, Taylor JS. Bacitracin: allergen of the year. Am J Contact Dermat 2003;14:3–4.

60. Morris SD, Rycroft RJ, White IR, Wakelin SH, McFadden JP. Comparative frequency of patch test reactions to topical antibiotics. Br J Dermatol 2002;146:1047–1051.

61. Iijima S, Kuramochi M. Investigation of irritant skin reaction by 10% povidone-iodine solution after surgery. Dermatology 2002;204(Suppl 1):103–108.

62. Goon AT, White IR, Rycroft RJ, McFadden JP. Allergic contact dermatitis from chlorhexidine. Dermatitis 2004;15: 45–47.

63. Murray JC. Keloids and hypertrophic scars. Clin Dermatol 1994;12:27–37.

64. Grimes PE, Hunt SG. Considerations for cosmetic surgery in the black population. Clin Plast Surg 1993;20:27–34.

65. Roques C. Massage applied to scars. Wound Repair Regen 2002;10:126–128.

66. Gold MH, Foster TD, Adair MA, Burlison K, Lewis T. Prevention of hypertrophic scars and keloids by the prophylactic use of topical silicone gel sheets following a surgical procedure in an office setting. Dermatol Surg 2001;27:641–644.

67. English RS, Shenefelt PD. Keloids and hypertrophic scars. Dermatol Surg 1999;25:631–638.

68. Berman B, Villa A. Imiquimod 5% cream for keloid management. Dermatol Surg 2003;29:1050–1051.

69. Manuskiatti W, Fitzpatrick RE. Treatment response of keloidal and hypertrophic sternotomy scars: comparison among intralesional corticosteroid, 5-fluorouracil, and 585-nm flashlamp-pumped pulsed-dye laser treatments. Arch Dermatol 2002;138:1149–1155.

70. Pickett BP, Burgess LP, Livermore GH, Tzikas TL, Vossoughi J. Arch Otolaryngol Head Neck Surg 1996;122:565–568.
71. Knize DM. Periauricular facelift incisions and the auricular anchor. Plast Reconstr Surg 1999;104:1508–1520.
72. Brink RR. Auricular displacement with rhytidectomy. Plast Reconstr Surg 2002;109:408–409.
73. Brink RR. Auricular displacement with rhytidectomy. Plast Reconstr Surg 2001;108:743–752.
74. Mowlavi A, Meldrum DG, Wilhelmi BJ, et al. The "pixie" ear deformity following face lift surgery revisited. Plast Reconstr Surg 2005;115:1165–1171.
75. Eisenberg E, Yaari A, Har-Shai Y. Chronic, burning facial pain following cosmetic facial surgery. Ann Plast Surg 1996;36:76–79.
76. Borah G, Rankin M, Wey P. Psychological complications in 281 plastic surgery practices. Plast Reconstr Surg 1999; 104:1241–1246.

Index

Hypopigmentation
  cryotherapy-related, 91
  dermabrasion-related, 121, 122
  postoperative, 149–150
  skin resurfacing-related, 169, 172–173, 187, 189
Hypoxia, smoking-related, 6

I

Imiquimod, 92
Immunosuppression, as wound infection risk factor, 46–47
Immunosuppressive drugs, effect on wound healing, 6
Impetigo, 183, 184
Implanted cardiac devices (ICD), 7, 16–17
Incisions, surgical
  as hypertrophic scaring and keloid cause, 87, 89
  as pigmentary change cause, 149
Infections. *See also* Wound infections
  botulinum toxin injection-related, 211
  facelift-related, 230–231
  liposuction-related, 197–198
  skin resurfacing-related, 169, 170–171, 188–189
  as wound dehiscence risk factor, 79
Informed consent, 183
Infraorbital defects, 96, 109, 111
Infraorbital nerve
  anatomy of, 28
  injuries to, 30
Insect bites, 87
Insight, lack of, 4
Interferon therapy, for scars, 91, 117, 119
International normalized ratio (INR), 39
Iodophors, 52, 62, 63
  adverse reactions to, 140–141
Ischemic heart disease, as mortality cause, 9
Isopropyl alcohol, 52, 53
Isotretinoin, 184, 187

J

Judgment
  evaluation of, 157
  lack of, 4

K

Keloids, 115, 116, 118
  burn-related, 92
  comparison with hypertrophic scars, 87, 88
  facelift-related, 232–234
  as facelift-related complications risk factor, 224

isotretinoin-related, 184
prevention of, 87, 89, 90, 116, 232–234
as pruritus cause, 148
recurrence of, 119
treatment of, 87–94, 116, 120, 232–234
Keloid surgery, as hematoma cause, 43
Kenalog, 120, 184, 226
Klebsiella infections, 67

L

Lacerations, as scar and keloid cause, 87, 88
Laser therapy, 167–182
  ablative
    for scar revision, 121, 123, 124
    for skin resurfacing, 167–173, 178–179
  for hyperpigmentation, 216–217
  for hypopigmentation, 187
  for keloids, 91
  nonablative
    for scar revision, 120–121
    for skin remodeling, 174–176, 178
  as pigmentary change cause, 150
  preoperative patient evaluation for, 167
  for scars, 91, 118, 120–121, 173
  side effects of, 91
  technical basis for, 167
Latex allergy, 13, 14
Lentigines, 167–168, 187
Lidocaine
  allergic reactions to, 12, 14
  hepatic dysfunction and, 7
  intraincisional, 65
  toxicity of, 193
  use in liposuction patients, 193, 194
Linezolid, 56
Lip
  free margin distortion on, 95, 111–113
  soft tissue filler injections into, 201–202, 203
Lipoatrophy, 204–205
Liposuction, 192–198
  in combination with facelifting procedures, 224, 226, 227, 229
  under general anesthesia, 192–193
  under local anesthesia, 192, 193
  tumescent
    as infection cause, 197–198
    local complications of, 195–197
    preoperative assessment for, 193–195
  ultrasonic, 193
Liver disease, 7
Local anesthesia, use in liposuction patients, 192, 193
Local anesthetic injections, patients' tolerance to, 147
Lorazepam, 11, 15

M

Malnutrition, as wound infection risk factor, 47
Mandibular nerve, marginal
  injuries to, 26–28, 33–34, 228–229
  location of, 228
Mania, evaluation of, 157
Manic-depressive disorders, 162
Marfan's syndrome, 40–41
Massage therapy, for scars, 117, 118–119
Medical and surgical histories, 4–8
Melanocytes, cold sensitivity of, 149
Mental nerve
  anatomy of, 28, 30–31
  injuries to, 31
Mental status examinations, 157
Microscopic epidermal necrotic debris (MEND), 178–179
Milia, 145, 169, 170, 189–190
Minnesota Multiphasic Personality Inventory, 155
Mitral valve prolapse, 69
Mohs' micrographic surgery
  as alar crease defect cause, 108
  as ear wound infection cause, 50–51, 68
  endocarditis prophylaxis in, 71, 72
  free margin distortion associated with, 99
  as herpes simplex virus infection risk factor, 58
  infection rate in, 64
  intraincisional antibiotic prophylaxis for, 65
  as nerve injury cause, 24, 26, 229
  in patients with implantable cardiac devices, 17
  preoperative questionnaire for, 5
Molecular mimicry, 201
Mood, evaluation of, 157
Mupirocin, 64
  as contact allergy cause, 141
  intranasal application of, 66
Muscle twitching, botulinum toxin injection-related, 211
Mycobacterial infections, 57, 197, 198, 230
Myonecrosis, clostridial, 58, 59

N

Nares, *Staphylococcus aureus* colonization of, 66
Nasal tip, ptosis of, 96
Nasal valve, compromise of, 148–149
Neck
  anatomic "danger zones" of, 22, 23–33
  excessive liposuction of, 196, 197
Necrosis, cutaneous tissue
  collagen injection-related, 200
  definition of, 81

Printed in China